What Others Are Saying About
The Kidney Patient's Book

A public policy leader ...

"Tim Ahlstrom puts it all on the line. This is not another disinterested observer, but a patient who has seen the entire system from the inside with the stake no less than his own life. To Tim, this is not an abstract argument. He has thus written a book not only to guide other patients with kidney disease, but having a broader applicability to all society. The lessons that he learned individually are going to have to be learned collectively. **The tide of events is with Tim Ahlstrom. Our whole society is going to have to follow him down this path.**"

Richard D. Lamm
Former Governor of Colorado
Director of Center for Public Policy and Contemporary Issues
University of Denver, Colorado

Doctors and scientists ...

"...an important contribution...a much needed work that will provide support and information for people with kidney disease and their families. **I believe this book will be of great benefit to a great number of patients.**"

Saulo Klahr, M.D., Nephrologist
Past President, *National Kidney Foundation*
Simon Professor of Medicine, Physician-in-Chief
The Jewish Hospital of St. Louis
Co-Chairman, Department of Medicine
Washington University School of Medicine, St. Louis

"Compared to the host of books that address the scientific aspects of kidney disease, there are few detailing kidney disease from the perspective of the patient. Tim Ahlstrom has written such a book in terms that are easily understood. **This book is more than an explanation of kidney problems; there are valuable lessons for physicians and others involved in the care of 'kidney' patients.** ... a brief glimpse of a chronic illness as perceived by a patient is a valuable experience."

William E. Mitch, M.D., Nephrologist
Garland Herndon Professor of Medicine
Director, Renal Division
Emory University School of Medicine, Atlanta

"This book is unique in many respects, as is its author. **Unlike other laymen who have written about their illnesses, Tim Ahlstrom has progressed in his understanding of treatment options for his disease far beyond the norm.** His kidney function has also improved more than any of the patients I have treated in the last twenty years. There is clearly a connection between his own health and the content of this book."

Mackenzie Walser, M.D., Nephrologist
Professor of Pharmacology and Professor of Medicine
Johns Hopkins University School of Medicine, Baltimore

"The message of this book is that patients help themselves. Tim Ahlstrom sees, as do I, the outlines of a 'new relationship' between doctor and patient—cooperative, advisory, turning on persuasion rather than prescription. **He is on to something important for patients and for doctors.**"

Alan G. Wasserstein, M.D., Nephrologist
Associate Professor of Medicine, Director of the Dialysis Program
University of Pennsylvania School of Medicine, Philadelphia

"Tim Ahlstrom's message is that conservative treatment may delay the need for dialysis or transplant for considerable periods of time. **This most interesting book is an important source of information for kidney patients and families.**"

Professor Giuseppe Maschio, M.D., Nephrologist
Professor of Nephrology, Chief of the Nephrology Division
University of Verona, Italy

"**This book is not only for patients, but also for doctors.** Tim Ahlstrom provides excellent practical instructions on how to change eating habits and lifestyle to combat the progressive loss of kidney function."

Norbert Gretz, M.D., Nephrologist
Clinical Researcher
University of Heidelberg, Germany

"This book has the great merit of informing kidney patients, their families and their doctors that conservative treatment can delay the need for dialysis for long periods of time. **I believe that kidney specialists around the world are slowly coming to an agreement on the usefulness of nutritional treatment for kidney disease.**"

Professor Sergio Giovannetti, M.D., Nephrologist
Professor of Medicine, Chief of the Nephrology Division
University of Pisa, Italy

Patients and families ...

"Like Tim Ahlstrom, I have followed the program in this book to control my own kidney disease. I have delayed dialysis for over two years. My wife and I were able to adopt an infant son—something we probably could not have done if I had been on dialysis. **Every kidney patient and his family need to know what is in this book.**"

Murray West, M.D.
Kidney patient and family practitioner
Baltimore

"My husband and I have maintained our normal lifestyle, despite his chronic kidney disease. **The ideas in this book have changed our lives.**"

Barbara Park
Wife of a kidney patient, director of a nuclear medicine laboratory
Joppa, Maryland

The Kidney Patient's Book

New Treatment, New Hope

Timothy P. Ahlstrom

With Forewords By:

William E. Mitch, M.D.
Emory University
School of Medicine, Atlanta

The Honorable Richard D. Lamm
Center for Public Policy and
Contemporary Issues, University of Denver

Mackenzie Walser, M.D.
The Johns Hopkins University
School of Medicine, Baltimore

Alan G. Wasserstein, M.D.
University of Pennsylvania
School of Medicine, Philadelphia

Murray West, M.D.
Kidney patient and family practitioner
Baltimore

Sergio Giovannetti, M.D.
University of Pisa
School of Medicine, Italy

Norbert Gretz, M.D.
University of Heidelberg
School of Medicine, Germany

Giuseppe Maschio, M.D.
University of Verona
School of Medicine, Italy

Great Issues Press
Delran, New Jersey

This book presents one patient's experience with his chronic kidney disease, describing his efforts to learn about his disease, about doctors and other kidney specialists, and about the treatments they offered. This book should not be substituted for the advice and treatment of a physician, but rather should be used to increase the patient's knowledge and therefore his ability to understand treatments recommended by a physician.

The author and publisher specifically disclaim responsibility for any adverse effects resulting from the information in this book.

The Kidney Patient's Book; New Treatment, New Hope

Copyright © 1991 by Timothy P. Ahlstrom

All rights reserved. Printed in the United States of America. No part of this book may be used or reproduced in any manner whatsoever without written permission except in the case of brief quotations embodied in critical articles and reviews. Address inquiries to Great Issues Press, P.O. Box 1336, Delran, N.J. 08075

Cataloging-in-Publication Data

Ahlstrom, Timothy P.
The kidney patient's book; new treatment, new hope/ Timothy P. Ahlstrom.
p. cm.
Includes bibliographical references and index.
ISBN 0-9629078-7-1
1. Chronic renal failure—Diet therapy—Popular works.
2. Kidneys—Diseases—Popular works. I. Title.
RC902   1991
616.61   91-72531
                                                CIP

First Edition

1 2 3 4 5 6 7 8 9 10

Edited by Susan J. Ahlstrom

Contents

Acknowledgements

The heroes of this book are the patients and families who are learning to live with their chronic disease, and the physicians and scientists who have dedicated their life's work to studying conservative treatment for chronic disease. They have something important to say, and they are saying it through their work. I am deeply grateful to them.

Dr. Mackenzie Walser of the Johns Hopkins University School of Medicine and Dr. Alan Wasserstein of the University of Pennsylvania School of Medicine have helped me learn about my chronic disease and deal with it. Dr. Saulo Klahr and Dr. William Mitch have encouraged me to tell this story. Professor Sergio Giovannetti, Professor Giuseppe Maschio and Dr. Norbert Gretz have helped me understand the European perspective.

My family has helped me every day—with my disease and with this book. Our daughter Susan has been my partner in researching, writing and preparing the book for publication. She is becoming an expert on living with kidney disease, and on the business of books. Our daughter Cindy worked on the illustrations. Our sons David and Marc made helpful suggestions, and my wife Cynthia provided the quiet support the family has always been able to count on.

Author's Note

This book is for patients, like me, and their families, like mine. Their doctors may find some new facts and insights, too. The message is simple: *If you are in the early stages of a chronic disease, you may be able to prevent it from threatening your life simply by making some lifestyle changes, and by adopting some new eating habits*. This book presents not a quack diet, but thoroughly respectable conservative treatment based on a substantial body of medical research. The treatment is used widely in Europe, but rarely in the United States.

I have terminal kidney disease. But the work of some physician-scientists in the United States and Europe has taught me how to stop my disease from getting worse, at least for now. These scientists have also taught me that some other chronic diseases, the biggest killers of late 20th century Americans and Europeans, may respond to conservative treatment—heart disease, high blood pressure, stroke, diabetes and cancer.

But what does a *patient* know about treating chronic disease? *A mere patient?* Doctors spend a lifetime studying disease and treatments. Can a book by a patient help other patients and families?

If I picked up this book in a library or a book store, I would want to know what some world-class kidney specialists thought of it. So, I asked several of the world's most experienced and respected kidney physicians and researchers to read *The Kidney Patient's Book.* You can read "book reviews" by six of the world's leading kidney specialists in the Forewords, plus the views of a physician who is living with his own kidney disease.

I hope the ideas in this book help you as they have helped me and my family. I hope that you will write to me about your own experiences.

Tim Ahlstrom
May 29, 1991

Forewords

William E. Mitch, M.D.
Garland Herndon Professor of Medicine
Director, Renal Division
Emory University School of Medicine
Atlanta

Compared to the host of books that address the scientific aspects of kidney disease, there are few detailing kidney disease from the perspective of the patient. Timothy Ahlstrom has written such a book in terms that are easily understood. The book is more than an explanation of kidney problems; there are valuable lessons for physicians and others involved in the care of "kidney" patients.

Kidney disease viewed through the eyes of a patient loses much of the technological trappings often associated with treatments for kidney failure. A viewpoint which is not based on complex strategies and nuances provides important insight and need not be trivial. Patients and their families may have considerable difficulty comprehending the meaning and limitations of technology. This book brings these issues to the forefront. The book also details important, if not startling, statistics on morbidity and survival associated with current therapies.

While one might disagree with the author's conclusions about the usefulness of different types of therapy, none would disagree that new ideas are needed. Stated differently, other strategies including a limitation of dietary protein must be explored even though advances in dialysis and transplantation therapy have saved many patients. The author argues for this conclusion in a compelling manner and I believe he succeeds. Even if others disagree, a brief glimpse of a chronic illness as perceived by a patient is a valuable experience.

Richard D. Lamm
Former Governor of Colorado
Director of Center for Public Policy and Contemporary Issues
University of Denver
Denver, Colorado

It is often said that American medicine has a heavy bias towards high technology. While most thoughtful people concede the point, an argument soon develops as to the extent of this bias, the solutions to it and, of course, "what would you do if it were your mother?" The conversation, in other words, is fraught with almost equal amounts of light and heat, done largely in hypothetical settings.

Tim Ahlstrom puts it all on the line. This is not another disinterested observer, but a patient who has seen the entire system from the inside with the stake no less than his own life. To Tim, this is not an abstract argument. He experienced the bias first hand, thought and read deeply about the medical advice he was given, and came up with an alternative.

To paraphrase Ambrose Bierce, "Nothing focuses a man's mind as the sentence of his own death." Some people give up; most people throw themselves on the experience of the medical profession; and a very few people, like Tim, question, explore, research, evaluate, and triple check the advice that they have been given. If everyone would put the time and talent into evaluating their medical choices, perhaps competition would truly work in the American health care system. But, while we may wish for educated patients, we should do nothing to diminish the truly magnificent and thoughtful work of one who did.

No trees grow to the sky, and no element of a nation's budget can continue to grow at two and a half times the rate of inflation. Something must be done and done soon to dampen the runaway medical costs lest we leave our children with an overbuilt health care system on top of a shattered economy. Controlling health care costs is a hydra-headed problem. Everyone agrees that part of the problem is the bias towards high technology. The United States has five percent of the world's population, yet we have half of the CT scanners and two-thirds of the MRI machines. Virtually every doctor from abroad looking at the American health care system comments on our bias towards high technology medicine, and how it ends up being counterproductive to the total health of the nation. What other country would take 90 year olds with congestive heart failure out of nursing homes and put them in intensive care units to die expensive deaths, and yet not give pre-natal care to all of its pregnant women? In almost every stage and every segment of American medicine, we have invented magnificent technology, but often do not have the wisdom to use it properly. "Can do" has become "must do" in the brave new world of American medicine.

Tim has thus written a book not only to guide other patients with kidney disease, but having a broader applicability to all society. The lessons that he learned individually are going to have to be learned collectively. In many areas of American medicine, there is an alternative that is equally or more effective, but because of our medical culture or the national bias towards technology, or the fact that a doctor has an economic interest in one alternative over the other, it is often ignored and occasionally disparaged. Volcanic health care cost increases are going to force us to make some hard choices. The tide of events is with Tim Ahlstrom. Our whole society is going to have to follow him down this path.

Mackenzie Walser, M.D.

Professor of Pharmacology and Professor of Medicine
The Johns Hopkins University School of Medicine
Baltimore

This book is unique in many respects, as is its author. Unlike other laymen who have written about their illnesses, Tim Ahlstrom has progressed in his understanding of treatment options for his disease far beyond the norm. Indeed, his book contains hard data and analyses, particularly concerning the outcome of dialysis and transplantation, that are not readily available in the literature, as well as a thoughtful presentation of these and other results.

Tim is also unique in another way: his kidney function has improved more steadily and more significantly on the ketoacid supplement than any of the many patients I have treated since 1970. I have no idea why.

Clearly there is a connection between his own health history and the content of this book. Like all of us, he is biased, which is simply to say that his experience has lent an emotional coloration to his views. A totally unbiased approach to the question of alternative therapies for chronic renal failure (or any other potentially fatal disease for which alternative treatments exist) would be hard to find.

Those who are dedicating their careers to dialysis and transplantation feel, with ample justification, that these techniques have permitted long-term survival with an acceptable quality of life for thousands of patients who would otherwise have died.

Likewise, the small number of individuals who, like me, have spent most of their careers attempting to prevent end-stage renal disease, instead of treating it, are biased in favor of this alternative approach.

That is not to denigrate in any way the value of what Tim calls "high technology treatment." Every patient on nutritional therapy is grateful that, down the road, if his disease reaches end-stage, these options are available.

Tim's point is simply that the nutritional approach has received short shrift. How could I fail to agree?

The controversy revolves around whether nutritional therapy is (1) tolerable and (2) effective in slowing progression (that it reduces symptoms is uncontested). My own experience has convinced me that it is both tolerable and effective in most cases. I, like Tim, am troubled by the fact that the brain power and resources being devoted to improving this alternative approach are dwarfed by the efforts devoted to end-stage therapy. Perhaps this book will serve to persuade some readers that we need to redirect our priorities in this field.

Alan G. Wasserstein, M.D.
Associate Professor of Medicine, Director of the Dialysis Program
University of Pennsylvania School of Medicine
Philadelphia

Tim Ahlstrom is my patient, but not a typical one. At his first office visit he brought some thirty or forty computer printouts of his laboratory studies, going back several years. Here was a man who wanted to be in control, I thought; and, I suspected, not in a helpful way. I thought of patient control in the negative way in which doctors tend to imagine it: intellectualizing his illness, failing to come to terms with it emotionally, running away from "realities" he would have to face sooner or later, challenging his doctors. But I quickly found that Tim did not have confrontation in mind. Nor was his studious approach only a way of coping. He genuinely wanted to find out what was best for himself, and he had the independence of mind and the distrust of technology to question what we doctors were telling him.

Tim's message is that patients help themselves. They need not settle for the passive role that the technological model sets for them: the role of a "field" on which the competing forces of disease and medical intervention play. Tim has shown his independence in two ways: in adopting a dietary treatment plan in which his own performance is required for success, and in discovering, by his own efforts, the very existence of such treatment. His success consists both of preserving his health and of taking control of his life; not only a physical but a moral success. One recalls that the ancient Greeks thought of dietary regimen not so much as a means of extending life—Plato thought that the term of life was fixed by fate—but as moral training in the conquest of the appetites.

Tim raises the possibility that contemporary American medicine has been slow to recommend dietary treatment for the progression of kidney disease. Most nephrologists would disagree. They would point out, rightly, that the efficacy of dietary treatment remains to be proved. And they might add that some doctors, even in the absence of proof, do recommend such treatment. Nevertheless, I think that Tim is on to something. The parallel with coronary artery bypass grafting is instructive. That operation was introduced in 1967 and was received enthusiastically by the medical community. About a decade passed before the first controlled trials were performed, and these trials have come to show that the procedure was not uniformly helpful. Some subgroups benefitted; others did not. The use of bypass grafting has since become more selective. With dietary protein restriction for kidney disease the same interval has passed, roughly a decade before a definitive controlled trial has begun. But there is this crucial difference, that in the intervening years dietary therapy has not been taken up widely. The need for the controlled study of dietary protein restriction is not to limit its unscientific use but to get it going. So we see that it is more than scientific standards of proof that account for the different receptions of bypass grafting and of dietary protein restriction, and for physicians' practice styles in general.

Well, what else then? We could say that Americans (doctors and patients both) love high technology, but that begs the question: *Why* are we more taken by bypass grafting than by dietary therapy? Tim suggests that economic interest plays a part and, while I hesitate to admit that physicians put it ahead of the best interests of their patients, I have a feeling he is right. But I don't think the calculation is even conscious for many nephrologists: Dialysis and kidney transplant are the "established" (and establishment) therapies, and they are automatically to be preferred to an upstart dietary approach that may turn out to be no more than a fad. Of course, one need not believe that nephrologists are conscious of profit and loss to assert that these considerations play a determining role in the rationalizations that they give for their preference. But, proving this assertion would be difficult.

Certainly the large and costly controlled study that the government requested and is now funding has an economic motive. The cost of the dialysis program, paid for with public monies, has become enormous. A tactic that would delay dialysis would save millions, but nephrologists have been slow to try it. So the government has invested millions in a controlled study in the hope of getting an affirmative answer. If it is forthcoming the prestige of the scientific result will compel nephrologists to adopt dietary therapy. The reimbursement for dietary instruction could be increased, that for dialysis reduced. The government is not merely promoting good science here. It is trying to change medical behavior in the interest of saving millions.

My own suspicion, however, is that the economics don't entirely account for the matter, not even for physician behavior. Like the notion that "Americans like high-tech," the economic argument is also tautological: if reimbursement for dialysis and kidney transplantation is high and that for dietary counseling is low, well, the reimbursements could have been reversed. The question is why these activities have been valued as they have up to now. My guess is that matters of control and mastery are at the core of the problem. That is, after all, what science is about: control and mastery of nature. Medicine is thought most powerful (certainly in the minds of its practitioners) when it has control over the phenomena of disease and treatment. Technological control of the passive patient seems surer, and more rational (in Max Weber's sense of more calculable), and, finally, *better* medicine than that which depends on the vagaries of patient understanding, agreement, and compliance. And, incidentally, don't imagine that there is some conspiracy on the part of the doctors here: what happens to patients depends a great deal on what patients themselves want, as any physician knows who has had to give antibiotics for a viral upper respiratory infection for which he or she knows they will be useless. Patients like the technological model as much as their doctors do.

How things have changed since the ancient Greeks, and not for the better. Plato recommended that physicians treat freemen and slaves differently: prescribe to slaves but instruct freemen. The Hippocratic writings list rhetoric as one of the skills of the physician, so that he shall be able to persuade his patient to adopt a recommended regimen. By ancient standards the patients of today are slaves!

I do not agree with everything that Tim has written, especially about doctors. I take exception, for example, to the tone of anomie that grips his hypothetical dialysis doctor in thinking about a new patient. And I don't believe that life on dialysis is so bad as he makes it out to be. But the issue transcends any adversarial relation between patients and doctors, any talk of "liberation" from medical power. Both patient and doctor are caught in the technological ethos, both are not only constrained but created by its articulations. The doctor herself is a "field" in which technical knowledge and particular situations play, not more free than the patient. Let us say, rather, that the freedom of one is the freedom of the other. We can see the dim outlines of a "new" relationship of doctor to patient, cooperative, advisory, turning on persuasion rather than prescription, taking shape around the lowly issue of diet. Even if the dietary protein hypothesis turns out to be wrong, this relationship (which is really an old idea) is worth keeping in mind.

Murray West, M.D.
Kidney patient and family practitioner
Baltimore

Tim Ahlstrom and I are fellow end-stage renal disease patients participating in Dr. Mackenzie Walser's research on keto and amino acid supplementation of low protein diets. We share very personal hopes for the success of dietary therapy and I am pleased that we are both benefitting from it. Tim has organized a support group which has been enthusiastically attended by the patients in the study.

As a family practice physician I approach renal disease and its treatment somewhat differently from Tim. I do not reject the technological achievement of dialysis and transplant nor do I view diet therapy as a panacea. Dietary therapy has given me some control over what I felt was an inexorable decline towards dialysis. For this I am thankful. The year or more that dietary therapy has delayed the need for dialysis has allowed me to learn to accept the fate that I will one day be on dialysis. The importance of this reprieve should not be underestimated. It cannot be measured simply in terms of money saved on delaying dialysis. I suspect that those who experience some measure of success on dietary therapy are better able to adjust to dialysis itself.

I do not see a conspiracy by the medical community to promote dialysis over diet therapy. Diet therapy is not adequately promoted by physicians because of a fatalistic sense that the time devoted to dietary instruction is not well spent. Low compliance rates with much less difficult diets such as diabetic or low-fat diets makes physicians doubt that effective diets are efficacious in practice. However, a subset of patients who are highly motivated should greatly benefit from this therapy.

This book starts from the premise that patients *should* be motivated to participate in the treatment of their disease. I hope this book will help more end-stage renal patients realize that they do have a third option in the early treatment of their disease. I hope it will motivate some patients who would otherwise have taken a passive role in their treatment. And I hope that this book will encourage doctors to help those motivated patients to receive the instruction necessary to adhere to low protein diet therapy.

Sergio Giovannetti, M.D.
Professor of Medicine, Clinical Researcher
Clinica Medica Generale e Terapia
University of Pisa, Italy

Timothy P. Ahlstrom is a patient suffering from chronic renal failure who, when diagnosis was made on December 26, 1988, was told that nothing could be done for his disease until the terminal stage had been reached, when dialysis and transplant could be done. He reacted in a quite unusual manner. He decided to learn as much as possible about his problem. He started to spend time in libraries looking for a third treatment for chronic renal failure.

He found that, beside dialysis and transplantation, a third treatment exists for the pre-dialysis stage when nothing is usually done: dietary therapy. He started dietary treatment and, contrary to the pessimistic prognosis of doctors, his renal function remained stable.

He has written this book over the last months with the specific purpose of informing patients and families (and doctors) that chronic renal failure can be treated effectively and safely with conservative measures.

I do agree on this point with Mr. Ahlstrom. I believe that dietary treatment of chronic renal failure is not only a way to relieve and prevent uremic symptoms, but also to slow down the rate of decline of the residual renal function. I also believe that a general agreement on this is slowly being reached in the nephrology community.

I do believe in dietary treatment for chronic renal failure, but I do not believe that it is an alternative to dialysis or transplantation. I have no doubt that many patients on dietary therapy have a lower rate of decline of renal function, even stabilization for long periods of time, and may live in a symptom-free condition with extremely low levels of kidney function. The moment will eventually arrive, however, when replacement of their lost kidney function becomes mandatory. The purpose of dietary treatment is to help the patient to reach this moment as late as possible, in good nutritional, hormonal and psychic condition—nothing more.

Mr. Ahlstrom is then perfectly right when he maintains this and his book has the great merit of informing patients and families, and of stimulating doctors.

There are some points, however, on which I do not agree with Mr. Ahlstrom. I cannot refuse, as he does, all he has called *high-tech medical care*, including dialysis. I too remember well, as many of my colleagues do, the condition of chronic uremic patients when kidney replacement therapy was not yet available, and I accepted high-tech dialysis with enthusiasm. I also do not agree with Mr. Ahlstrom's opinion about the quality of life of patients on dialysis. They are almost always well rehabilitated, and, if there are no other superimposed diseases, they can enjoy several decades of almost normal life.

Norbert Gretz, M.D.
Clinical Researcher
Nephrology Clinic
University of Heidelberg
Mannheim, Germany

When Mr. Ahlstrom asked me quite a while ago to write a foreword to his book, I was slightly hesitant. The reason was that books written by patients about the decision for a certain mode of treatment are quite unusual in Europe, and if they are published, they might be something like a crusade. Despite the fact that I do not agree with everything Mr. Ahlstrom has written, I really appreciate the way he outlines his decision for the type of treatment he has chosen. His point of view toward dialysis and transplantation is rather pessimistic. Most doctors probably have a more optimistic view, especially with the availability of cyclosporine for treating transplant rejection. However, the data he presents are absolutely correct and are reported in a straight-forward way.

In our own medical center in Germany, the use of a low protein diet has a longstanding history. As early as 1918, Dr. F. Volhard—the Nestor of German nephrology and at that time director of our Medical Hospital—advised giving only 20 grams of protein and at least 2000 calories per day to patients suffering from uremia. This was recommended in the Handbook of Internal Medicine. In a later edition he wrote that he could also delay the occurrence of uremic symptoms for several years just by prescribing a low protein diet. However, as pointed out by Mr. Ahlstrom, the problem of malnutrition arose, as doctors ignored that protein restriction also means that a high energy intake has to be provided in order to prevent the use of protein of the body for energy synthesis (gluconeogenesis).

In our hospital, it is good practice to recommend dietary management to any patient exhibiting discrete signs of chronic renal failure. In a first step, we recommend that the patient should stick to a vegetarian diet, which is a quite popular recommendation due to the ecological movement in Germany. Such a diet is low in phosphorus, as meat is the major supplier of phosphorus. In general, a vegetarian diet provides 0.7 grams of protein per kilogram of body weight, which is a bit higher than the 0.6 grams per kilogram of body weight needed for normal life. In our unit we prefer prescribing a diet according to body weight; otherwise, for example, a woman weighing 40 kilograms might be prescribed a 45 gram protein-restricted "diet," which in reality, however, is an overfeeding with protein. If creatinine rises and therefore a further decline of renal function occurs, we institute a 0.6 gram protein-restricted diet, providing in addition 35-40 calories per kilogram of body weight. The compliance of patients with such a prescription is rather good and, as recently published, most European patients overdo it, coming up with a calculated protein intake of roughly 0.55 grams protein per kilogram of body weight.

The basis of the 0.6 gram restricted diet again is the vegetarian diet. Furthermore, a slightly higher phosphorus restriction occurs than with the normal vegetarian diet. When a further decline in renal function occurs (for example, a serum creatinine of 6 milligrams/deciliter), we recommend a 0.3 gram protein-restricted diet supplemented with amino acid or ketoacid supplements. Again, the basis is a vegetarian diet. In any of these diets dairy products are prohibited. Thus, in reality, these are *vegan* diets. Thus, our treatment recommendations for our patients differ from what most American centers would recommend. One should, however, be aware that in spite of the fact that quite a number of German centers claim to provide patients with the opportunity to try to delay the progression of their chronic renal disease by dietary management, the quality of such treatment differs widely from center to center.

In my opinion, one of the major obstacles for good nutritional therapy is that most doctors and dietitians are not adequately educated for such treatment. We recently examined the contents of nine German dietary cook books intended to be used by renal patients.We looked closely at recommendations for protein and energy intake. To our surprise, despite the fact that the books were written by specialists, an enormous calorie deficit occurs if the patients stick to such a diet. Thus, even the experts need further training. In my opinion, this deficit in knowledge and in skills explains the unwillingness of quite a number of doctors to recommend certain dietary therapies. One should also be aware of the fact that a good dietary therapy is related to the availability of suitable food. Thus, for example, it might be difficult to obtain fresh broccoli in Norway during wintertime. There are, thus, some regional limitations to such treatment modalities.

Furthermore, one could observe that good eating habits and an excellent cuisine are the basis for modifying the eating habits of the patients. I would assume that it is not possible to introduce a renal diet in the United Kingdom because the British are not used to eating many fresh vegetables. This is well outlined by Mr. Ahlstrom, too. On the other hand, the French are probably not willing to give up their excellent food in order to preserve their renal function. These are the two extremes of the broad spectrum. In the middle, probably, is Italian cooking, which is absolutely excellent for renal patients, as also outlined by Mr. Ahlstrom. Thus, if a patient is not able to really stick to a vegan diet, we would recommend at least an Italian type of diet leaving out most of the meat. In my opinion, it is not reasonable to include small amounts of meat in the diet. Two ounces of any meat shrink so much in cooking that you need a microscope to dissect it. Thus, in our medical center, we stopped the use of the so-called Swedish type of diet inaugurated by Dr. Jonas Bergström of Stockholm.

In addition to these difficulties, there is another problem. With nutritional therapy, the responsibility for the treatment is given to the patient. I am quite sure that some patients are not willing to accept that it is their own responsibility to stick to the diet, or that it is their own responsibility to reduce or prevent progression of their renal failure. This is also described in this book in an excellent manner. In my opinion, it makes no sense to try dietary management without instituting a cooperation between patient and doctor. And again, such treatment requires considerable skills and knowledge of the patient. The patient has to be ready to learn quite a bit. An excellent idea, I think, is the organization of patient support groups to help with this task. This is a phenomenon not often found in Europe; however, I think it is worthwhile trying it.

In summary, this book describes arguments for the decision to start with a low protein diet. Furthermore, it provides excellent instructions in how to change eating habits and life style to combat the progressive loss of renal failure. This book is not only suitable for patients, but also for doctors.

References:

Gretz, N., et al. Protein/amino acid composition of low protein diets. *Contrib Nephrol*. 72:11-20, 1989.

Gretz, N., et al. Low protein diets: Mineral and electrolyte contents. *Contrib Nephrol*. 72:36-41, 1989.

Volhard, F.: Die doppelseitigen hämatogenen Nierenerkrankungen (Bright'sche Krankheit); in Mohr und Staehelin (eds.), *Handbuch der Inneren Medizin*.Berlin: Springer, 1918. pp. 1149-1722.

Volhard, F.; and Suter, F.: Nieren und ableitende Harnwege; in Mohr und Staehelin (eds.), *Handbuch der Inneren Medizin, Bd. 5/1*. Berlin: Springer, 1931. pp. 804-811.

Giuseppe Maschio, M.D.
Professor of Nephrology
Chief, Division of Nephrology
University of Verona, Italy

I read with great interest *The Kidney Patient's Book,* written by Timothy P. Ahlstrom, which deals mainly with dietary treatment of chronic renal failure.

As a matter of fact, the role of diet is not new in clinical medicine. In the early 12th century, the first Italian school of medicine, established in Salerno, advised that:

"Fortior est meta Medicinae certa dieta quam si non curas, fatue regis et male curas." [A suitable diet is the strongest point in Medicine; if you neglect it, you will act foolishly and be a bad doctor.]

In the last 15 years, some points have been established concerning dietary treatment of chronic renal disease.

First, the deleterious effect of excess protein and phosphate on renal structure and function has been confirmed both in experimental and clinical studies.

Second, dietary protein and phosphate restriction reduces renal injury in all models of experimental renal disease.

Third, virtually all clinical reports have concluded that protein restriction slows the progression of chronic renal disease.

Admittedly, a rigorous statistical confirmation is not yet available, and might also prove to be impossible due to the many variables that should be considered when randomized clinical trials are planned. However, a moderate restriction in protein and phosphate has proved to be safe and well accepted by the large majority of patients. It should not be forgotten that low protein diet may exert favorable metabolic and clinical effects beyond its supposed efficacy on progression.

Clearly, an adequate dietary composition is only part of the conservative treatment in patients with chronic renal failure. Appropriate pharmacologic intervention is now available and looks especially promising when administered early in the course of chronic renal failure.

A kidney patient is now offered a conservative treatment that may delay dialysis for considerable periods of time. This message is contained in Ahlstrom's book and therefore the book should be regarded as an important source of information for patients living with chronic renal disease and for their families.

Introduction

On the day after Christmas in 1988, a prominent kidney specialist told me that my kidney disease had gotten much worse. He advised me to start thinking about dialysis or transplant because my kidneys were likely to fail entirely by the summer of 1989. I asked him what I could do. "Nothing," he said. "Kidney disease is progressive; there's nothing we can do until your kidneys have stopped working. Then we have two treatments—dialysis and transplant. Eighty or ninety percent of kidney transplants are successful now. It's a proven treatment."

I asked him what I could read to learn about my kidney disease. "There aren't any good books," he said. "You could try the National Kidney Foundation. They have some pamphlets for kidney patients." The pamphlets, I found, delivered the same message.[1,2]* There were two treatments for chronic kidney disease—dialysis and transplant. Both worked, and Medicare would pay most of the cost.

I felt frightened and confused. The specialist was confident that a kidney transplant was the best way to treat my fatal kidney disease, but my twenty-five years working with high technology as an inventor and entrepreneur had taught me to be cautious about new technology. I knew that technology sometimes created as many problems as it solved.

I learned that the average person going on the artificial kidney machine at my age could expect about four years of not very healthy life.[3] I also learned that three of four transplanted kidneys "harvested from a brain-dead organ donor," as the transplant surgeons say, would fail within ten years.[4] I wanted another way to treat my kidney disease, and I set out to find one.

I was astonished to learn, after a morning's work in the medical library, that there was a *third treatment for my chronic kidney disease*. It was a simple and natural method developed in leading medical research centers

* Notes start on page 357.

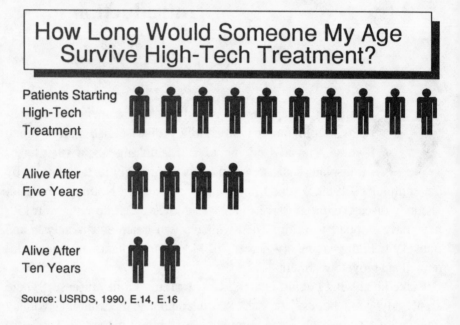

Source: USRDS, 1990, E.14, E.16

Figure 1 Survival Probability, Patients Age 50-54

I learned that the government had studied records of 372,000 patients enrolled in the Medicare End-Stage Kidney Disease Program since 1976. Experts had calculated survival probabilities for all patients on dialysis or with transplants. Six of ten patients starting high-tech kidney treatment between the ages of 50 and 54 were likely to die within five years. Eight of ten would die within ten years. I didn't like the odds, no matter how confident the high-tech doctors were. (You will find survival probabilities for other age groups in Appendix 1. You will also find many other facts from the most comprehensive study ever made about American kidney patients, their disease, and the treatments they receive. Your doctor may not know much about the results of dialysis and transplant because many of these facts were published by the government for the first time in late 1990. Many of the facts have not been published in the medical journals, and I haven't found any of them in popular books, magazines or newspapers. You may find them important as you consider what to do about your own kidney disease.)

in the United States and Europe. It was not a quack cure promoted by somebody trying to sell something. It was a conservative treatment, using nutritional therapy, a method doctors have recommended for over a century to treat the symptoms of kidney disease. For the last thirty years a few prominent physicians and scientists have been accumulating scientific proof that *conservative treatment can stop kidney disease from getting worse*. They have observed that the third treatment has given people with chronic kidney disease an opportunity to avoid the risky and expensive high technology treatments with their often undesirable side effects.

I wrote this book for people like me, people with chronic disease, and for the families who help them, because I believe they need to know about conservative treatment. I believe they need to know that they may be able to control chronic disease without submitting to the drugs, scalpels and artificial organs that have become the "treatments-of-choice" for some doctors.

Kidney patients may have heard and read, as I did, that there are only two ways to treat kidney disease—dialysis and transplant. Heart patients may have heard that there are only two ways to treat their heart disease—bypass surgery or a transplant. People with high blood pressure, stroke or cancer may have heard that there are no alternatives but surgery and powerful drugs whose long-term effects are not well understood. I want you to know *that there are alternatives.*

This book is about *a thoroughly mainstream conservative treatment* for kidney disease, not a fringe theory, but the product of three decades of research in some of the world's leading medical centers. The details are about chronic kidney disease, but people whose lives are affected by other chronic diseases—patients, their families, and their doctors—will find here the story of how some patients and their doctors learned to *work in a new partnership to control chronic disease*. Other patients, families and doctors have found that conservative treatments can also be powerful tools against other chronic diseases—heart disease, high blood pressure, stroke, diabetes and cancer, the biggest killers in America and Europe in the late 20th century.

I have described my efforts to understand my chronic disease, and to understand the professionals who tried to help me. I have worked to understand why, as a patient, I thought, felt and behaved as I did. I have worked to understand why my doctors behaved as they did, and what they may have been thinking and feeling. Most of all, I have tried to describe *the new partnership* between patient and doctor that may be medicine's oldest and most powerful tool. The ideas and facts in this book have changed my life; they may change yours.

1

The Good News

This book is an attempt to spread the good news about kidney disease to those who can benefit most—the people who have learned about their disease early enough to do something about it. Early enough, that is, to prevent kidney failure—the condition government researchers have called "a devastating medical, social and economic problem to patients and their families." [1]

If you or someone close to you are among the thirteen million Americans who have kidney trouble,[2] this book will tell you the good news that kidney specialists may not have told you: *You may be able to prevent kidney disease from getting worse by changing some eating habits, and perhaps making some other simple lifestyle changes*. You may be able to stop kidney disease from killing you. You may be able to prevent the disease from progressively weakening your kidneys until they stop working, the life-threatening condition doctors call end-stage kidney disease, or end-stage renal disease.

Like heart disease and some other chronic conditions, kidney disease is often far advanced by the time symptoms appear. You may have lost two thirds or even three fourths of your kidneys' capacity before you and your doctor recognize the symptoms.[3] Then he may send you to a kidney doctor, an internal medicine specialist concentrating on the study and care of the kidneys, a nephrologist. A blood test may confirm that you have a kidney problem, but if you are in the early stages of your disease, the specialist may tell you there is nothing you can do until it gets worse. He may tell the doctor who referred you, "There's nothing I can do for him now. Send him back to me when he is vomiting." What he means is, "Wait

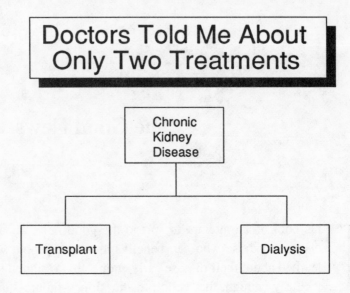

Figure 2: The Treatments-of-Choice For Kidney Disease

The nephrology establishment considers dialysis and transplant as the accepted "treatments-of-choice" for chronic kidney failure. Kidney specialists advised me to do nothing (except control my blood pressure) until my kidney disease reached end-stage. Then they said I could use one or both of the high technology treatments to save my life.

until the patient is in end-stage kidney disease, then we'll put him on dialysis, and maybe get him a transplant."

Some kidney doctors are so committed to high technology treatments that they don't even try to help their patients prevent kidney failure. A kidney patient like me may spend months or years after learning about his disease simply waiting for the disease to get worse, doing nothing to prevent it from threatening his life. Then, when he reaches end-stage, he faces the devastating medical, social and economic problems of kidney failure.

Kidney failure is not a problem for the doctor—in fact, it's an opportunity. He can often extend the kidney patient's life for a few months or years by performing high technology "medical miracles," and in the proc-

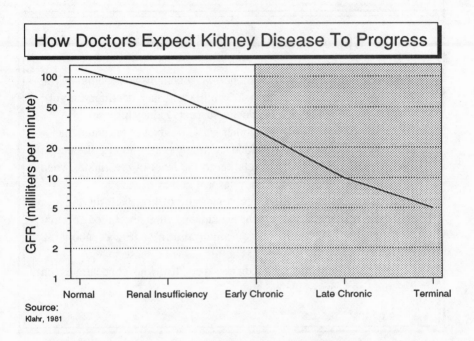

How Doctors Expect Kidney Disease To Progress

GFR (milliliters per minute)

100 · 50 · 20 · 10 · 5 · 2 · 1

Normal   Renal Insufficiency   Early Chronic   Late Chronic   Terminal

Source:
Klahr, 1981

Figure 3: The Expected Progression Of Kidney Disease

As the GFR — glomerular filtration rate — declines, the kidney patient passes through the phases of what doctors call progressive kidney disease. (GFR is a measure of how much blood the kidneys are filtering and therefore how well they are working.) People with normal kidneys have a GFR of about 120 milliliters per minute (ml/min). A person with diseased kidneys usually needs dialysis or transplant to stay alive when his GFR falls below about 5 milliliters per minute.

ess earning handsome fees. I don't mean to say that kidney doctors are greedy, although some surely are. They are simply doing what their training, experience and culture tell them to do. "Let the patient get to end-stage disease, then replace his lost kidney function with an artificial kidney or a transplant. That's the accepted way."

If kidney failure is not a problem for the doctor, it is often, as the government says, "a devastating problem" for kidney patients and their families. When I learned how close I was to kidney failure, I wanted a way to prevent the disease from getting worse. I didn't want to wait for the devastating consequences. I found a thoroughly mainstream third treat-

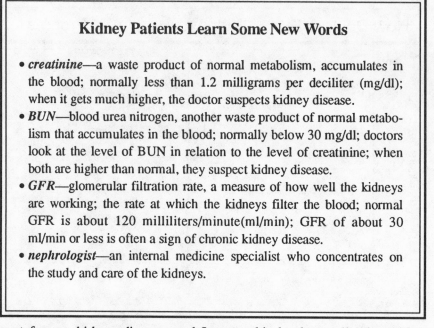

Kidney Patients Learn Some New Words

- *creatinine*—a waste product of normal metabolism, accumulates in the blood; normally less than 1.2 milligrams per deciliter (mg/dl); when it gets much higher, the doctor suspects kidney disease.
- *BUN*—blood urea nitrogen, another waste product of normal metabolism that accumulates in the blood; normally below 30 mg/dl; doctors look at the level of BUN in relation to the level of creatinine; when both are higher than normal, they suspect kidney disease.
- *GFR*—glomerular filtration rate, a measure of how well the kidneys are working; the rate at which the kidneys filter the blood; normal GFR is about 120 milliliters/minute(ml/min); GFR of about 30 ml/min or less is often a sign of chronic kidney disease.
- *nephrologist*—an internal medicine specialist who concentrates on the study and care of the kidneys.

ment for my kidney disease, and I wrote this book to tell other kidney patients what the doctors often don't tell them.

There is not yet a known cure for kidney disease, nor is there a known way to prevent the disease from getting started. But there is a way to stop the disease from progressing. Even though the kidney doctor may not have told you so, kidney patients and their families have lived nearly normal lives without the risky "medical miracles" of dialysis and transplant and the devastation of kidney failure.

THE OLD VIEW: KIDNEY DISEASE ALWAYS GETS WORSE

Until the 1960s, doctors believed kidney disease got inevitably worse, month by month, year by year, until the patient needed a medical miracle to stay alive—an artificial kidney or a transplant. They believed there was an underlying disease process causing this relentless progression to the condition they called end-stage kidney disease. It might take a very long time, years or even decades, to reach end-stage. The symptoms might be minor—fatigue, tiredness, frequent urination—easy to ignore, easy to live

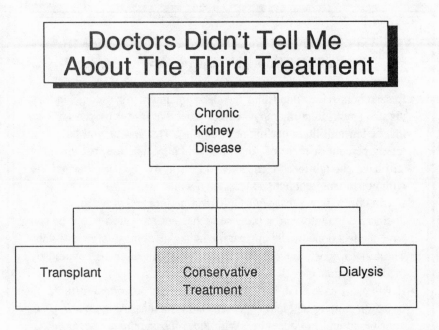

Doctors Didn't Tell Me About The Third Treatment

Figure 4 Three Treatments For Kidney Disease

Two prominent nephrologists had advised me to wait until my kidney disease reached end-stage. They didn't tell me that physician-scientists had developed a widely-used third treatment that could stop my disease from getting worse.

with. The patient's kidneys would continue to deteriorate progressively until he reached the point where they would stop working. He would have the condition doctors called uremia. His blood would be contaminated with the chemical waste products of everyday living that normal kidneys would have filtered from the blood. His body would be bloated with water the kidneys failed to remove. He would lack a vital hormone preventing him from becoming anemic. Without a medical miracle, he would die.

For the last thirty years some physicians and scientists in the United States and Europe have challenged that old view of kidney disease.[4] They have observed in thousands of patients that kidney disease can be stopped before it becomes life-threatening. Dr. Mackenzie Walser, a kidney specialist, professor and researcher at the Johns Hopkins University School of Medicine in Baltimore, observed in the 1970s that nutritional therapy

How Do I Know If I Have Discovered My Chronic Kidney Disease Early Enough For The New Treatment?

- Researchers have found that the third treatment for chronic kidney disease—nutritional therapy—can be effective if you have a GFR as low as ten milliliters per minute (ml/min). That means you have lost ninety percent or more of your normal kidney function, but you may still have enough reserve capacity to let you live a nearly normal life with nutritional treatment, at least for a while.
- If you don't know what your GFR measurement is, you can ask your doctor. He may not know because he has not measured it, but he can have the test done by the nuclear medicine lab at most large hospitals. The test can cost about $100 or more, and can often be covered by medical insurance.
- If you can't have a lab measure the GFR, your doctor can estimate it based on simpler and less expensive lab tests measuring *creatinine* in your blood and in your urine. With those measurements he can use a formula that will give a working estimate of the GFR.
- If the GFR is low—below thirty ml/min or so—you may want to have an actual GFR measurement done every few months to see how you are responding to conservative treatment.
- Kidney specialists at The National Institutes of Health say that people most at risk for kidney disease—those with high blood pressure, diabetes, or a family history of kidney disease—would benefit from a more accurate measurement of their kidney function than simply the measurement of creatinine in the blood.[5]
- If you ask a kidney doctor about this, don't be surprised if he tells you a GFR measurement isn't necessary. That's the accepted way.

slowed progression of kidney disease.[6] His theory is that a common mechanism causes the progression of all or nearly all kidney disease, and that the process can be slowed or stopped by diet or drugs. Dr. Walser and many other physician-scientists in the United States and overseas have tested this theory by treating thousands of kidney patients during the last thirty years, and although most researchers admit they have not yet provided solid scientific proof of the theory, they have accumulated substantial evidence that the progression of kidney disease can be stopped.

What this means to someone who has just learned of his kidney trouble is that the disease does not have to be a crippler, requiring one or both of the high technology treatments—transplant or dialysis. There is a simple and natural treatment that may prevent kidney disease from progressing to kidney failure. It is what doctors call the conservative treatment for kidney disease.[7] I call it the third treatment—nutritional therapy. It's not a quack scheme, but the product of some of the world's leading medical research centers in the United States and Europe. It is simple, natural and it works for many people. The third treatment may give kidney patients and their families the chance to live normal lives, without risky and expensive high-tech medicine.

The medical label for my kidney disease is chronic renal failure. When a kidney specialist gave my condition that ominous name, he told me there was nothing I could do except wait for the disease to destroy more of my kidneys until I reached end-stage, the life-threatening condition when I would need dialysis or transplant. He said kidney disease usually progresses relentlessly to complete failure, that there was nothing he could do to help me; nothing I could do to help myself. Kidney disease was progressive; it was a fact of life; I could only wait for the worst to happen.

Even though my disease would soon become life-threatening, he said, I shouldn't worry because I was a likely candidate for a kidney transplant. I was only fifty, younger than many transplant patients, and my other diseases were not yet serious. I might wait a year or two until a kidney became available from an organ donor. About 15,000 people were on waiting lists in the United States for kidney transplants in 1989 and only about 9,000 kidneys were donated.[8] (I could avoid the wait if I asked one of my two brothers to give me one of their healthy kidneys, and if their tissue types and blood type matched my own. I wasn't ready to ask my brothers to risk that, so I would have to wait for a donor.)

While I waited, the specialist said, I could go on dialysis. The artificial kidney would do the job my own diseased kidneys could no longer do. I wouldn't have to worry about paying for the treatment. Medicare would pay most of my dialysis and transplant costs under the End-Stage Renal Disease Program. Transplant almost always worked—"a ninety percent success rate," he said. Even though I had a fatal disease, the kidney specialist had a way to keep me alive with dialysis, and an even better way to

What Doctors Recommended For Me

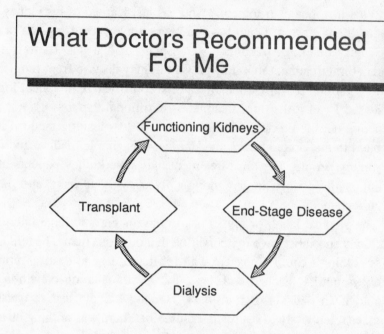

Figure 5 How Doctors Wanted To Treat My Kidney Disease

When my disease reached end-stage, they told me I could go on dialysis while I waited for a transplant that might return me to reasonably good health.

get me back to reasonably good health with a transplanted kidney. He was proud and happy that he could help me. I was frightened and confused.

The kidney specialist (by now I had learned to call him a nephrologist) had been following my case for four years since a neighborhood doctor had discovered some signs of my kidney disease. Dr. Robert Grossman was the director of the transplant program at the Hospital of the University of Pennsylvania, one of the most respected research and teaching hospitals in the country. Dr. Grossman was one of the pioneers of organ transplantation. He had been trying to help me control my blood pressure with drugs and lifestyle changes. He had been attentive to my condition, experimenting with various combinations of drugs that would produce the best control of my high blood pressure with the mildest side effects. He even became almost a family doctor for us, helping us find the right specialists

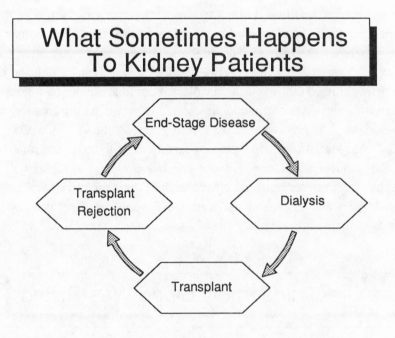

What Sometimes Happens To Kidney Patients

End-Stage Disease

Dialysis

Transplant

Transplant Rejection

Figure 6 A Cycle: Transplant-Rejection-Retransplant

I learned that transplants are often rejected by the body's immune system, forcing the patient back to dialysis to await a second transplant—"a retransplant." Sometimes the body rejects the second kidney.

for routine surgery on my wife and our oldest son, helping us recognize in our youngest daughter a case of extended mononucleosis that some other doctors wanted to treat with surgery. Some doctors in Philadelphia referred to Dr. Grossman as "the internists' internist," and *Philadelphia Magazine* had called him the best internist in town in 1984.

Dr. Grossman had been monitoring my blood tests for the signs that might indicate progressive kidney disease. He was watching two measurements in my blood chemistry most closely, creatinine and BUN (blood urea nitrogen). Both measurements are easily and inexpensively made as part of a routine blood test, and both are considered reliable indicators of kidney trouble. If the creatinine gets much over 1 milligram per deciliter (mg/dl) and the BUN gets over about 30 mg/dl, the nephrologist often suspects the start of progressive kidney disease.

That day after Christmas 1988, Dr. Grossman saw a big jump in the measurement of creatinine in my blood and concluded that I was entering the final stages of the disease. His guess was that I could stay alive for about six months with my own diseased kidneys, and then I would be in uremia. I would need dialysis or a transplant. I could make my own guess, he said, with a simple formula doctors used to estimate the progression of kidney disease. "I'll give you the data from your blood tests since 1985," he said, "and you can plot the graph yourself. It will show you that in about six months your kidneys will have failed almost completely." I plotted the graph on my personal computer, and the conclusion was inescapable. If he was right about the formula, I would be dependent on a dialysis machine by the summer of 1989, waiting for a transplant.

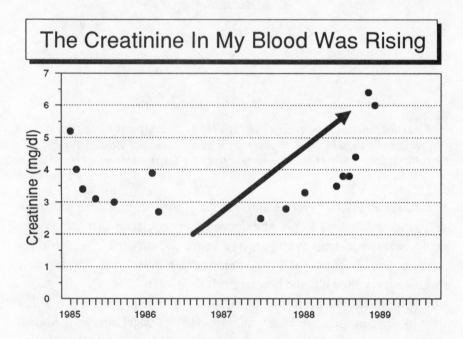

Figure 7   The creatinine in my blood

As my kidneys became progressively weaker, they were losing their ability to filter my blood. Creatinine is one of the waste products normal kidneys filter. When the doctor saw the creatinine in my blood rising (the "serum creatinine"), he suspected that my kidney disease was progressing to end-stage.

I felt frightened and angry that I would have to depend on high technology medical procedures to stay alive. I had worked with high technology as an inventor and entrepreneur for twenty-five years, and I had learned to be skeptical of technologists who promise high-tech miracles. I had made some technological promises of my own that didn't work quite the way I planned. I understood that troubles happen in all complicated high-tech undertakings—from the space shuttle and the space telescope to nuclear power plants and toxic waste dumps. I knew that some new technologies created as many problems as they solved. I believed that dialysis and transplant could appear successful in the view of the doctor—the doomed patient stayed alive—but I suspected that the risk was high and the quality of life was not good. I hoped there was another way, a simpler and more

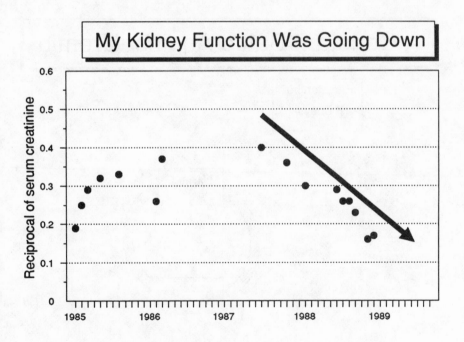

Figure 8 The reciprocal of my creatinine

Nephrologists often calculate the value of the reciprocal of the serum creatinine to predict the progression of kidney disease. Because of the way the mathematics works, the reciprocal goes down as the creatinine goes up. The result is a simple chart showing how the kidney function is declining.

natural way, a treatment that didn't depend on machines, drugs and surgery. I set out to find one in the medical library.

A SEARCH FOR A THIRD TREATMENT

Although I had never used a medical library, I hoped that I could find
some new research that would show me another way to deal with my
kidney disease. I had asked Dr. Grossman if there were other treatments.
"No," he said. "There is only dialysis and transplant, and that's it. There is
nothing else you can do. Transplant is the treatment-of-choice for kidney
disease. You could get a new kidney and be quite healthy." He had been
working in kidney transplantation for fifteen years, since the days when
most transplants failed within months. He believed in his work, and be-

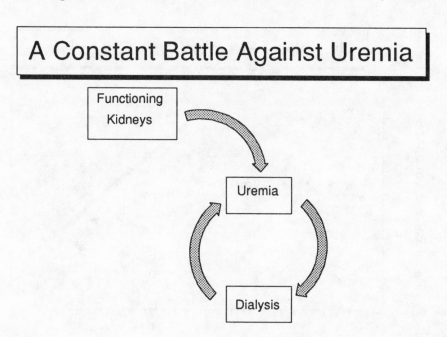

Figure 9 Dialysis As A Constant Battle Against Uremia

*When I reached end-stage kidney disease, I would be in the condition
known as uremia. Dialysis would relieve some of the symptoms by doing
some of the work of my diseased kidneys, but my body would drift back
toward uremia when I was not on the dialysis machine.*

lieved he could not only keep me alive, but restore me to good health. He was committed to transplant as the best way to treat my disease. I respected him and wanted to believe him, but I also wanted to find another way, a third treatment as an alternative to dialysis and transplant.

To my surprise I learned that the medical library is an accessible place. The computerized catalogs and extensive indexes made it easy for me to find the pertinent research. Since I have no medical or scientific background (my high technology experience was with computers, software and telecommunications), I had a language barrier. The technical terms in the research literature baffled me, but a medical dictionary and encyclopedia helped.

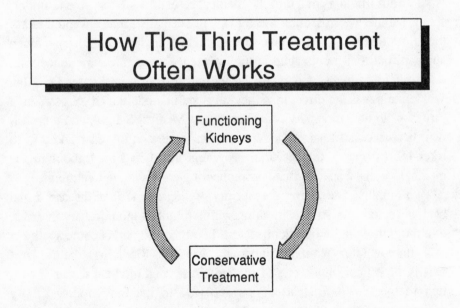

Figure 10 Nutritional Treatment Can Control The Disease

If it was successful for me, nutritional treatment would help me preserve some of the kidney function I still had. I could delay or even avoid the need for dialysis and transplant by controlling my disease.

After a morning in the medical library, I had found books and papers by highly-respected medical researchers and physicians in the United States and Europe who were working to prove their theory that conservative treatment could prevent, or at least slow down, the progression of kidney disease. I even found a 1988 medical reference book for kidney doctors, *Nutrition and the Kidney*, edited by two of the most prominent nephrology practitioners and researchers in the world, Dr. William E. Mitch of Emory University in Atlanta and Dr. Saulo Klahr of Washington University in St. Louis.[9] The book collected articles from leading nephrologists, dietitians and other researchers in the United States and Europe. It was thoroughly mainstream, not a fringe theory. The book recommended conservative nutritional treatment for most people with kidney disease. The book cover said, "Nutrition is now a primary tool in the treatment of renal disease."

After absorbing as much of the medical research as I was able to understand, I told Dr. Grossman, the transplant specialist, that I wanted to try the third treatment, nutritional therapy. He said he didn't know much about it, but that a colleague at the university had some experience with nutritional treatment, and might be willing to follow my case. Dr. Alan Wasserstein was the director of the dialysis unit, and, like Dr. Grossman, a professor in the University of Pennsylvania Medical School, and a prominent nephrologist. I asked Dr. Wasserstein to take on my case and also to refer me to one of the research programs that I had read about in the medical journals, a study that was pioneering conservative treatments.

Two months after learning about my progressive kidney disease, I had been accepted as a volunteer, along with two dozen other kidney patients, in a program to help the scientists test their theory. I had become a subject in a study at Johns Hopkins University School of Medicine, like the University of Pennsylvania, one of the most respected medical research centers in the world. Instead of surrendering to the inevitability of my progressive kidney disease, I would have an opportunity to work on stopping it from getting worse. With the help of Dr. Wasserstein at Penn and Dr. Walser and his team at Johns Hopkins, I would learn to follow a program so simple and natural that I would have the chance to avoid being dependent on high technology medicine. I would feel more in control of my own life; perhaps I would be able to live normally despite my disabling disease.

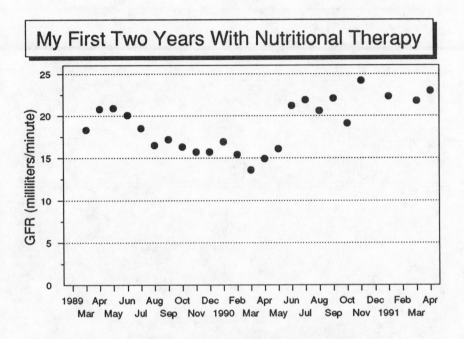

Figure 11 My First Two Years With Nutritional Therapy

I started nutritional therapy for my own chronic kidney disease with a GFR of about 18 ml/min in March, 1989. Two years later my GFR was over 20 ml/min. That doesn't prove anything to anybody but me, of course. It may even be a coincidence. But obviously nutritional treatment agrees with me, at least for now.

The third treatment has worked for me so far (about two years as I write this in early 1991), and for many others. It shows promise of working for most kidney patients. But even if it doesn't work, most kidney specialists experienced with nutritional therapy have observed little risk for the patient in trying, maybe no risk at all. The good news is that there is a third treatment for kidney disease. The prognosis is good.

2

Please, Doctor, No Miracles

People with end-stage kidney disease once needed miracles to stay alive. No longer. All three treatments for kidney disease are routine in the 1990s. No miracles; simply routine medical care. Two are high-tech and risky, but the third treatment for kidney disease is simple, low-tech and natural, holding out the promise of *preventing* kidney failure, not just treating it.

The most widely-used high-tech treatment is *dialysis*, either the artificial kidney, the *hemodialysis* machine, or a method known as *peritoneal dialysis*, using a natural membrane in the abdomen. Dialysis is so routine that there were about 110,000 people on dialysis in the United States in 1988. The other high-tech treatment, *transplant*, is also routine. About 37,000 people were living with a functioning kidney transplant in 1988.[1] Surgeons performed kidney transplant operations an average of 25 times a day in the United States in 1988.[2] They claim "a ninety percent success rate," although some transplant scientists are not sure about that. (More about "success rates" in Chapters 7 and 8.)

The two high-tech treatments carry with them the risks of any high technology. Riding in a car or in an airplane has risks; using electricity in your house has risks; walking on a city street at night has risks. But there were 172,506 kidney patients in the Medicare End-Stage Renal Disease program at some time in 1988, the last year for which complete Medicare statistics have been published,[3] and about 150,000 Americans were alive at the end of 1988 because they used some form of dialysis, or they were living with someone else's kidney transplanted into their bodies. The two

How Many Kidney Patients Survived Dialysis And Transplant?

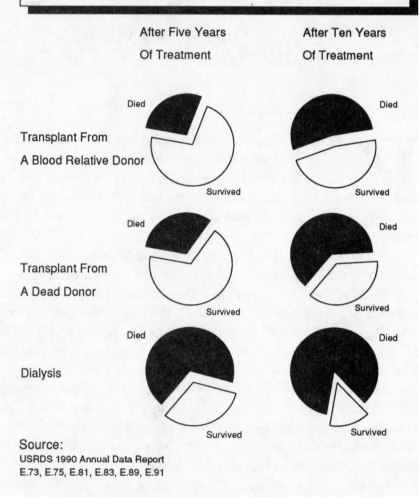

Source:
USRDS 1990 Annual Data Report
E.73, E.75, E.81, E.83, E.89, E.91

Figure 12 Patient Survival Probabilities

The government's U.S. Renal Data System has gathered facts about 372,000 patients in the Medicare End-Stage Renal Disease Program since 1976. I found that the study painted a grim picture of the effectiveness of high technology treatment for my kidney disease.

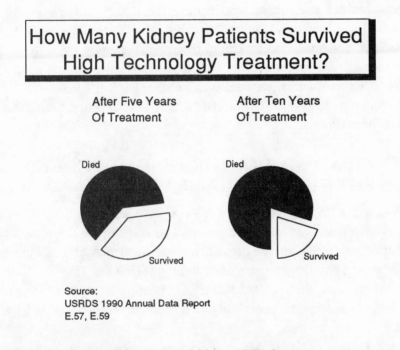

Source:
USRDS 1990 Annual Data Report
E.57, E.59

Figure 13 Patient Survival Probabilities, All Patients

When the statisticians measured the survival of all patients in the program, they found that six of ten had died within five years. Eight of ten died within ten years. I wondered how "miraculous" the high technology treatments were, especially when there was a simple alternative that had worked for many people.

high-tech treatments are common and routine, no matter how expensive, complicated and risky they may be.

The third treatment for chronic kidney disease—nutritional therapy—is as simple as the high-tech treatments are complex. *When the kidneys aren't working well, give them less work to do.* The patient eats a diet low in protein and phosphorus to reduce the amount of waste products the kidneys must filter from the blood. He tries to control his blood pressure, and he tries to achieve a good balance of the important constituents of his blood chemistry, like calcium, potassium, cholesterol and blood fats.

Nutritional therapy for kidney disease is not accepted by the medical establishment, and many doctors question whether it is effective.[4] Some doctors and scientists have observed that nutritional therapy slows or stops progression, but even those who believe the theory will eventually be confirmed say that they have not yet provided scientific proof.[5] Some researchers and many doctors think nutritional therapy isn't worth the bother, because they believe the diet is too difficult for most people to follow.[6, 7] Other doctors, especially in Europe, think it's unethical *not* to treat kidney patients with nutritional therapy before committing them to dialysis or transplant.[8]

WHY DIDN'T MY DOCTOR TELL ME I COULD PREVENT KIDNEY FAILURE?

When the kidney doctor told you, "You have serious kidney disease," he may also have said that there was no known cure, but there were two effective treatments—dialysis and transplant—and that your fellow tax-payers would pay for your treatment through Medicare. If you have read the booklets from the National Kidney Foundation or the American Kidney Fund, you learned about only two treatments—dialysis and transplant.[9, 10]

Some kidney professionals—the doctors, nurses, social workers and technicians who help kidney patients—may not have told you about the third treatment because they believe the new theory has not been scientifically proven. Some believe the evidence is not only incomplete, but is also

---

**Some Reasons Doctors Give
For Not Recommending Nutritional Treatment,
Sometimes Not Even Telling Patients About It**

- "The studies are not conclusive."
- "Too difficult for patients to follow."
- "May cause malnutrition."
- "Transplant is 'the treatment-of-choice,' although dialysis may be better than transplant for some patients."
- "Transplant can return a kidney patient to nearly normal kidney function."
- "Nutritional treatment is merely a 'rearguard action' against kidney disease."

Some Other Reasons Why Doctors May Ignore Nutritional Treatment For Kidney Disease

- "I don't know much about nutritional treatment. My medical training included little about nutrition because modern medicine is skeptical of the connection between nutrition and disease."
- "Throughout medical history, much nutritional treatment was nonsense, quackery and charlatanism, with no scientific basis."
- "Kidney disease, like other diseases, should be *removed* from the body by *aggressive medical treatment*—drugs, surgery, artificial organs."
- "Nutritional treatment for kidney disease has never been proven by a well-designed scientific study—a prospective randomized controlled trial."
- "There are no such trials proving the value of dialysis and transplant either, but the results of these aggressive therapies are intuitively obvious. No trials are needed."

---

contradictory. They point out that research on animals provides conflicting evidence: dietary restriction seems to stop progression in rats, but not in dogs.[11] They note that nearly all the studies on humans have not included *controls*, that is, untreated patients whose condition can be compared to that of the treated patients to judge the effectiveness of the condition. Many of the scientists working hardest to prove the theory agree that they have not yet presented the conclusive scientific evidence that would come from a *prospective randomized controlled trial.*[12] As I listened to this scientific debate, I wondered if the doctors demanding conclusive proof before they would recommend conservative treatment for kidney disease were relying on the argument the tobacco companies used for twenty years when they ridiculed claims of a connection between cigarette smoking and disease.

There isn't any conclusive scientific evidence proving dialysis and transplant as the "treatments-of-choice" for kidney disease either, but when doctors *want* to do something, they can often find ways to do it. For example, in 1960 doctors learned how to use the artificial kidney machine to keep diseased patients alive for years instead of days. Dr. Belding H.

Still More Reasons Why Doctors May Ignore Nutritional Treatment For Kidney Disease

- Medicare and insurance companies pay $5 billion a year to the doctors, hospitals, dialysis centers, equipment, drug and supplies makers, nurses, technicians, social workers and others who are the "kidney business." It would not be surprising if this special interest group wanted to keep the $5 billion a year flowing with no change in the way kidney disease is treated.
- Medicare and insurance companies may not pay for nutritional treatment.
- Nutritional treatment requires skills and interests that kidney doctors may not have because their training largely ignored nutrition, and because they may be skeptical of nutritional causes of disease.
- It may be far easier for a kidney doctor to prescribe dialysis or transplant than to help the patient use nutritional treatment—easier for the *doctor*, but far more difficult for the patient and his family.
- The kidney doctor may face the prospect of attempting nutritional treatment that is more difficult for the doctor, and less rewarding than the high technology treatments.
- A convenient, comfortable and safe position for the kidney doctor is to say, "Nutritional treatment is not proven."
- Nobody can criticize a kidney doctor for recommending dialysis and transplant, not even a medical malpractice lawyer.
- The kidney patient may want to decide for himself whether he wants treatment that is easy and financially rewarding for the *doctor*—dialysis and transplant—but often devastating for the *patient and his family*.

Scribner had invented a way to get the patient's contaminated blood out of his body into the artificial kidney machine for cleansing and back again into the body. He used the new method on a kidney patient in Seattle, Clyde Shields, who eventually survived on dialysis for 11 years. Dr. Scribner wrote in 1990:

"Successful treatment of Clyde Shields represents one of the few instances in medicine where a single success was all that was required to validate a new therapy."[13]

Dr. Scribner says that dialysis became a treatment-of-choice because of *a single success*. There was no conclusive scientific evidence of the kind doctors are demanding for nutritional treatment. There was simply the fact that dialysis worked, as Dr. Scribner says, *in one patient*. Nutritional treatment has worked in *thousands of patients over the last thirty years*, but many kidney doctors continue to ignore it. I wondered how doctors could have accepted dialysis so quickly after it worked *on a single patient*, yet scoff at nutritional therapy that has worked for thousands of patients over thirty years. Could there be something here beside the best interest of the kidney patient? Could the kidney doctors be so influenced by their high technology, aggressive treatment, drugs-and-surgery culture that they *deny the kidney patient a chance to prevent his disease*?

THE DREAM OF KIDNEY REPLACEMENT

Some kidney professionals may not know much about nutritional therapy for kidney disease. For the last 50 years, the medical establishment has been pursuing the dream of *renal replacement therapy,* kidney replacement therapy. When a patient's kidneys failed, doctors wanted to replace their function with an artificial organ (dialysis) or, better yet, give him a completely new organ (a kidney transplant). Dialysis machines began to work in the 1960s, keeping people with kidney failure, like Clyde Shields, alive for a while, sometimes for years. Transplanted kidneys functioned more often, and for a longer time. For the last half century, the medical establishment has put most of its energies and money into renal replacement, little into helping people prevent the disease from getting worse. Dialysis and transplant fit in neatly with the "aggressive treatment" many American doctors seem to favor.[14] Disease is something alien to the human body, they say, something to be removed aggressively, with drugs or surgery, not with nutrition and lifestyle changes. Perhaps some doctors feel uncomfortable suggesting lifestyle changes, instead of prescribing a drug, surgery or three days a week on the artificial kidney.

In 1972, the multi-billion dollar kidney business was launched when Congress decided that taxpayers should pay for renal replacement for 90 percent of Americans who needed it. Henceforth there would be virtually unlimited taxpayers' money to pay for artificial kidney machines, transplant operations and drugs. An army of kidney specialists, transplant surgeons, dialysis center owners, technicians, nurses, dietitians, social workers, drug companies, medical equipment manufacturers, supplies vendors, patients and families became dependent on Medicare-paid renal replacement therapy. By the 1990s, the kidney business was a $5 billion a year industry, and growing, most paid by taxpayers. There were almost twice as many Medicare-certified profit-making dialysis and transplant centers in 1989 as there had been in 1981.[15] Even the most zealous medical crusaders, like the pioneering transplant surgeon Dr. Thomas E. Starzl, were saying that kidney transplantation was no longer a crusade. It had become a *business*.[16] In 1990 two transplant surgeons won the Nobel Prize for medicine; one for his work in transplanting kidneys, Dr. Joseph Murray of Harvard; the other for work in bone marrow transplants, Dr. E. Donnal Thomas.[17]

With the best of motives—saving the lives of dying victims of kidney disease—the kidney establishment had become committed to what the physician, scientist and philosopher Dr. Lewis Thomas called the "half-way technology" of renal replacement. He called it *half-way* because the technology does not *prevent the disease or stop it from getting worse*, but simply deals with the consequences. A classic example of half-way technology is the now-forgotten artificial lung, the "iron lung," a machine of the 1940s and 1950s that helped paralyzed polio victims breathe when otherwise they might have died. Using half-way technology to keep polio patients alive, entombed in an iron lung, was surely better than letting them die. But a far better solution for the patient was a technology that would *not* be half-way—the polio vaccines *that prevented the disease from getting started in the first place*. People who grew up in the 1940s and 1950s, as I did, can remember the movie newsreel pictures of Sister Kenny raising money for hospital wards filled with iron lungs to keep polio victims alive. By the 1960s, the half-way technology of the artificial lung was no longer needed because doctors had used the new vaccines to eliminate polio almost completely as a threat to Americans.

While Medicare was pouring billions into renal replacement, only a few kidney researchers worked on the problem of *preventing* the ultimate failure that was the normal result of kidney disease. It was like pouring money into iron lungs, and not trying to find a vaccine to prevent polio.

Are the dialysis machines and the kidney transplant operations of the last half of the 20th century like the iron lungs of the middle decades? Can a patient prevent his kidney disease from getting worse, eliminating the need for dialysis and transplant? Can the dialysis machines and the transplant scalpels be junked along with the iron lungs? Is there even a way to prevent kidney disease from getting started? I hope scientists will find the answers to those questions in the 1990s, and as a volunteer subject in the government studies I hope to do my part.

A SLOW BUT RELENTLESS KILLER

Despite all the scientific research in the United States and Europe over the last thirty years, many doctors think kidney disease is a certain death sentence unless they intervene with high-tech dialysis or transplant. By the time kidney disease is serious enough to be noticed, it has often started what doctors believe is a relentless and inevitable progression. No treatment would work. No medicine. No surgery. Kidney disease was hopeless. The disease would progress from mild to serious and then on to complete kidney failure and death. The medical terms the doctors use show how they believe the progression, once started, proceeds inexorably to death. The most widely-used physician's reference, the *Merck Manual of Diagnosis and Therapy*, says "progression of underlying chronic renal disease generally is not susceptible to specific treatment."[18]

The kidney establishment believes nobody knows how to stop the progression of kidney disease—the nephrologists, medical school professors, scientific journal editors, association executives, dialysis center owners, drug companies, machine and supplies manufacturers who influence and probably control the way doctors treat kidney patients like me. For example, in 1989 a prominent nephrologist from the Cleveland Clinic, Dr. Phillip Hall, reviewed the current state-of-the-art in treatment of kidney disease for a medical journal widely read by non-specialist doctors. He asked the question: Can progression of renal disease be prevented? His answer: Maybe, but nothing is proven yet. Controlling blood pressure and cholesterol, restricting protein in the diet, using certain drugs may help, but "whether such interventions will significantly alter progressive renal disease in humans is as yet uncertain."[19] Such has been the conventional medical wisdom throughout the twentieth century. Once it starts, kidney disease keeps getting worse. We don't know the cause. We can't prevent it. We can't cure it. The best we can do is treat it, try to keep the patient alive after his kidneys have failed, try to cheat death by extending the patient's life for a while with technology.

A DIFFERENT APPROACH FOR AN INCURABLE DISEASE

Believing that they did not know how to prevent or cure kidney disease, doctors tried a different approach. They searched for high-tech ways to replace the kidneys that no longer worked. *Renal replacement* would use high technology to replace the function of the damaged natural organs. If the patient's kidneys didn't work, doctors would give him a new kidney, somebody else's healthy kidney transplanted into his body, an artificial kidney machine three days a week, or some other form of dialysis. They would save his life with this half-way technology that didn't prevent or cure the disease. But it did the next best thing, something vitally important. It kept the patient alive.

It was a widely shared dream, something worth working on. Twentieth century scientists and engineers had solved dozens of problems with high technology. Why not medicine? Everybody looked for solutions in technology. Doctors working in the 1940s, 1950s and 1960s had grown up with the coming of the car, telephone, airplane, radio, television. Why not high-tech artificial organs to replace those that no longer worked because of injury or disease? The iron lung was the way to deal with polio, until the vaccine prevented the disease. For the doctor himself, high technology offered a chance to be a hero, help people and make a good living at the same time, maybe even win a Nobel prize, the ultimate recognition for scientific achievement. Doctors who developed high-tech treatments or drugs could become famous, command high fees, earn valuable patents, found companies to develop the technology. What ambitious researcher wouldn't try?

The most prominent pioneer of organ transplantation, Dr. Thomas Starzl, a surgeon now at the University of Pittsburgh, saw transplantation not only as a way to treat diseases of the kidney, liver, heart, lung, pan-

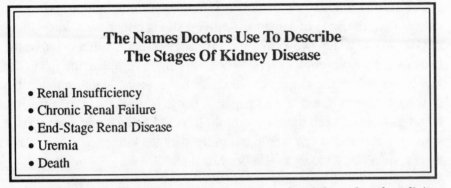

**The Names Doctors Use To Describe
The Stages Of Kidney Disease**

- Renal Insufficiency
- Chronic Renal Failure
- End-Stage Renal Disease
- Uremia
- Death

creas and other organs, but as *a way to change the philosophy of medicine.*
No longer would doctors

> **"...preside over lethal disease powerless to provide much more than a
> priestly function. Suddenly, with the advent of transplantation, it be-
> came possible for the first time in human history to provide exactly what
> was needed, a completely new organ."**[20]

Dr. Starzl saw himself working on not merely an ordinary problem—
like a cure for cancer or a way to prevent polio. *His work would change
the art and science of medicine forever.* He would teach doctors how to be
more than just priests, presiding powerless over disease. He would teach
doctors how to give the patient the ultimate gift—a new organ. How
miraculous it would be if a diseased person could come to his doctor for
exactly what was needed, a new kidney, a new heart, a new anything. The
transplant surgeons, led by Dr. Starzl, would father a new kind of medicine. It was a thrilling dream.

Doctors saw two ways to do renal replacement, either of which some
people would call "miracles" in the middle decades of the 20th century. In
the first miracle, a machine would perform some of the functions no
longer handled by the diseased kidneys. The patient's arteries and veins
would be attached to the machine. His blood would pass through the
machine over a membrane that would remove some of the unwanted substances his kidneys no longer filtered. The machine would then return the
cleansed blood to his veins. It would be an *artificial organ*, a man-made
kidney, a miracle that would keep the patient alive even though his own
organs had failed.

The second miracle was even better. Surgeons would remove a healthy kidney from the body of someone—either a living donor, who was willing to give up one of his two kidneys to save someone else's life, or, from the body of a dead person, a cadaver. Then, rushing to complete the job in the few hours before the kidney tissue died, the surgeons would implant the healthy kidney in the diseased person's body. It would start filtering the blood as if it had been there from birth. It would be an organ transplant, a surgical intervention that would return the doomed kidney patient to a life that his own failed kidneys were denying him.

EARLY RESULTS WERE POOR. NOW THEY ARE BETTER

In the last half of the twentieth century, doctors worked to make the high-tech treatments common and routine, no matter how risky and expensive. By the 1990s they had succeeded in convincing the medical establishment that dialysis and transplant were the "treatments-of-choice." In 1988, the 110,000 people on dialysis in the United States numbered more than a hundred times as many as there were twenty years earlier.[21] About nine thousand people got kidney transplants each year during the last half of the 1980s in the United States. About three-fourths of the transplanted kidneys were still functioning after one year. Only five percent of the patients died within a year after transplantation.[22, 23] During the 1970s, there had been only one third as many transplants each year in the United States, and the success rate had been much lower.

In the 1980s researchers had gained a better understanding of the *rejection phenomenon* that made transplantation so difficult in the early years—the body's effort to reject the foreign tissue of a transplanted organ. They were able to do a better job of identifying the tissue types of the donor and the recipient. (Some people have compared the concept of *tissue types* to the vastly more simple *blood types* that make possible routine blood transfusions from a blood donor to someone who needs new blood.) The better understanding of rejection also led to new drugs, particularly *cyclosporine*, and more effective *drug cocktails*, mixtures of several drugs intended to prevent rejection. Although the results were much better in the 1980s, they were still not good. Few dialysis or transplant patients were well enough to return to work, and life expectancy was not long. (Much more about the outcome of high technology treatments, *the results for the patient,* in the chapters on dialysis and transplant, Chapters 6, 7 and 8.)

A CHALLENGE TO
THE CONVENTIONAL WISDOM

While some medical researchers worked on the two high-tech kidney replacement treatments, others were asking themselves a different question. *Can the progression of kidney disease be prevented?* Can the patient preserve enough kidney function to stay alive without expensive and risky technology? Many doctors were skeptical of this research. Kidney disease is progressive, they said, and we don't know how to prevent it or stop it from progressing. But we do know how to replace kidneys that don't work, with an artificial kidney or, better yet, a transplant.

Some scientists nonetheless challenged this conventional medical wisdom. One of the therapies they tested was nutritional treatment. Medicine had known for over a century that nutritional treatment might be useful in treating the symptoms of kidney disease, but nobody believed it would *slow or stop progression.* A medical textbook by a British doctor published in London and Philadelphia in 1869 recommended dietary treatment for the symptoms of kidney disease.[24]

Despite the skepticism and while the kidney establishment was pursuing renal replacement therapy, some scientists were exploring *nutrition and the kidney* in both animals and humans. One of the leaders was Dr. Mackenzie Walser, a nephrologist, pharmacologist and professor of medicine at Johns Hopkins University in Baltimore whose work I had discovered in the scientific journals on my first trip to the medical library in 1988. Dr. Walser had first suggested in 1974 that there is a common mechanism underlying progression in all or nearly all kidney disease, and that the process can be successfully treated with diet and drugs, or both. He had observed that some patients on very low protein diets supplemented with a form of essential amino acids had a temporary stabilization, or even some improvement in their kidney function.[25] He developed (and patented the formula for) a form of amino acids known as *keto acids* that supplemented a kidney patient's low protein diet, and which he suspects may contribute to slowing down or stopping the progression of the disease.

Dr. Walser has treated hundreds of patients since 1974, exploring nutritional and other factors in the progression of kidney disease. Although he doesn't know how to cure kidney disease, he believes he knows how to prevent it from getting worse. He can't yet prove why his treatment works, but he is working to understand the mechanism. He believes restricting protein and phosphorus in the diet, controlling blood pressure, cholesterol and blood fats, and maintaining a good balance of other blood chemistry constituents can slow or stop the progression of kidney disease for most people.[26] (Chapter 9 describes the work of Dr. Walser and other researchers.)

A FEDERAL STUDY TO FIND OUT IF NUTRITIONAL THERAPY WORKS

Although most scientists admit that nutritional therapy is not yet proven, the evidence is accumulating rapidly. The federal government has launched a study intended to test the new theory conclusively. The National Institute of Diabetes and Digestive and Kidney Diseases, one of the National Institutes of Health, has organized sixteen medical centers nationwide for this major study to be completed by 1993.

The $50-million study—Modification of Diet in Renal Disease—is often called the "MDRD study." The research centers were trying to recruit up to 800 patients whose kidney disease they plan to study through 1992. In 1993, the scientists will analyze the data and report the results of

---

Questions The $50-million Government Study Hopes To Answer

- Will a diet low in protein and phosphorus retard the rate of progression of renal failure in patients with chronic kidney disease?
- Will a low-protein, low-phosphorus diet cause malnutrition?
- Will such a diet be acceptable to patients over the long term?

Source: Klahr, 1989.

the study.[27] Dr. Walser believes the study will conclusively prove the benefits of dietary treatment in slowing or stopping progression of kidney disease.[28]

The director of the study, Dr. Saulo Klahr, has apparently already concluded that even if nutritional therapy is proven to slow or prevent the progression of chronic kidney failure, it will not be a practical treatment. In an article published in December, 1990—two years before the study is scheduled to be completed—Dr. Klahr wrote:

> "... compliance will persist as a major limitation of the use of such dietary approaches on a wide-scale basis, thus pharmacologic approaches will emerge as the preferable future therapy."[29]

When doctors say *compliance,* they mean, "Will the patient follow doctor's orders? Will he *comply* with doctor's recommendations?" What Dr. Klahr said in this 1990 article, I think, is that the early results from the big study have convinced him *that most kidney patients will not comply* with the doctor's recommendation for nutritional treatment, and that dietary treatment is therefore not practical. A better approach, he apparently believes, is to find a drug—"a pharmacologic approach"—that will stop kidney disease from progressing. I wondered, as I read this prediction, why taxpayers' money was being spent on a $50 million government study whose director had already made up his mind about the results.

Dr. Klahr told me a few months after his article was published that he had not pre-judged the results of the MDRD study. He said that the preliminary phase of the study had showed "poor compliance," but that in the final phase, patients seemed to be adapting well to the dietary changes.

> "We have learned a lot and have developed training methods that result in good to excellent compliance. Although compliance to a diet may still be a problem in a general population, I do not believe in doing a study in which the results can be predicted in advance. Since dietary modification represents for many people a major change in lifestyle, I still feel that besides dietary restriction and its potential role in preventing the progression of renal disease we should continue to explore the role of potential pharmacological agents that may slow or halt the progression of renal disease."[30]

Some people may feel threatened by the new treatment. Some powerful economic interests may be at risk if the treatment proves useful. Congress's decision in 1972 that taxpayers should pay for treating most Americans with end-stage renal disease provided $5 billion a year guaranteed revenue to the renal replacement industry. Medicare pays as much as $32,000 a year for treatments for each dialysis patient, who is often also eligible for Social Security disability and other medical expenses provided by law specifically for end-stage kidney disease patients. A new drug to treat dialysis patients' anemia, erythropoetin, can cost $10,000 a year.[31] Transplant costs can be $50,000 to $60,000 if there are no complications with another $10,000 to $20,000 a year for anti-rejection drugs. Medicare pays most of the treatment costs of most Americans with end-stage renal disease, over 147,000 of them in 1988.[32]

The result is $5 billion a year—much of it from taxpayers—going to dialysis centers, consulting nephrologists, artificial kidney machine manufacturers, dialysis supplies providers, the army of technicians who keep the dialysis centers running, the transplant surgeons and centers, the drug makers. That combination of personal financial interests is a powerful incentive to keep the $5 billion flowing just as it is today, from the same taxpayers and insurance premium payers to the same dialysis and transplant providers. It would not be surprising if some members of the kidney establishment were tempted to think, "Don't change the system by claiming there is another way to treat kidney disease, perhaps reducing the need for dialysis and transplant. Don't stop the flow of $5 billion a year."

If you are early enough in the course of your kidney disease, you may be able to avoid the high-tech treatments, or at least to delay the need for dialysis or transplant. If so, you will save yourself the risk of high-tech treatments that sometimes don't work as well as doctors hope. You may save yourself and your family from the expense of those treatments, and you may save your fellow taxpayers the tens of thousands of Medicare dollars that would be spent on your treatment. The third treatment for kidney disease may be worth a try for you. It was for me. The risk, the down-side, for a patient is very low, maybe none. The possible benefit is a chance to live normally despite your disease.

3
Who Gets Kidney Disease and Why?

Nobody knows for sure how many people have kidney disease in the United States, but the National Institutes of Health says that 13 million Americans are affected by kidney disease and related disorders. The best estimate comes from scientists studying the statistics from Medicare's End-Stage Renal Disease Program and the U.S. Renal Data System, records on 372,000 Medicare patients who have been treated for end-stage kidney disease since 1976.[1] The figures for 1988, the latest available, show that about 150 people out of a million population reach end-stage kidney disease each year in the United States. Ten times as many people get cancer—about 150 out of 100,000. If you live in a city of a million people, there are about 150 whose kidney disease reaches end-stage each year. If your town has 10,000 people, there are one or two new cases a year. In 1988, 36,160 kidney patients entered the Medicare program for end-stage kidney disease.

(I have taken many of the facts in this book from the U.S. Renal Data System Annual Report published in late 1990. Your doctor may not know many of these facts, particularly about the less-than-hoped-for results of dialysis and transplant. You may want to show him some of the charts in this book and the detailed statistics from the government reports included in Appendix 1. You may also want to consider that these facts are from a detailed, patient-by-patient study of the 372,000 patients who have passed through the Medicare Program since 1976, not from a a study sample. These are the real facts about kidney disease and treatments. I found them to be grim, not at all like the rosy picture some doctors have painted about the "miracle treatments for kidney disease.")

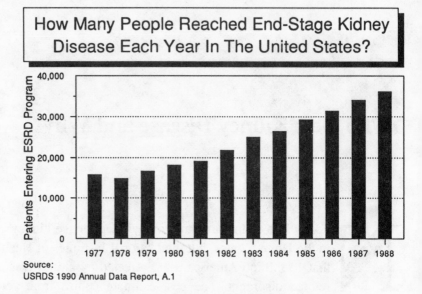

Source:
USRDS 1990 Annual Data Report, A.1

Figure 14 New Cases of End-Stage Kidney Disease (Count)

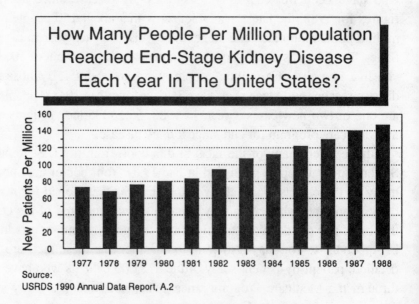

Source:
USRDS 1990 Annual Data Report, A.2

Figure 15 New Cases Of End-Stage Kidney Disease (Rate)

Some groups are more at risk of kidney disease than others. Blacks are four times more likely to reach end-stage disease than whites, and researchers have found that people living in some parts of the United States are far more likely to get kidney disease than those living in other areas. Blacks had 404 cases per million population while whites had only 109 per million.[2] Residents of New Jersey—the state with the highest rate of kidney disease—were twice as likely to get the disease as residents of North Dakota, the state where the disease is most rare. People in the southwestern states (Texas, New Mexico, Arizona and California) were much more likely to have kidney disease than people in the deep south states (Arkansas, Louisiana, Mississippi, Alabama and Tennessee.) Nobody knows why the regional differences are so big.[3]

Experts found that only two of the demographic and environmental factors they studied seemed to have a relationship to the occurrence of kidney disease—the percentage of a state's population living in a metro-

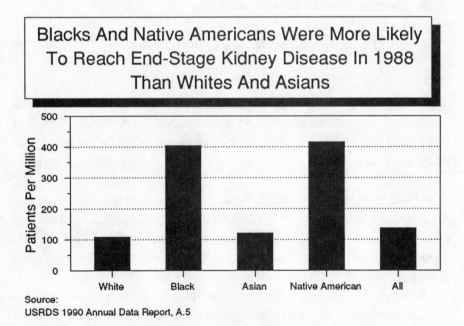

Figure 16 New Cases Of End-Stage Disease, By Race, 1988

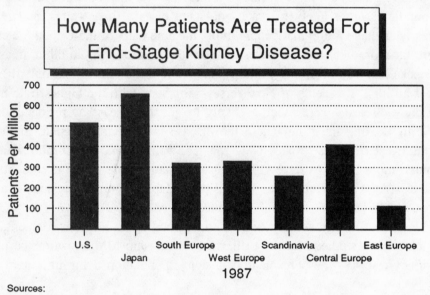

Figure 17 End-Stage Kidney Disease In Other Countries

politan area (high in New Jersey and low in North Dakota), and, in a minor way, the gallons of gasoline used by an average person. Whether this means that city living, or something about gasoline or the amount of time spent driving increases the chances of kidney disease, nobody knows.[4]

In Europe, about 300 persons per million population were being treated for end-stage kidney disease in the late 1980s.[5] In Japan, the number was twice as high, 658 persons out of every million.[6] In the United States, about 515 patients per million persons were being treated for end-stage kidney disease. Nobody knows why there is such a wide variation.[7]

Life expectancy for an end-stage kidney patient is much shorter than for the average American—about nine years for a 40-year-old kidney patient compared to 37 years for an average 40-year-old. A kidney patient's life expectancy is even less than that of many cancer patients, despite the "miracles" of the artificial kidney and the transplant.[8]

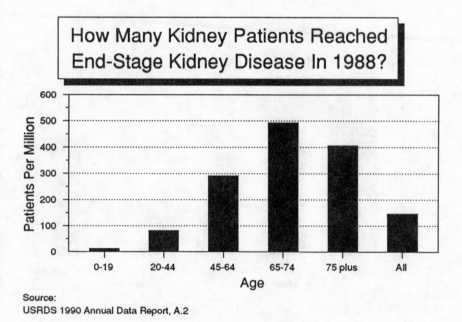

Figure 18 End-Stage Kidney Patients On Medicare, 1988

WHAT CAUSES KIDNEY DISEASE?

Just as we don't really know how many people have kidney disease, we often don't know the cause of the disease either. In the vast majority of cases, there are no symptoms until the disease is advanced. There may be clues, like high blood pressure, anemia, or a slight elevation of BUN or creatinine, two of the blood chemistry items a routine blood test measures. There may be slight changes in the retina, something the doctor looks for when he examines your eyes with a bright light. There may be minor abnormalities in the urine, perhaps protein in the urine. When I had an insurance company physical examination as a 25-year-old, the doctor found a trace of protein in my urine. The insurance company wrote the policy anyway, but at a slightly higher rate than they would have given somebody else. They knew I was at risk for kidney disease, but the symptoms were very slight until I reached middle age.

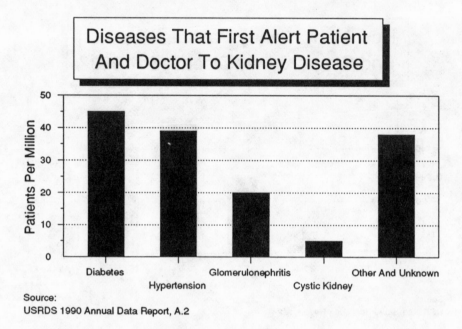

Figure 19 Diseases Diagnosed Before End-Stage Disease

The causes of kidney disease are complex and largely unknown. Dr. Walser calls my kidney disease *analgesic nephropathy*, caused by the excessive amount of aspirin I took for many years, six or eight tablets a day to deal with my persistent headaches that disappeared, perhaps coincidentally, after I lost 75 pounds, altered my high-fat, high-protein diet, and brought my high blood pressure under better control. Other nephrologists who have considered my case are not so sure of the cause of my disease, and in my case, it may not matter anyway.

High blood pressure may cause kidney disease, or kidney disease may cause high blood pressure. Nobody knows for sure, except to suspect that high blood pressure—and probably low blood pressure too—are problems for kidney patients. Nobody is sure what the proper level of blood pressure should be to help prevent the progression of kidney disease.[9]

Some scientists see an analogy between *atherosclerosis*—disease of the arteries—and *glomerulosclerosis*—disease of the kidneys. They suggest

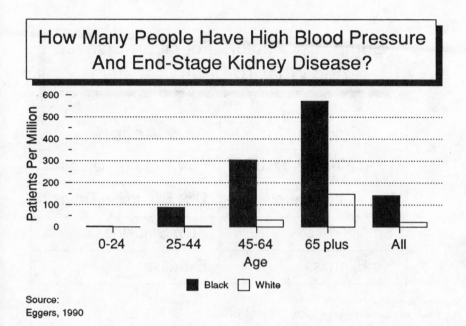

Source:
Eggers, 1990

Figure 20 High Blood Pressure and End-Stage Kidney Disease

that as high cholesterol and blood fats may clog the arteries, they may also damage the kidneys. Some studies have shown that increasing cholesterol in the diet can increase the likelihood of kidney disease in laboratory animals. Lowering cholesterol with drugs in laboratory animals has shown an improvement in kidney disease. Nobody knows for sure what this means about humans, if anything.[10, 11]

Dr. Saulo Klahr, the Washington University scientist leading the government study of nutritional therapy, has compiled a list of possible "risk factors" for kidney disease, similar to the familiar risk factors for heart disease—high blood pressure, high cholesterol, smoking and lack of exercise. Risk factors for kidney disease, he says, are high blood pressure, high cholesterol, high protein diet, inflammatory cells invading the kidney, protein in the urine.[12, 13]

What can a patient do about those risk factors? Some doctors think he can control his blood pressure with diet, exercise and perhaps drugs, and by not smoking. He can control his cholesterol, again, with diet, exercise

Some Risk Factors For Heart Disease And What To Do About Them

Risk Factor	Action
High Blood Pressure	Diet,Exercise,Drugs
High Cholesterol	Diet,Excercise,Drugs
Smoking	Stop Smoking
No Exercise	Exercise

Source:
American Heart Association, 1990

Figure 21

and perhaps drugs. He can moderate the amount of protein he eats. Nobody knows yet what to do about the invasion of the kidney by the potentially destructive cells.[14, 15]

The latest government studies show that people with diabetes and high blood pressure are the most likely to develop kidney disease, with glomerulonephritis and polycystic kidney disease the next most prevalent. The causes of all these conditions are poorly understood (except for polycystic kidney disease—many cysts and fibrous tissue replacing normal kidney tissue—which is believed to be hereditary.)[16]

WHAT ARE THE SYMPTOMS OF KIDNEY DISEASE?

The bad news about kidney disease is also good news. You can live for years without knowing that you have kidney disease. With your kidneys functioning even at 25 percent of normal, you can be free of symptoms.

Some Risk Factors For Kidney Disease And What To Do About Them

Risk Factor	Action
High Blood Pressure	Diet,Exercise,Drugs
High Cholesterol	Diet,Excercise,Drugs
Inflammatory Cells	Unknown
Protein In Urine	Diet

Source:
Saulo Klahr, 1990

Figure 22

That is also bad news, because you may not know how badly your kidneys have deteriorated until three-quarters or more of your kidney function is gone.[17]

The first real symptoms of chronic renal failure, coming late in the course of the disease, can be very vague, like frequent urination, getting up often at night to urinate, itching, easy bruising, muscle cramps, fatigue. Sometimes a non-specialist doctor mistakes these symptoms of kidney disease for stomach or intestinal problems, resulting in a delayed or occasionally wrong diagnosis. Meantime the kidney disease may be getting worse without treatment.[18]

One of my most noticeable symptoms was making more urine, particularly at night, my kidneys having lost some of their normal ability to concentrate the urine while I sleep. High blood pressure was another early clue. I also had breathlessness and a tired, run-down feeling.[19] It may have been the beginnings of *uremia*—toxic substances in the blood—plus *anemia*—lower than the normal amount of red blood cells—combining to

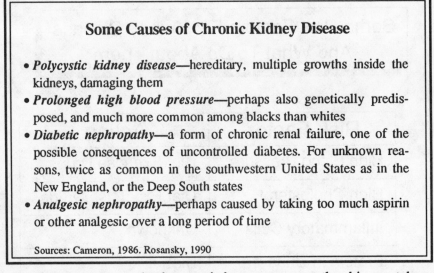

Some Causes of Chronic Kidney Disease

- *Polycystic kidney disease*—hereditary, multiple growths inside the kidneys, damaging them
- *Prolonged high blood pressure*—perhaps also genetically predisposed, and much more common among blacks than whites
- *Diabetic nephropathy*—a form of chronic renal failure, one of the possible consequences of uncontrolled diabetes. For unknown reasons, twice as common in the southwestern United States as in the New England, or the Deep South states
- *Analgesic nephropathy*—perhaps caused by taking too much aspirin or other analgesic over a long period of time

Sources: Cameron, 1986. Rosansky, 1990

cause these symptoms. As the uremia becomes worse, the skin can take on a muddy color. Sexual desire decreases, or even stops; impotence is common. Mental quickness declines or vanishes. As the disease progresses, the mouth takes on a foul taste and odor, appetite declines, there can be vomiting. Cramps at night and frequent twitching can occur. Itching develops. Sleep is disturbed. Eyesight may be impaired. Breathing may become difficult. Ankles may become swollen, the face bloated. Sores and bruises may not heal.

While the symptoms of early kidney disease are nearly invisible, the symptoms of end-stage disease are grim and unmistakable.[20]

4

Helping Yourself: Learning About
The Disease, Treatments

I paid $2.99 for a pound of oat bran in the summer of 1988. I wanted an easy way to reduce my high cholesterol, so like millions of other Americans, I bought some oat bran, running the price up to nearly ten times its usual level. Looking for a *silver bullet* to cure my high cholesterol, I had become part of the oat bran mania of the late 1980s.

I was a eager for a simple, one-step, almost mechanical cure for my health problems—a *silver bullet*. A best-selling book had recommended a lifestyle of sensible nutrition, moderate exercise and oat bran, a thoroughly common sense plan.[1] Like many readers, plus people who had not read the book, but only heard about it through the media, I missed the three point program—good nutrition, exercise, oat bran—and heard only the part about the oat bran. Television talk show hosts joked about hot fudge sundaes with oat bran, hamburgers with oat bran. For me, and perhaps a few million other Americans, oat bran had become *a cure for high cholesterol.* I overlooked the recommendations about lifestyle changes; it was the silver bullet I wanted.

Silver bullet medicine was an important tradition for me, and judging by the price of oat bran, for some others of my generation. After all, hadn't we seen some silver bullets before? Why not now? I could remember when polio had been a feared disease during my childhood, a crippler of thousands. My parents tried to keep me away from the public beaches during the "polio season." Then came the silver bullet—the polio vaccines—and the disease vanished. Measles, diphtheria, whooping cough, small pox, tuberculosis were common when my parents were growing up; but suddenly the diseases were gone, eradicated by silver bullets. My children were no more threatened by these diseases than they were by yellow fever or malaria. Like many Americans, I came to believe firmly in *aggressive* medical treatment. The doctor could be a miracle worker. His vaccines, drugs and surgery eliminated diseases that had killed people prematurely throughout human history. In 1910 the doctor might have been limited to watching helplessly as a patient died with a ruptured appendix, but 65 years later the surgeon could remove my daughter Cindy's ruptured appendix in a routine procedure and treat her infections with "wonder drugs." I was not the only 20th century American who believed in silver bullets.

When I first learned about my progressive kidney disease in 1988, I wanted one of those silver bullets. Although I had avoided polio and the other scourges of my parents' generation, I had grown up with my own diseases, as I discovered in my forties: heart disease, hypertension, clogged arteries, obesity, addiction to tobacco—afflictions that have not yet yielded to silver bullets. I knew that my diseases were aggravated, perhaps caused by my high-tech lifestyle: little exercise, poor food, not enough sleep, too much stress on the job. I called them my *high-tech diseases*. Some people, like the British physician, Dr. Hugh Trowell, call them "the Western diseases" because people in poorer places (like Africa) are less likely to have heart disease or cancer than people from Europe or North America.[2] While my head knew that my lifestyle was probably causing my diseases, my emotion yearned for silver bullets. The place to get them was the doctor's office.

In 1983 our youngest son, Marc, had shown the first signs of his chronic disease, starting our family on the search for another silver bullet. He attempted suicide at the age of 21. He was in his second year at New York University, studying mathematics, computer science and creative writing. He was bright, good looking, athletic, a member of the elite NYU Scholars program for undergraduates, but he had been depressed for several years, treated by a neighborhood therapist. The suicide attempt almost succeeded, and it launched Marc and the rest of our family on a seven-year journey through the wards of psychiatric medicine, with no end yet in sight.

Marc was confined to a locked unit in a private mental hospital in Philadelphia for six months in 1983. Then, calmed somewhat and drugged with anti-psychotic and anti-depressant medications, he emerged and tried to live on his own. The psychiatrist had labelled his condition *schizo-affective*, a half-step above the ominous *schizophrenia*. In our ignorance of mental illness, my wife and I wanted a silver bullet that would help Marc get well. We wanted the doctors *to do something*, as they had done when they took out his sister's appendix. Perhaps they could give him some pills that would make the mental illness go away, or use psychoanalysis to uncover the childhood conflicts that they said were causing Marc's episodes of psychosis. We wanted to lift the suffering his depression was inflicting on him, and through Marc's bizarre behavior, on the family.

Seven years later, after countless hospitalizations, repeated suicide attempts, psychiatrists in four states, and hundreds of thousands of dollars of mostly unreimbursed doctor and hospital bills, we finally came to understand that the doctors had no silver bullet. We were on our own. The doctors could help with medications. The mental hospitals were there when Marc needed temporary protection from himself. The community mental health center was caring and effective, but Marc's mental illness was a fact of his life and the family's. His illness was chronic; it would last for a long time. We had to learn to adjust to his chronic illness. (Despite his mental illness, Marc made it through college, graduating from Rutgers University with a degree in computer science, and getting halfway through a masters degree in computer science at Temple University before another trip to the mental hospital interrupted his studies.)

A SEARCH FOR SILVER BULLETS

When I first heard the diagnosis of my own chronic illness—*chronic renal failure*—my instinct sent me for a silver bullet. The nephrologist had one; in fact, he had two. He could give me a new kidney to replace my own diseased kidneys or he could send me to the dialysis clinic. As a fan of silver bullets, I suppose I should have been pleased that doctors had such magical ways to treat my kidney disease. Yet I vaguely knew that dialysis patients often didn't do well, that transplants sometimes failed and even successful transplant patients were often kept alive with debilitating drugs. I also feared becoming dependent on medical treatment. If there was another way, I wanted to find it. Our experience with a mentally ill son had taught me to have more realistic expectations of medical treatment. I wasn't quite so ready to turn myself over to the professionals without understanding what they were doing.

First I looked for laymen's books on kidney disease. I needed a book like this one, but it didn't exist. I started with the bookstores, and found nothing. The public library had a few books, but they repeated what the nephrologist had told me—let the kidneys get worse until you are ready for dialysis or transplant. The National Kidney Foundation and the American Kidney Fund booklets and pamphlets about kidney disease described only dialysis and transplant.[3, 4] They told me there was nothing I could do about my disease except wait for it to get worse, then go on dialysis while I waited for a kidney transplant. It wasn't the message I wanted to hear. I had to look elsewhere.

I started digging in the medical literature, looking for the latest scientific research on kidney disease. I found that the computerized catalog at the Thomas Jefferson University medical library in Philadelphia was easy to use. In five minutes I had a printed list of the newest books on kidney disease, including a 1988 book that attracted my eager attention—*Nutrition and the Kidney*. The book was published by a major publisher and edited by two prominent nephrologists. It contained articles by leading kidney researchers from the United States and Europe. I had found what I was looking for: a thoroughly mainstream description of the latest research on kidney disease.

The editors were Dr. William E. Mitch, a physician and professor of medicine at Emory University in Atlanta, and Dr. Saulo Klahr, also a physician and professor of medicine at Washington University in St. Louis. They recommended conservative treatment for all kidney patients in the early stages of their progressive disease—nutritional therapy before dialysis or transplant.[5] I had found another way to treat my disease.

Armed with my newly acquired knowledge of alternative treatments for my chronic disease, I wanted a second nephrologist to look at my case. I had always used the referral method of finding a specialist—asking a respected friend to recommend a doctor somehow conferred some legitimacy on my choice. This time I called Thomas Jefferson University, another leading medical school in Philadelphia, and asked for the office of the chairman of the renal division, Dr. Michael Simenhoff, to make an appointment. On my first visit, he took a thorough history from me, did a careful physical exam, and studied the results of comprehensive blood and urine tests he had ordered. He reached the same conclusion Dr. Grossman at Penn had reached: chronic renal failure, progressing rapidly. He drew a graph of the reciprocal of my creatinine (the $1/creatinine$ mathematical formula we saw in Chapter 1). His guess was that I would be on dialysis in 1991, two years later than Dr. Grossman's estimate. But the difference in timing was insignificant; the outlook was the same. My chronic renal failure would reach end-stage soon. There was nothing I could do but wait.

My wish for a silver bullet left me vulnerable to excessive hopes. I had found in the medical library reports of some serious medical research that showed the possibility of *preventing* kidney failure. Now I wanted the opinion of another respected member of the nephrology establishment, the renal division chairman of a second major university medical school and the chairman of the National Kidney Foundation branch in the Philadelphia area. I asked Dr. Simenhoff, "What about nutritional therapy?" Do you agree with the conclusions of the book *Nutrition and the Kidney* by Mitch and Klahr?" Dr. Simenhoff hadn't read the book, and, in fact, didn't know about it. After all it was a new book, published just a few months earlier. But Dr. Simenhoff did know about nutritional therapy for kidney disease, and he didn't think much of it. "Not proven," he said, "and I'm not sure it ever will be proven. You're hearing what you want to hear when you read the research about arresting the progression of kidney disease. They haven't proven their case. The best bet for you is to control your blood pressure and get yourself prepared for dialysis and perhaps someday a transplant." So much for the second opinion. It was the same as the first, although the timing estimate was different.

My next step, recommended by Dr. Grossman, the transplant specialist, was an evaluation by the transplant team at the University of Pennsylvania, one of the most experienced and respected programs in the country. On the morning of my evaluation, the staff was buzzing with news of the liver transplant that had been done a few days before—a heroic procedure including a chartered jet to transport the liver that had been "harvested

Some Books In The Public Library

- *The Kidneys; Balancing the Fluids*, in the series *The Human Body*, Torstar Books, New York, 1985. A well-written, beautifully-illustrated and authoritative volume in a respected series describing the state of the art in modern medicine as of 1985. Apparently intended for schools and libraries. Not much practical information, but clear descriptions of physiology, disease, treatments. Dr. Lewis Thomas, the scientist, clinician, administrator, and philosopher of medicine was a member of the editorial board overseeing this series.
- *Kidney Disease; The Facts*, Second Edition, by Stewart Cameron, Oxford University Press, New York, 1986. A prominent British nephrologist writes for laymen seeking to understand their kidney disease. Little practical information. Recommends transplant as the ultimate treatment. The dust jacket illustration is a sketch of an organ donor's card. Notes the existence of research on nutritional treatment, but ignores it as a practical possibility.
- *Coping With Kidney Failure*, by Robert H. Phillips, Avery Publishing Group, Inc., New York, 1987. An easy to read handbook by a psychologist experienced in helping people deal with chronic conditions. The first two sentences describe the author's view of kidney disease. *"Your kidneys are an important part of your anatomy. But if they happen to lose their functions, there are two alternatives: dialysis, in which a machine takes over the work of your kidneys; or transplantation, in which someone else's kidney replaces your own."*

from a cadaver in the mid-west." I suppose it's perfectly natural for a transplant team to use jargon like "harvest an organ from a cadaver," but my ears were not yet ready for words like that. The image conveyed to me was of a midwestern corn field giving up its harvest of grain. I wasn't ready to think of a human being "raising a liver for harvest by the transplant surgeons." Perhaps it was the language that troubled me, or could it have been the idea of "harvesting organs?"

The Penn transplant team was proud that they had found a donor's liver, kept it alive on the trip, surgically installed it in the little girl's body, giving her a chance at life. Yet beneath their optimistic chatter I could hear an undertone of the desperation of the whole process: searching for a

---

Some Books In The Medical Library

- *Nutritional Treatment of Chronic Renal Failure*, edited by Sergio Giovannetti, Kluwer Academic Publishers, Boston, 1989. Intended as a standard medical reference for nephrologists, collecting articles by leading physicians and scientists in the United States and Europe. The most recent medical text on conservative treatment of kidney disease, edited by a physician-scientist from a university medical center in Italy who pioneered the treatment thirty years ago and has been studying it in hundreds of patients ever since.
- *Nutrition and the Kidney*, edited by W. E. Mitch and S. Klahr, Little, Brown & Co., Boston, 1988. This book for scientists and kidney professionals collects articles by leading kidney researchers in the United States and Europe. Includes chapters on exercise and menu plans for kidney patients. A complete review of the international scientific literature through 1987. Much practical information as well, such as a list of food values.
- *The Progressive Nature of Renal Disease*, guest editor, William E. Mitch, Volume 14 in the series *Contemporary Issues in Nephrology*, series editors Barry M. Brenner and Jay H. Stein, Churchill Livingstone, New York, 1986. A medical reference collecting articles from prominent physicians and scientists.
- *Nutritional Management*, edited by Mackenzie Walser, W. B. Saunders, Philadelphia, 1984. A handbook of nutritional requirements and treatments for a wide variety of conditions. A chapter about kidney patients includes tables of nutritional values, sample menus and other practical information.
- *The Kidney*, edited by B.M. Brenner and F.C. Rector, W.B. Saunders, Philadelphia, 1991. A major two-volume textbook of nephrology.

---

donor, getting consent to "harvest the organ," preserving the liver outside a living body, delivering it by chartered jet to Philadelphia in the middle of the night, preparing the little girl for her surgical ordeal, waiting for the rejection episodes that were sure to come. I sensed an unspoken fear that the transplant might not work, that the little girl would die in a few days or weeks anyway, despite the "heroism" she and the transplant team had shown. I was feeling the reality of the transplant ward, the narrow margin between sickness and health, life and death, the desperation of the whole transplant process. I wondered if transplant was simply a "business," as Dr. Starzl called it. Or was it a medical experiment that after thirty years was not yet successful?

Dr. Grossman was surprised that I had read some medical research. He knew the studies on nutritional therapy but had not seen the recently published book, *Nutrition and the Kidney*. He was as skeptical of nutritional treatment as the department chairman at Jefferson had been. He understood, however, that I had found a third treatment that I wanted to try, and he wanted to help. He told me that his colleague, Dr. Alan Wasserstein, a professor of nephrology, clinician, and director of the dialysis clinic at Penn knew more than he did about nutritional therapy, and would probably be willing to follow my case. I would be seeing a third nephrologist in a month, all distinguished university professors at leading medical schools.

While I launched myself into the experiment with nutritional therapy, the transplant team put my file in the follow-up drawer. I wondered if I would someday ask them to reopen my case. I wondered if they would ever consider me again, now that I had decided to try something other than transplant. I wondered if I would someday regret my decision to reject high-tech treatment for my kidney disease.

WHY LEARN ABOUT YOUR DISEASE? WHY NOT JUST FOLLOW DOCTOR'S ORDERS?

Kidney patients have used nutritional therapy to prevent their disease from getting worse, thousands of them over the last thirty years. End-stage renal failure need not be inevitable for people who have discovered their kidney disease early enough to do something about it. Nutritional therapy has delayed or even stopped the progression of kidney disease, but the nephrologist is not likely to tell you so because there is a subtle conflict between your interests and his. It took me a long time to glimpse the conflict, but it is very real.

The kidney specialist wants to help you—that's his job, his profession. But he has other motives as well. He wants to be a member-in-good-standing of the nephrology profession, accepted by his peers. That means not rocking the boat, following the accepted ways, the "treatment-of-choice" consensus reached by the elders of the profession. For chronic kidney disease, that means dialysis and transplant—not nutritional therapy. When I asked a prominent nephrologist to write a foreword for this book about nutritional therapy, he replied, "I may not be able to do it because the nephrologists' society might throw me out." I wondered if the culture of 20th century medicine may be teaching doctors to ignore conservative treatment for chronic disease, to prefer drugs, surgery or artificial organs. I wondered where I, *as a patient,* fit in with all this high technology. Did I have a role in my own health care, or was modern medicine expecting me to comply meekly with the recommendations of the drug-dispensing, scalpel-wielding doctors? And to pay the fees they demanded for their costly technology?

The nephrologist wants to earn a good living, of course; that's one of the reasons he worked so hard and long—until his mid-thirties, probably—trying to learn the profession. It takes little of his time to prescribe dialysis or transplant for a kidney patient, and he will be well-paid, often by Medicare, for providing the high-tech treatments. If he tries to teach his

---

What I Learned About My Chronic Kidney Disease

- Most nephrologists believe that kidney disease progresses inevitably to kidney failure, that transplant is the best treatment for most people, but that dialysis can help others.
- Many medical researchers—mainstream scientists, not fringe quacks—believe that conservative nutritional therapy can slow or even stop progressive kidney disease, delaying or eliminating the need for transplant or dialysis.
- Some European doctors believe that *not attempting nutritional therapy* in the early stages of the disease is unethical.
- The $50 million federal government study—Modification of Diet In Renal Disease—due for completion in 1993 is intended to evaluate the effectiveness of nutritional therapy.
- Conservative treatment for chronic kidney disease has little risk for the patient, maybe none.

patients nutritional therapy, however, he may spend much more time for a far smaller monetary reward. (More about this in Chapter 9.)

A very wise New England doctor, Dr. D.C. Jarvis, whose 1958 book on natural health care went to a 68th printing in 1989, wrote this:

> **"I believe the doctor of the future will be a teacher as well as a physician. His real job will be to teach people how to be healthy. Doctors will be even busier than they are now because it is a lot harder to keep people well than it is just to get them over a sickness."[6]**

Not many doctors in 1990 believe what Dr. Jarvis predicted thirty years ago about their roles as teachers as well as physicians. A survey of 4,000 internal medicine doctors published in 1990 found that the majority did not attempt to teach their patients how to *prevent disease.* In fact, they didn't even practice disease prevention for themselves.[7]

A physician and scientist with an international reputation, Dr. Alexander Leaf, found it necessary to write a long and carefully documented article in the *New England Journal of Medicine* in November, 1990 to persuade heart doctors that they should be thinking about *preventing* heart disease, not merely *treating* it.

> **"It would seem that a health care system that improved the health of the patient and of the public would be preferred to one that focused only on extending life."[8]**

Could it be possible, I wondered as I read Dr. Leaf's article, that a wise and experienced physician finds it necessary to remind his colleagues in 1990 that *prevention* may be more important than *treatment?* Do doctors need to be reminded that they should think about "health," and not merely about "extending life?" Healthful lifestyles, Dr. Leaf wrote, can reduce the risk of heart disease—"proper diet, physical exercise, smoking cessation, weight control, and other practices that promote health." Could that be *news* to doctors, I wondered, worthy of comment from an elder of the profession? Are doctors interested in *health,* or are they mostly interested in treating sickness? Do we have a "health care system," as the doctors and hospitals have taught us to call it? Or is it a "sick care system," a money-guzzling creature that asks us to spend much of our wealth on often-unsuccessful attempts to cheat death, while ignoring proven ways to prevent disease?

Conservative therapies for many diseases—heart disease, cancer, diabetes—are based on an enormous body of scientific research, much of it dating from the 1930s and 1940s before the start of the nearly limitless spending on high-tech medical care. A doctor who spent years studying this research and wondering why other doctors paid so little attention came to this conclusion:

> **"It took me years to figure why these nutritional studies were gathering dust on library shelves. This research has no economic value."** [9]

How can medical care providers—from doctors and hospitals to drug companies and equipment manufacturers—make money from recommending nutritional therapy? How can they tap the economic value of nutritional therapy for heart disease, diabetes, cancer, kidney disease? Nobody knows a good answer. It could be one reason the medical establishment has not paid much attention to nutritional therapies. It's not that doctors and hospitals are greedy (although, of course, some are.)[10] They are simply human, doing what they know, what is accepted, what will reward them, and what they believe will help their patients at the same time. When I finally began to understand this conflict between the nephrologist's interests and my own interests, I could begin taking responsibility for my own treatment, with the advice of the professionals, and I was ready to start recovering my health.[11]

There is still another reason why nephrologists are not likely to tell you about the new treatment for kidney disease. "Doctors hate to be wrong," Dr. Wasserstein says. "They hate to recommend something that later turns out to be useless or harmful. Nutritional therapy might end up in that category of useless or harmful treatments. We'll have to wait to see how the big controlled studies come out. But even if the trials are effective, nutritional therapy may be quite expensive: the cost of the supplements, the frequent clinic visits, the teaching and learning in the support groups. The cost in lifestyle might be very high too. Some people value eating as one of the great pleasures of life. Restricting it so severely with nutritional therapy may be a severe deprivation for some people."

Like Dr. Grossman, Dr. Wasserstein is a caring clinician, a teacher and a scientist. He wants to recommend what he believes is the best care for his patients, and in doing so, teach his students the best medicine. When I visit him, he often asks my permission for a student doctor, a resident, to sit in with us; his attention is properly as much on teaching the young doctor as it is on treating my illness. I am pleased to be part of a learning experience for young doctors at a leading teaching hospital.

Dr. Wasserstein teaches the young residents that he hopes my attempts to use nutritional therapy continue to work for me, that he will follow the research studies, particularly the big federal government MDRD study, but that he can't recommend nutritional therapy for all his patients because the theories are still unproven. I don't challenge him on that point, but I do wonder why he, like most nephrologists, is so reluctant to recommend a treatment that *may work and that has no significant risk for the patient.*

"It does have a downside for the patient," he says."The cost of nutritional therapy can be very high. The patient must come to the clinic frequently. We must measure his GFR [the *glomerular filtration rate* that some scientists say is the most accurate measure of how well the kidneys are working]. The patient must learn about nutrition and lifestyle changes. He may need to buy a form of amino acids and other supplements, perhaps special low-protein products. The patient must make changes in his behavior, including giving up things that may be important to him—like eating a thick, juicy steak. Nutritional therapy is not so easy and not so inexpensive. I want to make sure it is effective before I recommend it."

My research in the medical libraries and my consultations with three respected nephrologists had produced a conflict in my search for a way to deal with my chronic disease. It was finally obvious to me that I would not find a silver bullet, that I would have to struggle my way through my chronic disease as our son Marc was struggling through his mental illness. I hoped I would be as successful as he has been.

5
Getting Help:
Understanding the Specialists

A kidney patient in the 1990s, like me, has the curious problem of trying to understand the kidney professionals who are trying to help him with his disease. The professionals are telling us there are only two ways to treat kidney disease—and both involve high-tech renal replacement—while some researchers are saying they believe kidney failure can be prevented. A patient may feel confused, helpless and afraid. That's how I felt.

My first problem, and perhaps yours too, was learning to understand the professionals who help kidney patients. The problem, of course, is the difficulty a layman has understanding any professional. A newly diagnosed kidney patient does not have the same vocabulary as the specialist, and he has few easy ways to learn.

Although my life was threatened by my disease, I knew almost nothing about it. I knew more about my car engine or my personal computer software than I did about my kidney disease. I didn't know that a nephrologist was an internal medicine specialist who concentrates on kidney disorders. Words like creatinine and glomerular filtration rate meant nothing to me or, I suspect, to most people who have not yet learned much about their kidney disease.

Learning to understand at least some of the nephrologist's language is a big step forward in dealing with the disease. But compounding the language problem is that the nephrologist, like all medical specialists, has little time to spend with each patient. To meet his personal income goals, the nephrologist can afford to spend no more than 10 or 15 minutes with an individual patient, except on an extended visit like a first visit with a new patient when the bill can be $150 or $200 or more, allowing the specialist to spend a half hour or more with the patient.

How boring it must be for the nephrologist to explain the same basics over and over again to patient after patient, all day, every day. One nephrologist told me he has made the same speech about the pros and cons of kidney transplant, the risks and the benefits, the costs and the problems—the same speech four days a week for 15 years. Not many professionals have to do the same thing every day of every week for 15 years.

Some nephrologists (and most other specialists, in my experience) seldom make much effort to educate their patients about their disease. They seldom use teaching devices for their patients, not even the government or foundation pamphlets that could at least convey the basics to any patient who could read. I've never seen the National Kidney Foundation and the American Kidney Fund booklets on kidney disease in a nephrologist's waiting room, among the year-old copies of *Sports Illustrated* and *Readers' Digest*. Even my veterinarian has a video tape playing in his waiting room about various pet diseases. The tape is paid for, of course, by a company selling drugs to treat the condition, but at least I knew more about my cat's diseases than I did about my own.

The result of the language problem, the lack of time, the lack of teaching and learning tools is an extremely low level of communication between doctor and patient. The doctor may feel that he is wasting his time talking to a patient who can't understand him. The patient may feel confused and ignorant about an important topic. I learned more in the nephrologist's waiting room about cooking summertime meals or the prospects of the San Francisco 49ers than I learned about the reason both the nephrologist and I were there in the office in the first place—kidney disease.

Something that helped me in the early months of dealing with my kidney disease was my attempt to get a better understanding of the language, the ideas, and the motivations of the kidney professionals who had suddenly become so important in my life. The most important by far in the early phase of the disease is the nephrologist.

A PATIENT'S FIRST ENCOUNTER
WITH A NEPHROLOGIST

I was forty-six when I first consulted a kidney specialist. Never having missed more than a day or two of work in my life because of sickness, I suddenly had a serious health problem. Uncontrolled high blood pressure, the neighborhood doctors thought, had caused my congestive heart failure and kidney trouble. Two weeks in the local hospital with drugs to drain the excess fluid from my body and control my blood pressure had left me in more or less normal condition. But my creatinine was still five or six times the normal level, about 6.0 mg/dl. The neighborhood doctors thought I should consult a specialist at the university hospital in the city. I was apprehensive when I first visited him.

"I never heard of a 'nephrologist' until the neighborhood internist told me I ought to see one. Nephrologists specialize in kidney diseases, apparently, and high blood pressure, hypertension. My blood pressure was high, 190/100. The creatinine in my blood was high too. It was 6, he said, should be about 1 or less. When I asked him what that meant, he said I ought to see a nephrologist. He knew one at the university hospital. He said he'd refer me.

"The nephrologist has talked to his friend the local doctor who referred me. He has already looked at my blood tests. He takes a careful history from me. Mother with high blood pressure. Father died of heart trouble at age 59. Two brothers with high blood pressure. No kidney disease in the family, except that both my mother and wife had kidney stones. He says he needs to do a 'workup' on me. More blood tests, chest x-ray, ultrasound of the kidney to look for obstructions or cysts and measure the size. He says there's a little blood in my urine. Best to do a cystoscopy to look for bladder cancer, and a renal arteriogram looking for trouble in the arteries between the heart and the kidneys.

"A few weeks later, after the workup tests, he tells me his diagnosis: hypertension, renal insufficiency, atherosclerosis, enlarged heart. I never missed a day of work in my life for sickness, but now, age 46, I

have a bundle of diseases. His prognosis is not good, but there's hope. Kidney disease usually progresses to ESRD, end-stage renal disease. Thirty or forty thousand people a year get end-stage renal disease in the United States. But he can treat me with dialysis or a kidney transplant. He tells me he's old enough to remember when patients like me would be dead of uremia in a few months. Off in the back wards of the hospital somewhere with the hopeless cancer patients. But now, he says he can treat me. There is something he can do.

"His treatment plan is to lower the high blood pressure with drugs and diet. I will have to lose a lot of weight, all the fifty pounds I've gained since college."

I left his office happy that a smart, experienced guy was looking after my problem. It was serious, but treatable. If worst came to worst, there was dialysis, or even transplant. He told me that dialysis was routine now, and transplants were 90 percent successful. I was starting my new life as a kidney patient.

A NEPHROLOGIST'S FIRST ENCOUNTER WITH A NEW KIDNEY PATIENT

It took me four years to get a better understanding of what the nephrologist meant when he talked to me about my disease. He was a high-tech specialist, proud of the way he could help me once my kidneys had failed entirely. He was old enough to remember the days when the kidney patients were off in the back wards with the cancer patients, nothing to do but wait for uremia to kill them. Now he could keep me alive with dialysis and later, if all went well, with a transplant. He was doing what doctors most want to do—he was saving my life from a killer disease.

The problem was that he wasn't doing what I wanted him to do. I didn't even tell him what I wanted. I wanted to stop the disease from getting worse. I wanted to prevent the end-stage disease, not just deal with the consequences. But I never told him so during the four years he treated me. Neither of us did anything about it, especially me. Instead I went through the motions of a passive patient, learning nothing about my disease, doing nothing about it, except to take the blood pressure medications he prescribed. There wasn't much communication between us. I behaved like an *object of treatment,* not a participant.

Much later I could look back and understand better what the nephrologists who treated me might have been thinking as they followed my case. Here's my guess about what a nephrologist may be thinking as he meets a new kidney patient.

"When I decided to become a nephrologist in 1970, I was 28 years old and half way through my residency at the university teaching hospital. Nephrology was an exciting subspecialty of internal medicine. We were learning how to save terminally ill kidney patients, people who were sure to die without our help. We knew enough about dialysis to keep people alive with no kidney function, sometimes for years. Transplantation was experimental, but it occasionally worked and the experimenting was okay because the patients probably would have died anyway without the transplant. Some powerful people were pushing Congress to finance dialysis treatments for everybody who needed them. Insurance companies were starting to pay. It looked as though I could help save lives, manage interesting cases, and make a good living at the same time. I specialized in nephrology.

"But now, 20 years later, what I do mostly is treat artery and vein problems and infections. The dialysis unit runs itself, really, except for finding new patients to replace the ones that die, and worrying about more cutbacks in Medicare fees. We lose about 25 percent of our patients every year. They die from their other diseases, diabetes and heart trouble, mostly. Some just give up and don't come back for dialysis. The younger ones last longer, of course, because they're stronger and they usually don't have as many other diseases. But we're accepting older and sicker people now. We really accept anybody who needs dialysis. The federal government pays. For some reason, we have more diabetics than we used to have, and older people. Only about one third of the patients who start with us every year will last longer than five years.

"When we opened this new dialysis center fifteen years ago, we had six machine positions to fill. The state health department told us that there weren't enough patients around here to keep six stations busy. But we did it, and the hospital administration kept pushing me to expand, to get more revenue. Now I have 15 positions to fill. I wonder where I can find enough patients?

"About the only interesting part of the job now is getting a new patient. At least there's the hope of a diagnostic challenge, maybe something unusual to think about instead of hearing the endless complaints from the dialysis patients, things I can't do anything about. If I see one more collapsed artery, one more stomach infection . . . [1]

"This new patient I'm seeing this morning has some interesting symptoms. The neighborhood doctor who sent him to me was baffled. His creatinine was over 6, blood pressure 190/100. When I was in residency, if I saw somebody as close to uremia as this, the patient would surely be dead in a few months. Now we can keep him alive on dialysis. The federal government pays, so there's no hassle with the hospital administration over collections. I get a fee every time he comes in for dialysis, even if I rarely see him. I have to be on call, so I get the fee. I don't make as much money as the transplant surgeons, but then, I don't have to be in the operating room at midnight on Saturday when a cadaver kidney comes in from a teenager who was just killed in a motorcycle accident in Iowa.

"The transplant team is always pressuring me for candidates. But some of their transplant patients are just as sick as my dialysis patients, with all the immunosuppressive drugs they have to take. I'm not sure transplant is a good treatment unless the tissue match is about perfect and the patient doesn't have too many other diseases, like diabetes or heart trouble. I think sometimes my patients are better off on dialysis than going through the ordeal of transplanting, rejecting, transplanting again. I sent one guy over there who had three transplants, rejected them all despite buckets of steroids and cyclosporine. They finally sent him back here to me. He's pretty sick, but I think we can keep him alive for a while, at least for a few months.

"I prescribed blood pressure medication for this new patient. I hope he takes it. Most of my patients don't, although they say they do. I told him he should lose forty or fifty pounds. It would help with the blood pressure. This guy is pretty smart, and seems to be motivated. But what will probably happen is that he won't lose weight, and he won't take the blood pressure medications. His kidneys will get worse, and two or three years from now, he'll be coming to my dialysis unit every Monday, Wednesday and Friday. At least I'll be able to keep him alive for a while."

As a new kidney patient, I was passively putting myself in the hands of a nephrologist who was committed to the high-tech renal replacement therapies. If I had gone to the medical library in 1985, I may have learned about the new nutritional treatment then. I may have read a book like this one, if it had been available. I may have listened more carefully to the nephrologist's recommendations for blood pressure control. I may have preserved more of the capacity of my diseased kidneys.

THE CURIOUS DEBATE OVER NUTRITIONAL THERAPY.

For somebody with no medical training—like me and like most kidney patients and their families—there is an air of unreality to the scientific debate about nutritional treatment. The common sense questions seem to have simple answers.

> **Patient:** Does nutritional therapy slow or stop the progression of kidney disease?

> **Nephrologist:** We don't know. Nutritional therapy is helpful in treating the symptoms of kidney disease, but whether it stops progression, we just don't know yet. There is some evidence that it does slow or even stop progression for some people, but the studies are inconclusive. We just can't be sure.

Patient: If nutritional therapy can help treat the symptoms for most people and may stop progression for some people, why isn't it used routinely? Is it harmful?

Nephrologist: No, it has not been found to be harmful.

Patient: Then, why don't doctors routinely recommend nutritional treatment?

Nephrologist: Because scientific proof is not yet available that it works.

Patient: But if it's not harmful, and if it works sometimes, why not try it with everybody?

Nephrologist: Because it has not yet been scientifically proven.

Patient: If you're not willing to try it with everybody, will you try it with me?

Nephrologist: No. Because nutritional therapy has not yet been scientifically proven.

A CONVERSATION WITH YOUR DOCTOR

I was surprised that doctors are so reluctant to recommend something as simple and low-risk as nutritional therapy, while they routinely recommend the complex and risky dialysis and transplant treatments. After reading this book, you may have a similar experience. You may talk about this book with your doctor. If he believes that patients should be seen and not heard, as some doctors do, or if he believes the doctor should make all the medical decisions without consulting the patient, as some doctors also do, your conversation may go about like this:

Patient: I just read a book about kidney disease, **The Kidney Patient's Book.** It's by a kidney patient.

Nephrologist: A patient? What does a patient know about kidney disease?

Patient: He has been one of many volunteer subjects in a National Institutes of Health study of nutritional therapy to prevent chronic kidney disease from getting worse. He reports the results of the study he's in and many others. He says the therapy has worked for him and for thousands of others in many countries over the last thirty years.

Nephrologist: I have read those studies. They haven't proven anything yet. Even the researchers who proposed the theories say they have not yet been proven.

Patient: The book raised some questions I want to discuss with you. Does nutritional therapy work to slow down or stop the progression of kidney disease? Does it delay or eliminate the need for dialysis and transplant? Can a kidney patient live a more or less normal life if he follows the nutritional therapy?

Nephrologist: Nutritional therapy has been used for years to treat the symptoms of chronic kidney disease. It appears to slow or stop progression—sometimes for some people. But it doesn't work all the time for all patients. For some people it has delayed or even eliminated the need for dialysis or transplant. For others, it has not. A kidney patient on a low-protein, low-phosphorus diet may be able to live a more or less normal life, if he can adjust to the diet, which may not be easy.

Patient: If it works sometimes for some people, why don't doctors recommend trying the nutritional therapy? Is there some side effect, some hidden danger, some injury that the nutritional therapy can do to the patient?

Nephrologist: Most authorities believe there is no significant risk except the possibility of malnutrition caused by a diet too low in protein. That risk can be avoided with supplements of some form of essential amino acids, plus vitamin and mineral supplements. No researcher has found malnutrition to be a serious risk.

This confusing conversation may leave you where it left me. If nutritional therapy may work, if there is no downside, no risk, then you may want to try it. You may ask the doctor, "Will you help me?"

At this point, your doctor may be uncomfortable. He may be on unfamiliar ground. As a patient, you have asked him to undertake a specific treatment for your disease—nutritional therapy. He may not know much about it. He may not believe it is worthwhile. He may not want to try something experimental. He may be afraid you will sue him if it doesn't work out as you hope. So, he may take the comfortable, familiar and understandable way out, the way his culture has taught him to respond. He may say that he can't help you with an experimental treatment. He may say that if you want to try something experimental, you'll have to find a doctor who is willing to undertake it, as the author of the book did. "But if you want to stay with me, you'll have to follow my recommendations."

If he answers your questions about nutritional therapy this way, you may face a decision. Do you want to make an effort to prevent your disease from getting worse, despite the doctor's advice to do nothing until you are ready for dialysis or transplant? Do you want to try to avoid the high-tech kidney replacement treatments? Do you want to find a doctor who will work with you? If your answer is yes, this book could be the first step.

6

The Artificial Kidney: Dialysis

The nephrologist may have told you that you are a good candidate for a kidney transplant, but because of the shortage of organ donors, you may wait a year or two until the transplant program can find a kidney to match your tissue types. You may be too sick or too old to be a candidate for transplant, or you may choose not to have a transplant, preferring to remain a dialysis patient. In any of these cases, you can go on dialysis. Some people have lived on dialysis for over twenty years.

What are your chances with dialysis? How long are you likely to survive? How healthy will you be? How normal a life will you be able to lead? Will you be able to work? Travel? Exercise? Can you marry? Have sex? Have children? Does it make a difference what kind of dialysis you do? Does where you do it matter? How will you be able to pay for it? Will dialysis make you susceptible to other diseases? Will you develop heart trouble, diabetes? Will your mental health be affected? How disabled will you be? The doctors can probably keep you alive on dialysis, but for how long? And the most important question, by far, is *what kind of life?* [1] What quality of life can you expect on dialysis?

WHAT ARE YOUR CHANCES ON DIALYSIS?

Dialysis is a life-saving procedure for end-stage kidney patients, at least temporarily, and a newly approved genetically-engineered hormone, *erythropoietin*, is an important treatment for dialysis patients, reducing the anemia that troubles them, making them feel much better. But there are some troubling trends in dialysis.

About one out of four patients starting dialysis in the 1990s will die within a year. The average dialysis patient lives for three years.[2] The death rate among dialysis patients in the United States is higher than in other industrialized countries, and has been getting worse since the mid-1980s.[3] The older you are at the time of your kidney failure, and the worse your other diseases, the poorer your chances of surviving dialysis.[4] White people die sooner on dialysis than blacks, Asians and Indians.[5] Nobody knows why.

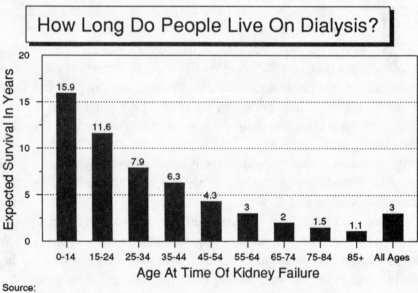

Figure 23 Life Expectancy of Dialysis Patients

The Health Care Financing Administration has calculated median life expectancy for dialysis patients based on Medicare records. The "median expectancy" is similar to the definition the federal government uses when it says "life expectancy for white males in the United States is 71.6 years." Half the dialysis patients will live longer than the median and half will die sooner. Younger people survive dialysis longer than older people.

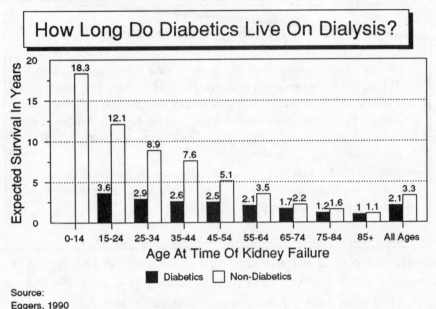

How Long Do Diabetics Live On Dialysis?

Expected Survival In Years

Age At Time Of Kidney Failure	Diabetics	Non-Diabetics
0-14		18.3
15-24	3.6	12.1
25-34	2.9	8.9
35-44	2.6	7.6
45-54	2.5	5.1
55-64	2.1	3.5
65-74	1.7	2.2
75-84	1.2	1.6
85+	1	1.1
All Ages	2.1	3.3

■ Diabetics ☐ Non-Diabetics

Source:
Eggers, 1990

Figure 24 Life Expectancy of Diabetics On Dialysis

Non-diabetics survive much longer than diabetic dialysis patients. The age at the start of dialysis has a major impact on the length of survival.

Over 110,000 kidney patients were on dialysis in 1988, the latest year for which complete statistics have been published.[6] The average age was 56 and about one-third of the patients were over 65. Twenty percent had diabetes and 6 percent of the diabetics were over 65. The total number of people on dialysis and their average age have been steadily increasing since the Medicare program started in 1972.

In 1978, 81 percent of patients survived for at least a year after starting dialysis. Nine years later, in 1987, the one-year survival rate was down to 77 percent, a steady and significant decline attributed by some analysts to the age and poor health of the patients starting dialysis. The average dialysis patient was older and sicker in 1987 than a decade before.

One way to judge your chances on dialysis is to consider the life expectancy of dialysis patients. Across all age groups, the median is two years for diabetics and about three years for all others. But you should look

---

Some Troubling Trends in Dialysis

- Among the industrialized countries, the United States has the highest dialysis mortality rate and it is showing a steadily increasing trend.
- The United States accepts a higher proportion of kidney patients for dialysis than other industrialized countries, but Japan and West Germany are approaching our acceptance rate and have significantly better survival rates.
- After surviving their first year on dialysis only six percent of Japanese dialysis patients die each year. The American death rate is twenty-five percent, four times as high.

Source: Hull and Parker, 1990.

---

closely at the table because your age *at the start of dialysis* makes a difference in the time you can expect to survive. If you are 45 to 54, the ages when most kidney failure occurs, you can expect 2.5 years if you have diabetes or 5.1 years if you don't. If you are over 75, the life expectancy is about one year for diabetics and just over 1.5 years for all others.[7]

DIALYSIS IN THE U.S. MAY BE LESS EFFECTIVE THAN IN OTHER COUNTRIES

Analysts are puzzled by comparisons between dialysis in the U.S. and in other countries. Forty people out of 100,000 were on dialysis in the United States in 1987, compared to about 67 per 100,000 in Japan. About one quarter of United States dialysis patients died in 1987, compared to less than 10 percent in Japan. The death rate among dialysis patients in the United States was over twice as high as the rate in West Germany and France, and three times as high as in Japan.[8] Nobody knows for sure why the dialysis death rate is so high in the United States compared to other countries.

Some researchers guess that Medicare accepts older and sicker patients than other countries do, particularly diabetics, accounting for the higher death rates. Others say that the United States does more kidney transplanting than other countries. The rate of transplanting is much lower in Japan, about 5 percent of the United States rate, which probably means that the healthier American patients leave dialysis to get a transplant while the sicker ones stay behind, die sooner, thus skewing the American death rate higher. Some say we may not manage dialysis as effectively in the United States as in some other countries. Dialysis professionals consider it a serious problem that needs to be understood. Two prominent nephrologists wrote in the *American Journal of Kidney Diseases* in May 1990:

> **"The United States dialysis community has a major problem: we need to know precisely why our mortality is as high as it is and precisely what to do about it."** [9]

Another comparison of dialysis in Japan and the United States has worried nephrologists. In the first year of dialysis about 17 percent of Japanese patients die compared to about 24 percent in the United States, not much difference. But after the first year, there is a big difference. Only six percent of Japanese dialysis patients die per year once they have survived the first year. The rate in the United States is four times as high.[10] Some analysts speculate that a Japanese dialysis patient has a better chance of surviving than an American because Japanese doctors often prescribe *longer dialysis treatments* than American doctors do.[11]

What all these statistics mean to somebody first learning about his kidney disease in the 1990s is that dialysis is a life-saving treatment for an end-stage kidney disease patient, at least for a while. The chances are three out of four that you will live for a year on dialysis, but *what kind of life*? To answer that question, we need to know more about how dialysis works, and about the early results from widespread use of erythropoietin.

THE DREAM OF ARTIFICIAL ORGANS

The artificial kidney was a miracle machine in the 1950s and 1960s. It was costly and risky, but it worked for a while. People who would surely have died of the body-poisoning effects of uremia were kept alive, miraculously it seemed, by the new technology that could do the work of the failed kidneys.

Some people thought the world was entering a new age of artificial organs—man-made heart, lung, kidney, joints; synthetic blood, veins and skin. Researchers were working on artificial eyes, lungs, hearts and bladders that they hoped could be implanted in the body to replace failed organs. A popular paperback book published in 1976 was called *No More Dying; the conquest of aging and the extension of human life*. The authors foresaw a future of medical miracles: transplants, bionic organs, cloning, a cure for cancer, a nuclear heart and so forth.

> "We are without doubt—for good or bad—standing at the gate of a new era, when *homo sapiens* will be medically transformed into *homo longevus*—extremely long-lived men and women who still retain their mental and physical vigor." [12]

It was the artificial kidney that became the most widely used and successful of the man-made organs after Congress acted in 1972 to provide Medicare-paid dialysis treatment for most Americans who needed it. Having thus provided an entitlement to costly treatment for end-stage kidney disease victims, the federal government had also provided the financing for what was to become by the late 1980s a $5 billion a year industry, with the 1,879 dialysis centers in the United States treating over 110,000 persons.[13] Dialysis had become simply another part of the $600 plus billion a year Americans were spending on medical care at the start of the 1990s, 12 percent of everything we were producing in goods and services.

WHAT IS DIALYSIS?

To understand the artificial kidney, we need to understand something about what the natural kidney does. Most people understand the job of the heart, the lungs, the digestive system, but may not be so sure of what the kidneys do. The heart pumps blood throughout our system. The lungs take in oxygen from the air and expel carbon dioxide. The digestive system processes what we eat and drink to sustain our body. The kidneys make urine, of course, but they are doing other work.

The kidneys have three main jobs, all helping maintain the balance of fluids in the body. They control the volume, the chemical composition and the distribution of fluids in the body. To do this work, the kidneys have an *excretory* function, that is, they excrete waste products the body doesn't need. They also have an *endocrine* function, producing hormones the body does need. And they have a *metabolic* function, working on the proteins and amino acids we need to sustain life. When we take in too much water, the kidneys excrete more of it in the urine. When we take in too little

---

Some Words I Learned About Dialysis

- *Dialysis*—a process used to remove some of the waste products of everyday living from the blood
- *Hemodialysis*—use of an artificial kidney machine to filter the blood, doing some of the work of normal kidneys
- *Semipermeable membrane*—a natural or artificial membrane with small holes that allow some waste products to pass through, but that prevent the passage of larger blood cells and proteins
- *Peritoneal membrane*—a membrane which lines the abdominal cavity and covers the intestines; blood circulates through the membrane
- *Continuous ambulatory peritoneal dialysis (CAPD)*—a type of dialysis in which the patient is free to move around unconnected to a stationery machine. Fluid, changed every four to six hours, is put into the abdomen to extract waste, using the peritoneal membrane itself as the dialyzing membrane.

---

water, the kidneys try to conserve it. If we eat too much salt or too little potassium, the kidneys try to balance the amount that remains in the body, excreting the excess or conserving to minimize the shortage. Normal kidneys also make *erythropoietin*, a hormone that stimulates the production of red blood cells, and that has now been created by genetic engineering and is available as a drug for treating kidney patients. The diseased kidneys produce less of the hormone and the number of red cells in the blood declines. The lack of the hormone is compounded by the toxic effect of the waste products accumulating in the blood, all of which results in the anemia that healthy kidneys prevent in normal people.[14]

Normal kidneys do this work continuously, twenty-four hours a day every day. The blood passes from the heart through the kidneys before circulating through the arteries to the rest of the body. The filtering action of the kidneys processes about 120 milliliters of blood per minute. Doctors measure this rate as an indication of how well the kidneys are working, and call it the *glomerular filtration rate* or *GFR* for short.

The diseased kidneys can do their job of fluid-balancing well enough to maintain the body in a good state of health until they have lost about

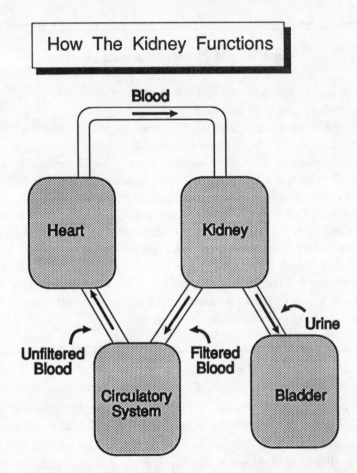

How The Kidney Functions

Figure 25 How The Kidney Functions

The kidneys are located near the heart and connected to the heart by a large artery. Blood is pumped from the heart through the kidneys before continuing on to the rest of the body. The kidneys remove waste products and water, making urine which they pass to the bladder for elimination.

three-fourths of their capacity. Often the body's chemical balance is not upset and no symptoms of kidney disease appear until the GFR drops below about one-fourth of the normal level, about thirty milliliters per minute (ml/min). At this point nephrologists often advise patients to start thinking about dialysis and transplant.

When doctors began working on the artificial kidney in the 1940s, they were trying to create a machine that would do the filtering job, the excre-

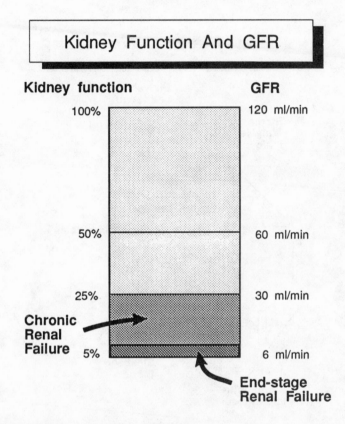

Figure 26 Kidney Function and GFR

The kidneys can lose three-quarters of their capacity before the symptoms of chronic renal failure appear. They can lose ninety-five percent of their capacity before the disease becomes life-threatening. This remarkable resiliency makes it possible for a living kidney donor to give up one of his two normal kidneys, losing half of his kidney capacity, and still remain healthy, although with a much reduced reserve.

tory job of the kidneys. They wanted to treat people with *acute renal failure*, the temporary loss of kidney function. It was much later that doctors began working on using dialysis for *chronic renal failure,* the long-term loss of kidney function that this book is mostly about.[15] Doctors hoped they could use the scientific principle of *dialysis*. A fluid containing impurities on one side of a membrane would let the small impurities pass through tiny holes in the membrane to a pure fluid on the other side. They

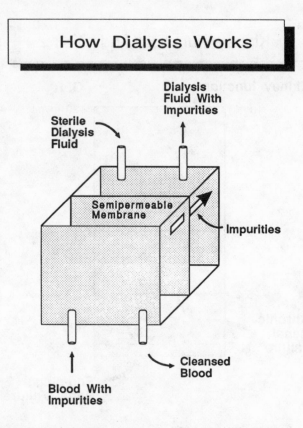

Figure 27 The Process of Dialysis

The impurity-containing blood is passed on one side of the semiperme-able membrane. On the other side is a sterile dialysis fluid, the dialysate. Small waste product particles pass through the membrane from the blood to the dialysis fluid. Larger blood cells are blocked, staying in the blood. The waste products, having permeated the membrane, are diluted in the dialysis fluid.

would need a special membrane, a *semipermeable membrane* with micro-scopic holes that would allow the small particles to *permeate* or pass through to the other side, but that would hold back the larger particles.

Scientists built devices to bring the blood containing impurities to one side of the membrane. On the other side would be the *dialysate*, the sterile dialysis fluid. The process of dialysis would let the unwanted small parti-cles from the blood pass through the tiny holes in the membrane to the

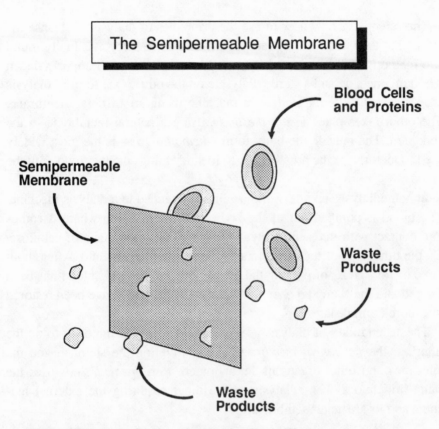

Figure 28 How the Semipermeable Membrane Works

The membrane may be artificial, as in the hemodialysis machine, or natural, the peritoneal membrane that covers internal organs including the stomach and intestines. Both membranes have small holes that allow the small waste product particles to pass through, but block the larger blood cells and proteins. They filter the blood, removing the unwanted small particles.

dialysis fluid, the dialysate, on the other side. The good particles, like blood cells, would be too large to pass and would stay where they were needed, in the blood. The wastes would be quickly diluted in the large volume of dialysis solution, allowing waste and water levels in the blood to become nearly normal in a few hours of treatment. The result was that the blood would be artificially filtered, cleansed of some of the impurities that had been making the patient sick.

The scientists knew how to use the principles of dialysis to cleanse the blood, but they had to find practical ways to do it. They eventually found two methods, both using a semipermeable membrane with impurity-laden blood on one side and a sterile dialysate on the other. One form of dialysis takes place *outside the body* in a machine using an artificial membrane. The other takes place *inside the body*, using a natural membrane in the abdomen. The outside-the-body form—*hemodialysis*—is the most widely used. (Doctors use the prefix *hemo* to identify things having to do with the blood.)

In hemodialysis, an artery and a vein are attached to a dialysis machine. The blood is pumped out of the body, into the machine where it comes into contact with the semipermeable membrane, often made of cellulose. On the other side of the membrane is the sterile dialysis fluid. After about three or four hours of passing the membrane, the patient's blood has been filtered and the fluid and chemical balance of the body have been restored to a more normal state.

The second kind of dialysis uses a membrane inside the body to do the filtering, the *peritoneal membrane*, a sac covering the stomach and the intestines and other organs in the abdomen. *Peritoneal dialysis* uses the same principle as hemodialysis, but without requiring the external machine and its artificial membrane.

HEMODIALYSIS: A BIG, EXPENSIVE, COMPLICATED MACHINE

The hemodialysis machine—usually called just a *dialysis machine*—is big and bulky, complicated and expensive, not at all portable. The machine needs a supply of water, dialysate and electricity. So while natural kidneys can work continuously, twenty-four hours a day, like all of the body's systems, the artificial kidney can only work when the patient is hooked up to a stationery machine. The dialysis machine can't be strapped on the patient's back or fastened to his wrist. He has to go to the machine, and spend several hours while it does its work. So the first problem with this new medical miracle was that the machine had to do in a few hours the filtering work that a normal kidney did continuously.

The dialysis schedule doctors settled on was to attach the patient to the machine for three or four hours every other day. Some patients have a dialysis machine at home and with the help of a partner, usually a family member, can learn to do their own dialysis. But most patients go to a dialysis center for treatment. A typical schedule is for the patient to go to the center on, say, Monday morning. He is hooked up to the machine for a three or four hour run while the dialysis machine does the filtering job, removing unneeded fluid and chemicals, bringing his body chemistry back toward a precarious balance. Then, the patient is on his own, with little or no kidney function—either natural or artificial—from Monday afternoon until Wednesday morning. The poisons build up in his blood; hour by hour he drifts back towards uremia.

Despite the patient's careful attention to his diet, the fluid and waste products build up Monday night and all day Tuesday as his blood flows through his body with little natural filtering, little urine being made, little kidney function. On Wednesday morning he returns to the center where the staff plugs him into the machine for another three or four hour run, bringing him back from uremia. He spends Thursday away from the machine, and goes back to the center on Friday to repeat the procedure.

Often the patient feels *washed out* after the intensive filtering run. Then as the waste products increase in the blood before the next run, he may have some symptoms of uremia—swelling, fatigue, easy bruising, itching, feeling bloated. Most nephrologists agree that daily dialysis would be far better for the patient than three times a week treatment.[16] But to be practical, daily dialysis needs two things that don't yet exist—a better way to plug the patient's veins and arteries into the machine and a simpler, cheaper machine that the patient can operate himself at home, without a trained partner or a technician to help him.

HOW TO GET THE CONTAMINATED BLOOD INTO THE DIALYSIS MACHINE

A big problem of dialysis is the method of getting the patient's blood out of his body into the machine and then back into his body. There are two ways to get *blood access*, neither of which is without problems. *Subcutaneous access* means puncturing the skin each time the patient must be connected to the dialysis machine. Doctors usually create a *fistula* in a minor surgical operation on the patient's arm. An artery and a vein are joined together. The increased flow of blood causes the vein to increase in size and develop a thicker wall. Dialysis technicians, or the patient himself, can then puncture the enlarged vein to provide access to the blood stream. Usually two needles are used: the *arterial needle* takes the blood out of the body and the *venous needle* returns the filtered blood to circulation. Many problems result from this kind of access to the blood, and from all of the cumulative effects of puncturing the skin in two places every other day.[17]

The other method is *transcutaneous access*. Doctors penetrate the skin permanently, implanting a device that can be plugged into the tubes of the machine repeatedly. The device is called a *shunt*. The important advantages of this kind of access is that, once implanted, it can be used without pain. The patient can be plugged into the machine quickly and simply, and no problems are created by frequent use. But the permanent devices are plagued by infection and clotting.

Neither of these methods of accessing the patient's blood is ideal. Researchers expect that the next step will be an *intravenous catheter,* a tube made of polyurethane or silicon rubber, implanted permanently in veins and arteries of the throat or neck. If eighty percent of such implants last for a year or more, which they don't do now, then they may become practical and daily dialysis at home may become possible.[18]

PERITONEAL DIALYSIS: CLOSER TO NATURE

While they were using the principle of dialysis across a semipermeable membrane, researchers realized that there is a *natural membrane* in the body that might do the same job. The external machine might not be necessary. They believed that this natural membrane might be made to do the filtering work of a natural kidney. They looked for a practical way to use the *peritoneal membrane,* a thin covering that helps protect many internal organs like the stomach and intestines. Some researchers began saying that the body really has *three kidneys*—the two natural ones and the peritoneal membrane. They saw the possibility of doing dialysis without the need for an external machine, without the disadvantages and inconveniences of cost, scheduling and blood access. They saw the chance to do the filtering continuously, while the patient continued his normal activities, much more natural and similar to the work of the normal kidneys.

They would make it work by applying the same principles that made hemodialysis work. Like all tissues in the body, the peritoneal membrane has its own blood supply. Blood is continuously circulated to the membrane. Every few hours all the blood in the body passes through the peritoneal membrane, just as it would pass through the dialysis machine during a three or four hour run. The peritoneum is also *semipermeable*, small molecules can pass through it, but the big ones are held back.

The researchers set out to find a way to get the special dialysis fluid— the dialysate similar to that used in the machine—*inside the body* where it could flood the peritoneal membrane. The impurities and water carried in the blood would pass through the membrane into the dialysis solution, cleansing the blood of unwanted chemicals and water. They could then remove the dialysis solution from the abdomen, taking with it the unwanted waste products.

The method the researchers developed—*peritoneal dialysis*—is now widely used all over the world. Ten percent of dialysis patients in the United States and higher percentages in other countries are being treated with chronic peritoneal dialysis in the 1990s.[19] Peritoneal dialysis is delivered in three different ways. *Continuous ambulatory peritoneal dialysis* or *CAPD* is the most common. (*Continuous* because it takes place all day, every day. *Ambulatory* because the patient is able to walk around, go about his normal activities without being tied down and connected to a machine.) The dialysis takes place inside his body, instead of outside in a big and expensive machine.

The doctors devised a method to get the dialyzing fluid into the abdomen, flooding the peritoneum so that the peritoneal membrane could filter the blood as the artificial membrane did in the dialysis machine. In a minor surgical procedure, they make a small incision in the abdomen and implant a small tube or *catheter* near the navel. The patient himself then hooks up a plastic bag containing about two liters of sterile dialysis solution to the catheter, and lets it drain into his body. When the bag is empty, he folds it up and leaves it attached to the tube in his abdomen, concealed under his clothing. Some of the newer catheter designs allow the bag to be

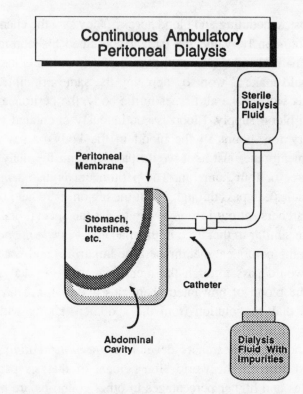

Figure 29 CAPD: Continuous Ambulatory Peritoneal Dialysis

The artificial membrane of the dialysis machine is replaced by the natural membrane of the peritoneaum. The CAPD patient drains 2 liters of dialysis fluid into his abdomen through a catheter that has been permanently implanted near his navel. Small waste products cross the membrane into the sterile dialysis fluid in the abdominal cavity. After four to six hours, the patient connects an empty bag to the catheter and drains the waste-containing fluid. He then connects a new bag of sterile fluid and repeats the process.

disconnected between the time the fluid flows into the abdomen and when it has to be drained.[20] The patient has filled his abdomen with two liters of sterile dialyzing fluid. The impurities in the blood start passing from the blood circulating through the peritoneal membrane into the dialysis solution.

Four to six hours after inserting the solution, the continuous ambulatory peritoneal dialysis patient reverses the process, draining the fluid out of

Types of Dialysis

- *hemodialysis*—the most widely-used; usually called simply dialysis; an artificial kidney machine with an artificial membrane often made of cellulose is used to filter the blood; the patient usually is treated for a three or four hour run on the machine three times a week.
- *continuous ambulatory peritoneal dialysis (CAPD)*—becoming more popular; allows the patient to dialyze without being attached to a stationery machine; the patient inserts two liters of sterile dialysis fluid into his abdominal cavity through a permanently implanted tube or catheter near his navel; the fluid floods the peritoneal membrane, a natural membrane covering internal organs including the stomach and the intestines; some people call this membrane "the third kidney;" the heart pumps blood to the membrane where the process of dialysis allows waste products to pass through into the dialysis fluid in the abdomen; after a few hours, the patient drains the fluid containing the waste products and starts the cycle again.
- *continuous cycling peritoneal dialysis (CCPD)*—uses the internal peritoneal membrane; an automatic machine inserts and removes several exchanges of fluid over an eight to twelve hour period while the patient sleeps
- *intermittent peritoneal dialysis (IPD)*—similar to CCPD, except that the exchanges are done more rapidly.

his abdomen into the empty bag. He then removes the old bag with contaminated fluid, plugs in a new one with clean fluid, and starts the procedure again.

One advantage of peritoneal dialysis is that there are no shunts or fistulas, the blood access methods that plague hemodialysis. There is no need to travel to the machine, to schedule life around being in the dialysis center, at the machine for three or four hours every other day. Peritoneal dialysis works continuously, much more like the natural kidneys. There is less need for a restricted diet or fluid intake.

A big problem with peritoneal dialysis is infection. All forms of peritoneal dialysis require a tube or catheter through which the fluid can be inserted into the abdomen and later removed. Whenever the catheter is opened to insert a new bag of fluid, there is a chance for contamination. No matter how carefully the patient tries to maintain the sterility of the catheter and the connection to the bag, the process of changing fluid four or five times a day, every day, exposes the patient to the inevitable contamination that causes infections. The skin around the catheter or the inside of the peritoneal cavity itself gets infected. One half of all peritoneal dialysis patients can expect to be hospitalized for complications of CAPD during their first year on the treatment. They can expect an average of eight days a year in the hospital for complications every year after that.[21]

Researchers have developed many devices to minimize the chance of infection. The best results have been found in Europe with the use of a catheter called the *Y-set*. The idea is simple: the new fluid bag is connected before the old fluid is drained. That way the draining fluid can flush the connection before the new fluid is inserted. The Europeans have been able to reduce peritonitis significantly, and American nephrologists are now beginning to use the Y-sets.[22]

There are other problems. The dialysis done by the internal membrane is sometimes not adequate, and the patient's blood chemistry as a result is not well balanced. There are sometimes problems with the high pressure in the abdomen caused by the constant presence of the fluid.

A variation of dialysis using the peritoneal membrane is *continuous cyclic peritoneal dialysis* (CCPD). The patient's catheter is attached to an automatic cycling machine that pumps the sterile dialysis fluid into his abdomen at night while he is sleeping and removes it after a few hours. The machine then pumps new fluid into the abdomen and repeats the exchange three times overnight. The next morning, the patient goes about his daily activities with the final fluid exchange in his body. That night the cycler drains the fluid and starts the cycle again.[23]

Still another variation is *intermittent peritoneal dialysis* (IPD). The patient is attached to an automated cycling machine for an eight to twelve hour treatment three times a week. The machine allows a measured amount of fluid to flow through the catheter into the abdomen where it stays for about ten minutes before being drained out over about fifteen minutes. This cycle of inflow and draining is repeated up to twenty-four times over a treatment that may last up to twelve hours.

LIFE ON DIALYSIS

Natural kidneys work all the time, cleansing the blood, balancing the fluids and the chemistry of the body. We don't tell them what to do. We are not even aware of what they are doing. But a dialysis patient has to do everything the natural kidneys would do automatically. With the help of the doctors, nurses, social workers, technicians and machines, he has to provide the equivalent of a natural function that no longer works. Either kind of dialysis is limited in what it can do in replacing the function of the kidney, so the patient must limit the work that needs to be done. The kidneys are no longer there to remove excess water, so the patient has to limit the amount he takes in. Most people can get rid of two or three cups of water a day through breathing or perspiring. The failed kidneys may produce some urine, getting rid of some more fluid. But a dialysis patient can usually take in no more than a few cups of fluid a day. Anything that's liquid at room temperature counts as fluid, so the restriction is very severe. Excess fluid causes serious problems like swelling, high blood pressure, and sometimes difficulty with breathing, making the limits on fluid important.

Nutrition is critical for a dialysis patient. Because the kidney can no longer balance the body's chemistry by conserving what it needs and getting rid of what it doesn't need, the dialysis patient must do the balancing job by taking in the right amount and the right kind of nutrients. The most critical elements are protein, sodium, potassium and phosphorus. Too much sodium causes the body to retain water and increases blood pressure. Too much potassium can cause heart trouble. Too much phosphorous can cause bone damage. Some dialysis patients find the fluid restriction harder to live with than the diet.

Dialysis patients have difficulty following dietary restrictions. Yet nephrologists prescribe dialysis routinely, while they scoff at conservative nutritional treatment that might *prevent* kidney failure "because it is too difficult for the patient to follow." How, I wondered, can nephrologists defend this strange logic. "Nutritional therapy is too difficult for the patient. Therefore I will prescribe dialysis." (With its own difficult nutritional restrictions.) Some nephrologists ignore nutritional therapy, yet they often prescribe a *vastly more difficult therapy*—dialysis. I wondered if conservative treatment to delay or avoid dialysis is too difficult for the *patient*. Or, is it too difficult for the *nephrologist*?

PSYCHOLOGICAL EFFECTS OF DIALYSIS

Some psychiatrists use a new word to describe the study of the psychology of kidney patients—*psychonephrology*.[24] The idea is that life with kidney disease is different enough to warrant a subspecialty drawing on both psychiatry and nephrology to study the mental and social condition of kidney patients.[25] During the early years of dialysis there was little academic interest in theorizing about psychonephrology. The issues were stark and well-defined in the 1960s. Without treatment, patients with kidney failure would die. Dialysis offered a way to keep them alive. But the treatment was very expensive. There was no government entitlement program guaranteeing to pay for dialysis treatment for anyone who needed it. Most dialysis was paid for by research and training grants from the National Institutes of Health. The only important questions of the 1960s for

---

A Physician With Kidney Disease Describes Life On Dialysis

- "... patients I have known on dialysis seem to be concerned about very real problems. To be held to an 800 ml total intake of fluids per day is most difficult. Restrictions on consumption of sodium and potassium make any kind of meal unpalatable. Restraints on travel even further constrain an already regimented, complicated and compromised life style."

- "A young woman wonders whether anyone will ever marry her, or whether she should even consider marriage. A young husband wonders whether he can, or even should, sire children and, if he does, who will support them. Older, more established patients on dialysis wonder if the struggle to live is worth the effort and money that must be put forth for the rest of their lives. Patients with growing children wonder whether these children's lives would be more damaged by continuing hemodialysis or by 'accidental' unplugging of the shunt, so that at least their family's future would be more financially secure."

Source: Calland, 1972.

A Physician With Kidney Disease Wonders If Dialysis Patients Have Unreasonable Fears?

- "I cannot emphasize strongly enough that [...] these fears are well founded and are based in reality. It is real, for example, that some employers will not lend money for necessary equipment, nor give time off for treatment. It is real that friends and neighbors, even when positively helpful, regard the dialysis patient as a marginal person—here today, gone tomorrow. It is real that the patient's own tenuous grasp on the future is reflected constantly in his own professional and financial dealings (promotions are delayed and arrangements for mortgages and insurances are difficult, if not impossible.)"
- "Patients on dialysis are accustomed to being told by the doctor, 'You are doing fine'—usually after the latest measurements of electrolytes and creatinine. The patient then thinks to himself, 'If I'm doing fine, why do I feel so rotten?' After undergoing correction of several days' accumulation of metabolites in a few hours, who could feel well [...]? Who [because of his anemia] feels well enough to function when he cannot climb his own stairway [...]?"

Source: Calland, 1972.

---

doctors trying to use dialysis to save the lives of uremic patients were "Who gets treatment? Who lives? Who dies? Who pays? Who makes the choice?" Some patients could pay for their own dialysis, but most could not. So the institutions ultimately responsible for the few dialysis facilities available were forced into the position of choosing some patients who would get the life-saving treatment, and others who would not. Nobody was thinking much about the *quality of life* of the patients who made it through the decision process to get on dialysis. Some kidney patients say doctors still don't think much about the quality of life.

In the 1970s and 1980s when Medicare and insurance companies started to pay for dialysis and later transplant, private and public entrepreneurs created a new industry—the kidney replacement industry. By the 1990s, with more than 150,000 people in the Medicare end-stage renal disease program, most of them on dialysis, the psychonephrologists began to focus on psycho-social issues important to kidney patients.

The psychiatrists, psychologists and social workers working with dialysis patients have observed three successive periods that most patients go through in adjusting to their dialysis treatments: *honeymoon, disenchantment and discouragement, and long-term adaptation.*

The *honeymoon* is a period of marked physical and emotional improvement as the symptoms of uremia are relieved by the dialysis. But this hopeful period includes repetitive and intense episodes of anxiety, insomnia, apprehension about life expectancy and the ability to return to work. Troubles with the blood access site are frequent—clotting and infections. Soon many dialysis patients enter the period of *disenchantment and discouragement,* a gradual change for some, abrupt for others. Contentment, confidence and hope decrease or disappear. They begin to feel hopeless, helpless and sad. This phase has been observed to last for a few months to a year or more. In the depressed patients repeated complications appear, particularly with blood access. Psychiatrists believe they have observed a connection between life stress, the change in emotional state, and troubles with blood access.[26]

A Nephrologist Looks Back On His Own 24 Years On Dialysis

- "Dialysis has served me well over the years. I completed my last two years of college, four years of medical school without loss of time, and I practiced for 17 years as a nephrologist in Brooklyn. I have never had to cancel a speaking engagement to date. I have been invited to several such meetings as this to speak of my experience but my local colleagues in Brooklyn, New York, have never asked me to share my experience with them. I think they have come to the point of accepting me as normal and to leave it at that."
- "Even though I have travelled over much of the Far East, through much of Europe and a bit of South America and the United States, every time I have to take a trip, it's always with trepidation as to what the dialysis is going to be like. I am not going to be able to enjoy the food as much as I would otherwise if I had good kidney function. There is still a sense of weakness, a sense of being ill."

Source: Lundin, 1990

Many patients eventually reach the period of *long-term adaptation,* an acceptance of their limitations, their dependence on dialysis, and the complications of chronic dialysis. Sometimes the life stresses of work and losses— real, threatened or fantasized—were thought to be related to dialysis problems. Patients become keenly aware of their dependence on the machine and the staff. They express anger at the inconveniences and hardships of life on dialysis, often directing their anger at the staff, demanding more help with jobs, housing, financial troubles, or relationship to spouse and family. They have been observed not trying to gain greater independence, but demanding more support.

A leading psychonephrologist, Dr. Norman Levy, considers the main problem of dialysis patients to be their dependency, and the most important task of the physicians and staff to help the patient with the transition from the *honeymoon* to *disenchantment,* recognizing the stressful nature of trying to return to work, and helping the patient work toward *long-term adaptation.* The patient may feel trapped, he says, between his desire to be dependent on the machine and the expectations of the staff that he return to productive work. Most dialysis patients don't return to work.[27]

ERYTHROPOIETIN MAY CHANGE
LIFE ON DIALYSIS

After years of research and clinical studies on human patients, the Food and Drug Administration in 1989 approved a new drug called Epogen, a genetically-engineered version of the hormone *erythropoietin* produced in proper quantities by normal kidneys, but deficient in patients with kidney disease. Doctors prescribe this very expensive drug—at least partially reimbursed by Medicare—to manage the anemia that goes with kidney disease, reducing the need for blood transfusions.

After a year of widespread use, doctors report that patients have more energy, better appetite, increased sexual interest, and a better sleep pattern. Some doctors are reaching the conclusion that symptoms they once thought were caused by *uremia*—the elevated levels of toxins in the blood—were in fact symptoms of *anemia* which could therefore be treated with erythropoietin. They have also found that the drug is effective and safe with nearly all patients. Some doctors consider erythropoietin a breakthrough in dialysis because it can help more patients attain the goal of rehabilitation, returning to productive work.

There are problems with erythropoietin, notably the cost and reimbursement. Medicare will pay about $40 a dose for a treatment most doctors prescribe three times a week. If all the 150,000 patients in the End Stage Renal Disease program got regular doses of erythropoietin, the cost to Medicare would be about $1 billion a year, in addition to the $5 billion already being spent annually. There is no reimbursement for patients who handle their own dialysis, either home hemodialysis or peritoneal dialysis.[28]

Erythropoietin has the potential to improve the quality of life on dialysis significantly, and the early indications are that it has done so for those patients who receive it regularly. Erythropoietin may change much about life on dialysis.

7
Replacement Parts:
The Kidney Transplant

What would your chances be with a kidney transplant? Would your new kidney survive, a living thing transplanted into your body like a rose bush in your garden? Would it live through the first year? The second? Longer? Or, would your body's defense mechanisms recognize it as an alien organ, something foreign and potentially dangerous, something to be destroyed like a virus, or expelled, like a wood sliver in your thumb, festering, swollen, and sore until you pick it out with a needle?

Would you need drugs to defeat your immune system, to prevent your body from attacking the new kidney, rejecting it? Would the anti-rejection drugs be so powerful that the drugs themselves would damage your new kidney they were intended to protect? Would they suppress your immune system so thoroughly that you would be susceptible to attacks on your system by other diseases, the way AIDS patients are attacked by diseases that penetrate the AIDS-weakened defenses? How long would your new kidney survive? How long would *you* survive, even if the kidney failed?

What kind of life would you have after a kidney transplant? How healthy would you be with a new kidney? Could you work? Travel? Exercise? Have sex? Even if the doctors consider your transplant "successful," how successful is a kidney transplant likely to be for you?

IF ALL GOES WELL, YOU'LL BE ALMOST LIKE NEW; IF NOT ...

In the best case, the transplant team will find a kidney well-matched to your own body, you will be in good health except for your kidney disease, and the transplant will be handled by experienced professionals with a good track record. The chances are seven or eight out of ten that your newly transplanted kidney will be functioning a year after the operation.[1] Your chances are even better if your new kidney came from a blood relative.[2] Best would be your identical twin, or a brother or sister, sometimes even a parent whose tissues closely match your own. You will take low doses of anti-rejection drugs. You may be able to work and live normally.

In a more common case, you will get your new kidney from a person who has just died, probably in an accident, a brain-dead person whose kidneys nevertheless remain healthy and able to function. This *cadaver kidney* will not be a perfect match to your own tissues. Your general health will not be as good. You may have heart trouble, for example, or diabetes. One out of four cadaver transplants is likely to fail within a year, and the success rate has been decreasing during the late 1980s. [3, 4]

I Learned Some New Words About Kidney Transplant

- *cadaver kidney*—a kidney that surgeons have removed from a dead person, often killed in an accident, but whose kidneys remain healthy
- *living related donor kidney*—a kidney that surgeons have removed from the body of a living person for transplant into the body of a close relative; usually a blood relative, like a brother or sister; sometimes a parent, and occasionally an even more distant relative (because cadaver donors are scarce)
- *transplant rejection*—the body's natural attempt to recognize the transplanted tissue as foreign, alien, something to be destroyed like a virus or bacteria threatening the body
- *immune system suppressing drug*—a drug used to reduce or defeat the body's attempt to reject the foreign tissue of the transplanted organ

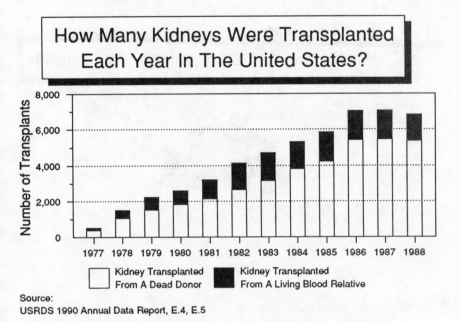

Source:
USRDS 1990 Annual Data Report, E.4, E.5

Figure 30 Kidney Transplants in the United States

U.S. Renal Data System records include information on most transplants done on patients in the Medicare End-Stage Renal Disease Program. Some transplants were also done on non-citizens and other non-Medicare patients. There were almost twice as many people waiting for a transplant in 1988 as there were kidney donors.

Overall, about 90 percent of transplants from a living blood relative, usually a brother or sister, are still functioning a year later.[5] Doctors call this a *living related donor* transplant, or, for short, an "LRD transplant." Transplants using a kidney from a brain-dead person who is not a blood relative are much more successful than they were as recently as the early 1980s, but the results are not as good as those with living related donor kidneys. Only about three out of four kidneys taken from a dead person, a cadaver, are still functioning a year after the transplant.[6,7]

What this means is that as many as three people out of ten who have kidney transplant operations in the 1990s will see their new kidney fail within the first year. They will then face the decision to have a second transplant, or to go back on dialysis. But these numbers also mean that

How Many Kidneys Transplanted From A Dead Donor In 1984 Survived Until 1988?

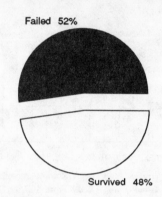

Failed 52%

Survived 48%

Source:
USRDS 1990 Annual Data Report, G.43

Figure 31 5-Year Survival Of Cadaver Transplants

Government experts studied records for all 372,000 Medicare End-Stage Renal patients since 1976. They found that less than half the kidneys transplanted from a cadaver, a dead donor, survived for five years.

seven or eight people out of ten will have a functioning kidney after one year. Many more transplants will succeed than will fail. (These statistics are for the kidney transplantations in the United States that have been recorded in government and university databases. You will find extensive government statistics on kidney disease and the outcome of treatments in Appendix 1, data published in late 1990. Some of the facts may be news to your doctor. You may want to show him this book.)

Some of the 219 transplant programs in the United States have much better records than the national averages, and some have much worse records.[8] If you are considering a kidney transplant, you may want to ask the program to tell you about its record. How long has it been in operation? How many kidney transplants has it done? The average center did 30 a year in 1989.[9] What is the survival rate—not just for one year, but how long have the *patients* survived? How many have had a second or third

How Many Kidneys Transplanted From A Blood Relative Donor In 1984 Survived Until 1988?

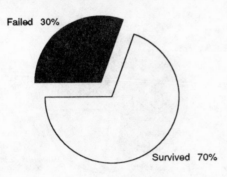

Failed 30%

Survived 70%

Source:
USRDS 1990 Annual Data Report, G.21

Figure 32 5-Year Survival Of LRD Transplants

Results for transplants from a living blood relative were much better. About seven out of ten transplants survived for five years. Some experts believe that the body is less likely to reject a transplanted kidney with a close match between the tissue types of the donor and the recipient.

transplant—"a re-transplant?" If they won't tell you, or if they say they don't know the answers, you may wonder why. Could it be that they don't *want* you to know? You may want to consult another transplant program.)

Most kidney transplant patients can expect to make it through the first year with their new kidneys functioning properly, but how long can they expect to live with their transplanted kidney? Five years after the transplant, seven of ten patients will still be alive; the other three will be dead.[10, 11] (About three of ten patients will be alive after five years on dialysis.)[12]

How Many Kidneys Transplanted From
A Dead Donor In 1979 Survived Until 1988?

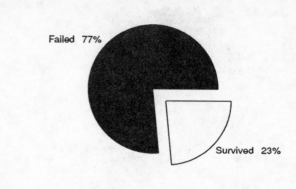

Failed 77%

Survived 23%

Source:
USRDS 1990 Annual Data Report, G.47

Figure 33 10-Year Survival Of Cadaver Transplants

When I learned that almost eight of every ten cadaver kidney transplants failed within ten years, I wondered how the transplant surgeons could claim a "90 percent success rate," and why the popular media often repeated their claim as fact.

KIDNEY TRANSPLANT IS NOT A MIRACLE IN THE 1990s, BUT IT IS RISKY

Kidney transplantation in the 1990s is a routine medical procedure that some doctors believe has a a high rate of success. But the risk of transplant failure or death is far higher than most technological risks we accept in our everyday lives. Experienced transplant teams are at work in 219 centers, 18 organ-finding and sharing networks are operating, tissue-typing techniques help assure a good match, surgical procedures are well-understood, anti-rejection drugs are more effective and less toxic, and, even if the transplant fails, dialysis is always there as a backup to keep the patient alive.[13] Kidney transplantation is not a "cure" for kidney disease. If the original cause of the kidney disease was related to diabetes, for example,

How Many Kidneys Transplanted From A Blood Relative Donor In 1979 Survived Until 1988?

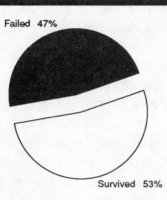

Failed 47%

Survived 53%

Source:
USRDS 1990 Annual Data Report, G.25

Figure 34 10-Year Survival Of LRD Transplants

About half of transplants from a living blood relative survived for ten years. This was the type of kidney transplant with the best chance of success. The tissue match was often good with less severe rejection. But even so, about half the transplants failed within ten years. Where was the "90 percent success rate?"

or high blood pressure, the newly transplanted kidney, like the original ones, may be damaged. Nonetheless, a kidney transplant can produce a better quality of life for someone with diseased kidneys.

The risks, though, are much higher than we expect from other technologies in our lives. For example, about 1,200 of the 5,000 cadaver kidneys transplants recorded in the U.S. Renal Data System in 1988 failed within the first year; about 170 of 1,400 living related donor transplants failed.[14,15] If other technologies in our lives were as risky, I wonder how widely they would be used.

Take the case of air travel, a 20th century technology once called a miracle. In 1987, 447 million passengers boarded commercial airliners in the US. Only *232* passengers were killed in aircraft accidents that year.

Scheduled flights took off from United States airports 6.6 million times in 1987. There were *four* accidents.[16] If the airlines had the same effectiveness as the kidney transplant teams, over *two million* of those flights would have crashed in 1987. If the airlines' "success rates" were the same as the "one year graft survival rates" the transplant teams claim, over *one hundred million people would have been killed in airline crashes in 1987.*[17]

Is it fair to compare other technological risks in our lives to the risk of transplant? An airplane trip may be a frivolous or unnecessary event while a kidney transplant may be a life-saving procedure undertaken only when the patient might die without it. If a transplant succeeds once out of ten attempts, or even once out of a hundred attempts, at least that one life will be saved. That certainly is true, and I don't question the motives of the transplant teams in trying to save lives and advance medical science. But, if there is an *alternative to transplant* that is far less risky, if the need for transplant *can be avoided*, is it right for the transplant advocates to describe their work as "routine?" *Newsweek* quoted Dr. Starzl in 1988: "We've gone from the unattainable to the routine." [18] Is it *routine* when so few transplanted kidneys survive beyond five years? The chance that the technology of the airplane will fail to accomplish its purpose is small. The technology of the kidney transplant is downright dangerous—*if there is an alternative.*

As I learned about the outcome of kidney transplant, I began to glimpse some reasons why the success rates are so poor. Prominent nephrologists wrote in 1990 that not much is known about the body's attempt to reject the transplanted kidney months or years after the transplant, about the long-term effects of the anti-rejection drugs. They also wrote that the drugs have powerful kidney-damaging and blood pressure-raising side effects, perhaps reasons why so many transplants fail after a few years.[19] Is transplant really a routine treatment? I had some doubts. The short-term results of transplant are not good. The long-term results are poor and poorly understood. Yet, transplant is the treatment-of-choice. I wondered if the transplant teams were being forthright and truthful with their patients when they presented the technology as "routine."

**Transplant Pioneer Dr. Thomas Starzl
On The Importance of Organ Transplantation**

"Until 50 or 60 years ago, practitioners of medicine observed and presided over lethal diseases powerless to provide much more than a priestly function. This began to change with increasingly specific drugs such as antibiotics but for most organ-specific chronic disorders, a rear guard strategy was all that could be offered. Patients with failing kidneys, liver or hearts could be treated with diet, medicines, or with operations that were often illogically designed. Suddenly, with the advent of transplantation, it became possible for the first time in human history to provide exactly what was needed, a completely new organ. Those who in small groups sat around tables in the early 1960s and discussed renal transplantation knew how high the stakes were or could be."

Source: Starzl, 1987.

THE IRRESISTIBLE DREAM OF INTERCHANGEABLE PARTS

Dr. Thomas E. Starzl is a giant of transplant science in the 20th century. Some of his colleagues thought he might win the Nobel prize, the scientist's most prized achievement, although his chances may have been diminished when the Nobel prize for medicine was awarded to two other transplant surgeons in 1990. Dr. Starzl has dedicated his life's work to making organ transplantation a routine medical treatment, a therapy instead of an experiment. But he is not simply a technician, a scientist seeking to add to human knowledge. He says he is working to revolutionize the practice of medicine. Some colleagues have called him a "cowboy" because of his obsession with undertaking transplants that other surgeons believe are impossible, and because of the agony many of his patients suffer while he tries out his experimental techniques and anti-rejection drugs.[20]

Dr. Starzl has said he wants to change the fundamental philosophy of medicine. He wants doctors to be more than merely what he calls "priests," powerless to help people with chronic troubles in their body's

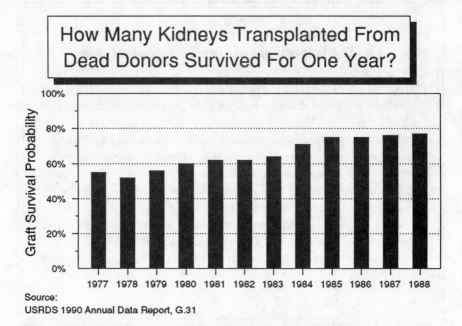

How Many Kidneys Transplanted From Dead Donors Survived For One Year?

Source:
USRDS 1990 Annual Data Report, G.31

Figure 35 1-Year Survival Of Cadaver Transplants

The transplant surgeons measure their own effectiveness by one year graft survival rates. For transplants from a dead donor, cadaver transplants, one year graft survival has improved from about 55% in 1977 to 78% in 1988. How can they claim a "90 percent success rate?"

organs. He wants to perform what he sees as the ultimate medicine. Dr. Starzl wants to give his patient a completely new organ, a new heart, a new liver, a new kidney, sometimes even a cluster of organs all at once, hoping he can find a way to give his dying patients the ultimate gift—new organs to replace the old. Like some other 20th century doctors, he is challenging death.

Dr. Starzl says he chose transplantation as his specialty because other doctors thought it was a hopeless cause, an alchemist's dream of turning lead into gold. He has often quoted the pessimistic views that prevailed among surgeons and basic scientists in the early 1960s when he began working on transplantation. He is particularly fond of quoting what the Nobel Prize winning scientist Dr. F. M. Burnet wrote in 1961:

"Much thought has been given to ways by which tissues or organs not genetically and antigenically identical with the patient might be made to survive and function in the alien environment. On the whole, the present outlook is highly unfavorable to success..." [21, 22]

Dr. Burnet made this pessimistic comment about transplantation, says Dr. Starzl, on the eve of the successful kidney transplantations the Starzl team did in Denver in 1962 and 1963. [23] Transplant, says Dr. Starzl, is now a treatment, not an experiment.

"What was a crusade when it was not a reliable way of treatment became a business when it turned successful." [24]

Although Dr. Starzl may consider transplant a "reliable way of treatment" and a "business," some doctors and many transplant recipients are not so sure. Consider the conclusion reached by two leading transplant

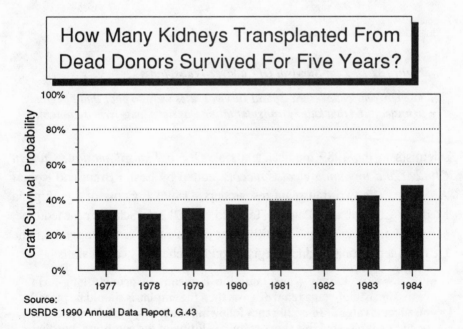

Figure 36 5-Year Survival Of Cadaver Transplants

The five-year cadaver transplant survival rates had improved since 1977, but they were still poor.

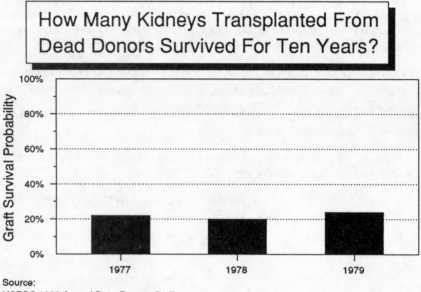

Source:
USRDS 1990 Annual Data Report, G.47

Figure 37 10-Year Survival Of Cadaver Transplants

The ten-year cadaver transplant survival rates were so poor that I began to understand that kidney transplantation was not a long-term treatment.

scientists in the 1989 medical textbook *Organ Transplantation: Current Clinical and Immunological Concepts*, edited by Leslie Brent and Robert A. Sells.[25] The two transplant researchers, Daniel J. Cook, of the Virginia Medical College and Paul I. Terasaki, of UCLA School of Medicine, surveyed the data from 70,000 kidney transplant cases logged in the UCLA International Kidney Registry, and reached this conclusion:

> "If, however, kidney transplantation is meant to provide long-term remission of end-stage renal disease, then the emphasis should be placed on success rates 5, 10 or 20 years following the transplant. Few patients would be interested in a short-term resolution of the condition, but that is all that has been offered to the recipients of cadaveric donor kidneys up to now." [26]

A practicing physician from Kentucky, Dr. Robert Yaes, was thinking about liver transplants, not kidney transplants, but he may have been expressing the views of many kidney transplant patients and their families when he wrote:

> "The fact that a single patient may require as many as six successive transplants suggests that this technique is not so much a cure for end-stage liver failure as it is an interim measure that must be repeated over and over to preserve a person's life. Is it any wonder that there is such a shortage of donor organs?" [27]

THE KIDNEY PATIENT'S DILEMMA—TREATMENT OR EXPERIMENT?

Confused, uninformed, afraid, as a newly diagnosed kidney patient I was tugged in opposing directions when I considered transplant. On the one side, world-class scientists and surgeons like Starzl were saying that kidney transplant is routine. Transplant is therapy, treatment. The odds are good. This is simply a business, not experimental medicine. On the other, my common sense was telling me that I probably wouldn't get into an airplane if two or three out of every ten airplanes that took off would crash. Is kidney transplant a treatment, a therapy? Or is it still experimental after thirty years and a Nobel prize? The answer is very personal. There is no objective truth here.

In 1989 Dr. Starzl looked back at the kidney patients he had transplanted in Denver from 1962 to 1964. Of 46 transplant patients, 14 were still alive a quarter century later; 10 with the first transplant still working. All of them had received their new kidney from a blood relative and 10 of the 14 still alive had been 18 years old or younger at the time of transplantation. None of the patients who received a cadaver kidney was still alive.[28] Is transplantation a treatment, or is it still experimental? Dr. Starzl commented after looking at the results of his own work on these 46 kidney patients over 25 years ago:

> "The follow-up provided in this report is less of a justification of the technology then available than a sobering description of its limitations. The treatment options available today continue to have many of the same risk factors for truly long survival as the methods of 25 years ago. The results provide a stark warning against complacency regarding what we have to offer transplant recipients today." [29]

This assessment of the limitations of transplantation in 1990 came from the man who has been the most determined advocate of transplant for the last thirty years. Was it really just a business, as Dr. Starzl has said, or were the physicians and surgeons still searching for a way to solve the rejection problems? Had the unattainable become the routine, as *Newsweek* had quoted Dr. Starzl two years before?

The surgical techniques for kidney transplantation have been refined and perhaps perfected over the last four decades. Most doctors agree there is not much experimentation there. But many kidney transplant specialists admit, however, that there is a good deal of experimentation in trying to defeat the immune system's attempt to reject the new kidney. Dr. Starzl is sensitive to the limitations of transplant. He has been testing a new anti-rejection drug—FK-506—that the government has approved for use by only a few university medical centers. He thinks it's a breakthrough, but, of course, it's experimental in 1990. (More on FK-506 in Chapter 8.)

One problem, I think, is that the *goals* of the kidney transplant specialist are very different from the kidney patient's goals. Like many surgeons, the transplant surgeon counts a success when the patient gets up from the hospital bed and goes home, no matter how sick he may be. The surgery was a success; the patient is alive; he survived surgery. He got off the operating table alive. The patient, however, wants something very different from the transplantation. *He wants the chance for the replacement part to work as well in his body as the old part did.* He is willing to undergo the ordeal of surgery, rejection, drugs and all the other complications in the hope that his new kidney will return him to reasonably good health. The patient doesn't want a "one-year success," but that's how the transplant specialists judge the effectiveness of their work. This difference in goals and in the perception of the results of transplantation can be a devastating problem between patient and surgeon. The surgeon can see "success" while the patient is mutilated and half-dead.

The experienced transplant specialist can remember when a kidney transplant could be expected to fail more often than it succeeded. In 1974, nearly six of ten cadaver kidney transplants failed within a year. The same year three of ten transplants from living related donors failed. In the 1990s, the same specialist sees much better results. He sees "success," which he measures as "one year survival rates." If the patient lives for one year, and the newly transplanted kidney functions reasonably well for one year, the transplant specialist declares the transplant a "success."

When *New York Times* medical writer Gina Kolata, an experienced and respected medical journalist, reported the award of the 1990 Nobel prize to the surgeon who performed the first successful kidney transplant at Harvard in 1954, she wrote "kidney transplants now have a success rate of 90 percent." [30] A kidney patient reading that article had reason to believe— as apparently Gina Kolata believed—that kidney transplant is simply a routine operation that almost always "succeeds." Her statement about "success rate" was accurate, if she had referred to one-year survival of living donor grafts, but may have been misleading to patients and their families. (I'm sure she didn't realize how misleading her statement was. She was actually quoting the *claim* of the transplant surgeons, although she presented it as a *fact*, and I am confident that when she studies the facts she will make her description of transplant "success" more accurate.)

A patient who lives for 12 months with his kidney still functioning, no matter how sick he may be, perhaps even near death, qualifies as a "success" by the surgeons' definition. You will read in Chapter 10 the story of a man who received a living related kidney transplant in early 1990, who was in a coma and very near death a few months after his transplant, who has undergone eight abdominal operations since the transplant, who has lost many internal organs because of complications of the anti-rejection drugs, and yet by the definition used by the transplant teams and repeated by the *New York Times*, his transplant is judged "successful," part of the "success rate of 90 percent."

It is easy to understand how the specialists and the popular media can consider kidney transplant "successful." The patient lives far more often than not. The specialist can be proud of the normal life led by some of the patients he transplanted 15 or 20 years ago; some for over 25 years. He can see anti-rejection drugs that work better with fewer harmful side effects, and far lower doses. He sees new "wonder drugs" coming, like FK-506. He sees what looks to him like "success." Compared to the disappointing results of the 1960s and 1970s, there *is* success.

When I first looked at these same results as a prospective candidate for my own kidney transplant, I saw something quite different. I saw a difficult operation, a life-long regimen of potentially toxic drugs, even if all went well. I saw that most transplant patients, no matter how successful the operation, were not able to go back to work. I wondered how successful a transplant was for the patient, even though the surgeons considered it successful.

Eventually I began to understand that what *success* means to a patient is very different from what *success* means to the transplant specialist. For Dr. Starzl, kidney transplant is routine and boring.[31] It's almost always successful by his definition. If the patient lives for a year—no matter how sick or disabled—the transplant was a success. Transplant succeeds far more often than it fails. The patient is alive, isn't he? Wouldn't he be dead without the transplant, or half dead on the dialysis machine?

Dr. Starzl is doing far more exciting things now, like *multiple organ transplants*— removing the stomach, liver, pancreas and other organs and replacing them with grafts of everything but the stomach and the spleen. The operation can take 12 hours non-stop. Not many patients have survived, but they would have died anyway.[32] He wants to treat a hopeless patient, trying to keep him alive; but perhaps more importantly, he wants to push transplant technology farther toward the dream of *interchangeable parts*. And that's where the trouble starts for a kidney patient.

Was I so desperately ill that I needed to submit to treatment that may have failed for me, the patient, even if the surgeons considered it successful? Was I ready to submit to a high-risk *experiment* to save my life, an experiment which may have left me mutilated and half-dead anyway, while the surgeons called it a "success?"

A PATIENT'S FIRST ENCOUNTER WITH THE TRANSPLANT PROGRAM

I was bewildered when I first encountered the transplant team at the University of Pennsylvania hospital. The transplant unit had been doing kidney transplants for twenty years, and was justifiably proud of the level of experience and success that the well-trained staff had demonstrated. The director of the program was a nephrologist, not a surgeon. There were nurses and social workers specifically trained and experienced in dealing with transplant patients. Even the technicians in the blood test laboratory were specialized in transplant. Some people considered it one of the best transplant units in the country.

I was there to be evaluated as a candidate for transplant. Did I have a blood relative who would give me a kidney, or would I wait for the year or two it might take for an organ donor to show up? Was I a likely candidate for a transplant at all? Was I healthy enough to undergo the operation and the rejection episodes that were sure to follow? Could I tolerate the immune-system suppressing drugs? This is about what I was thinking that day.

"When the nephrologist sent me to the transplant specialist, he told me I should be a good candidate for a kidney transplant. Not too old. Not too many other diseases. I might have to wait a long time because there aren't enough kidney donors to supply the demand, but I could go on dialysis in the meantime.

"The transplant specialist is a nephrologist too. He said it's a routine operation. Several a week in this hospital alone. Success rate 80 or 90 percent. Some people have lived for 20 or 25 years with a transplant. Some even had babies. Problem is there aren't enough donated organs to go around. He asked if I had a brother or sister who might give me one of his or her two healthy kidneys. There's almost no risk for the donor, he said. People can live with only one kidney. Occasionally something has happened during the surgery to remove the healthy kidney, but that's very rare.

"I told him I wouldn't feel comfortable asking either of my two brothers for a kidney. I wouldn't want to be responsible for trouble they might have from the organ-donating process itself, or from something that happened to them afterwards. Better think about a cadaver kidney then, he said. Results aren't quite so good, but much better than they used to be. The reason, he said, is that doctors can do a better job of matching tissues now. They understand better how to determine what tissue types I have, and to look for a donor with a good match. They also know a lot more about the immune system now, the body's natural attempt to resist the foreign kidney tissue. They have a new drug, cyclosporine, that is less toxic than the older drugs. They can give it in lower doses. It doesn't have as many side effects as the older drugs did."

I gave several blood samples for tissue matching. The social worker interviewed me about my personal life. The surgical resident took a medical history and gave me a brief physical. I had become a transplant candidate.

A TRANSPLANT SPECIALIST'S FIRST ENCOUNTER WITH A CANDIDATE

The director of the transplant program, a nephrologist, interviewed me. Looking back now, I can guess his thoughts as he considered me for a kidney transplant.

"This new patient is 50 years old. Kidney trouble for the last four years. High blood pressure, controlled by drugs, more or less, but still high. He's way over weight, probably 50 pounds or more. High cholesterol, but that's so common now. Some indications that he had a heart attack three years ago. Chest pains now and then, but not serious. He's on medication for that too. Some clogged arteries, not too bad. Some enlargement of the heart, probably caused by years of high blood pressure. But in general, he's in good shape, except for the kidneys.

"He says he doesn't want to ask either of his brothers for a kidney. Too bad, but not unusual. That means he'll go on our waiting list. It's already two years long. I doubt if his kidneys will last more than a few months the way they're going now. After he's been on dialysis for a while, he may change his mind about asking his brother for a kidney.

"I remember the days before dialysis and transplant when a patient like this would be dead in a few months. At least now we can keep him alive until we get a cadaver organ for him. Chances are seven out of ten we can make a good match, do a good transplant, get his kidney functioning almost normally. Maybe we can even get him back to work. And Medicare will pay for most of it.

"I used to run the dialysis unit in the 1970s. But it just wasn't right for me. The dialysis patients were alive, sure, but what kind of life? Some of them did well, but most were very sick, psychologically as well as physically. Not many could work. Most had troubles with their families. Their overall condition was poor. Sure, we were keeping them alive, but what kind of life? That's why I came over to the transplant program 15 years ago. Here we have at least the chance to return someone to a normal life.

"Some people say transplantation is not a panacea, but a disease that will stay with the patient forever. They say that when we put an alien organ in his body we are giving him many diseases in place of the one that he had. But I don't believe that. My patients may, in fact, have other diseases after the transplant, but at least we can treat them. If they get pneumonia or gout or heart trouble, we can treat that. We couldn't treat the kidney disease they had. All in all, they're better off after the transplant. And, with every transplant, we learn more about how to do it. The new immune system suppressing drug, FK-506, may be a breakthrough. Starzl thinks so.

"I know there are lots of problems with kidney transplants. But at least we can do something. At least we don't have to be helpless while the patient withers away on dialysis. Or we don't have to put him off in the back wards to die from uremia as we did when I was in medical school. I'm glad I decided to work in transplant. I'm proud of my work."

I left the transplant program that morning wanting to learn more about kidney transplantation. Was it just a routine procedure, even a business, as Dr. Starzl called it? Or, was organ transplantation still an experiment that after thirty years wasn't very successful for the patients? Was transplant a way to revolutionize medicine, as Dr. Starzl said, or had the Nobel Laureate Burnet been right in 1961 when he predicted that the outlook was not good for transplantation? Would Dr. Starzl himself be a Nobel Laureate for pioneering transplantation? Or, would he be a footnote to medical history, a dedicated surgeon and scientist who had tried, valiantly but unsuccessfully, to achieve the impossible?

8

Replacement Parts: Why Is Organ Transplant So Difficult?

In 1990 two American transplant surgeon-scientists won the Nobel Prize for achievement in medicine. Dr. Joseph Murray of Harvard had performed the first successful kidney transplant in 1954. Dr. E. Donnall Thomas of Seattle had done a successful bone marrow transplant in 1970. They shared the $703,000 prize and the recognition of their contributions to making organ transplantation what the Nobel committee called a major achievement of medical science.[1]

Medical men have dreamed about transplanting organs for centuries. There were sporadic attempts at kidney transplantation during the first half of the 20th century, none successful. In the late 1940s doctors in Paris, London, Edinburgh and Boston began working on transplant in an organized way despite the warnings and pessimism from the basic scientists.[2] Dr. Murray did the world's first successful kidney transplant at the Peter Bent Brigham Hospital in Boston, taking a kidney from a living donor and successfully transplanting it into his identical twin brother. Also in the 1950s, Dr. Murray removed a kidney from a living person and successfully transplanted it to a close relative, but not an identical twin. He later removed a kidney from a dead body, a cadaver, and transplanted it successfully to an unrelated person. The 1990 Nobel Prize recognized his achievements.

Dr. Murray had launched the transplant era. Transplant surgeon Dr. Starzl commended him and others at the Peter Bent Brigham hospital for not faltering "in their support of the quixotic objective of treating end-stage renal disease despite the long list of tragic failures that resulted from these early efforts..." [3] Transplant surgeons were beginning to push their new technology from experiment to treatment.

INTERCHANGEABLE PARTS, WHY NOT?

The idea of the organ transplant is so seductively simple. We do so many similar things. Why not do it with organs in the body? Is a diseased kidney like a broken leg? Set the fracture. Immobilize it in a cast for six weeks. The leg is as good as new. We do so much in our everyday life with "interchangeable parts." We grow a tomato seedling on our window sill. We transplant it into the garden on Memorial Day, water it, prune it, and wait; in July we have a large plant covered with tomatoes. When our car won't start, we remove the dead battery, install a new one, turn the ignition key. The starter cranks and the engine starts. A Hong Kong businessman emigrates to New York. He learns English, works at his business. Seven years later he's an American citizen. Are these all "transplants?"

Why can't a new kidney or heart be transplanted into a diseased body? Find a suitable organ donor. "Harvest" the heart or kidney. Implant it in the diseased body. Sew the patient up and let him heal. He has a new kidney or heart. He's healthy again. Such an attractive idea. Broken legs heal, tomato plants thrive, new batteries start the automobile, immigrants melt into the community in New York City. The process is so simple and attractive in so many other parts of our lives. Perhaps that's why the media and conventional wisdom have accepted the transplant surgeons' claims that the interchangeable body part, organ transplantation, is "routine"— despite the overwhelming evidence of failure.

Dr. Starzl has not yet convinced the human body that organ transplantation is routine. The body *rejects the transplanted organ*. It recognizes the transplanted organ as *alien tissue*, and it throws the strength of a billion years of evolution into the struggle to repel the alien. Trying to protect the body, it attempts to kill the foreign organ. Often it kills the patient.

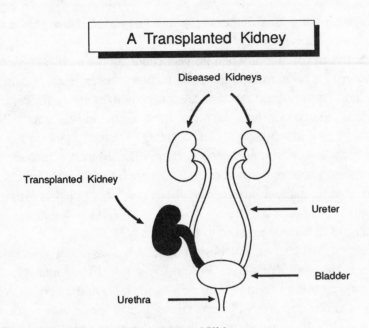

A Transplanted Kidney

Diseased Kidneys

Transplanted Kidney

Ureter

Bladder

Urethra

Figure 38 Location Of A Transplanted Kidney

A LIFE DEDICATED TO ORGAN TRANSPLANTATION

Dr. Thomas E. Starzl's office at the University of Pittsburgh is sparsely furnished. The most prominent accessories are a compact disk player and a stack of Mozart disks. He tells visitors he loves Mozart's music, and he asks them to consider how much more complete the world might have been if Mozart had not died of kidney failure, "if Mozart had been treated with renal transplantation instead of dying of glomerulonephritis at the age of thirty-four." [4]

He has also told the story of an event from his childhood that he has said influenced his career in organ transplantation. He was serving a requiem mass as an altar boy with an old Irish priest in his small home town in Iowa more than fifty years ago. The priest was unable to go on with the mass, overcome by grief for the death of a young girl. Her death, like Mozart's, had been caused by the failure of her kidneys. "The people who could be most helped by transplantation were those with the greatest potential, often at a young age, who had been doomed by failure of a single organ system but with all other organ systems intact. Now, they could be saved. It was like a miracle."

Dr. Starzl has said that when he was choosing his medical specialty in the late 1950s, he narrowed the field to two: cancer research and transplantation.[5] At the time, he has said, doctors thought a cure for cancer was just around the corner, but that organ transplantation was impossible. So Dr. Starzl chose to work on the impossible. He would work on a problem that nobody had been able to solve, despite Dr. Murray's few successes, and that many believed would probably *never* be solved. He would find a way to give the patient, hopelessly ill because of a failed organ, exactly what was needed—"a completely new organ." With the devotion common to saints and fanatics, he set out to find the way.

Dr. Starzl had chosen not only a formidable task, but an unyielding opponent. He would first have to find the surgical techniques to chop a usable organ out of a living donor or a dead body, find a way to preserve the organ during the hours of transporting it to where it was needed, then learn to attach the organ inside a diseased body so that it would perform the function a healthy organ had once performed. Those were the easy parts of the problem for a genius like Dr. Starzl—the surgical technique and the organ preservation. He solved many of those problems long ago. But his real opponent was not mere surgical technique or organ preservation, and would not yield so easily. His opponent was the human body itself.

THE BODY AS THE TRANSPLANT SURGEON'S ENEMY

During the millions of years while life has been developing on earth, the human body has learned to defend itself against the dangers of alien organs, the bacteria and viruses, the microbes that are everywhere. The transplant surgeon was introducing an *alien organ* into the body, an organ from another person. The body would mobilize to repel the organ it recognized as a threat, *to reject it*.[6] As Dr. Starzl and the other transplant pioneers searched for a way to save the Mozarts and the little Iowa girls of the 20th century, they were struggling against millions of years of biological evolution that had produced the human body's *immune system*, a superb defense against threats to life and well-being, but also a threat to the potentially life-saving transplant. The body recognizes the alien tissue and fights to kill it. This *rejection* is the body's way of protecting itself. After 30 years, Dr. Starzl and others have not yet found a good way to defeat the immune system. That's why so many transplants fail, why even "successful" transplant patients are often so sick.[7]

Our immune system protects us from the millions of microbes, bacteria, viruses that are constantly attacking us. It protects us against the infection and diseases that are everywhere around us. It also protects us against the foreign tissue the transplant surgeons have implanted in us, the transplanted kidney. It would be as if the garden had a system to repel the tomato plant. Or, if the Chevrolet's electrical system had been designed to recognize the Japanese battery and repel it as a foreign part. And, of course, New York City has as many ways to repel immigrants as it has to welcome them. The immune system has millions of years of experience on how to reject foreign organs.

AIDS has brought the words "immune system" to the front of our minds. We know that the AIDS virus prevents the immune system from functioning properly. It leaves the AIDS victim's body open to attack from diseases that a normal immune system would protect him from. We also know how little power we have to counteract the effects of the AIDS virus, how hard it is for us to reverse its action.

What we may *not* know is how little medical science understood about the immune system until the last few years. The body's other systems were much better understood. The cardiovascular system: heart, arteries and veins, moving blood around the body. The digestive system: from the mouth through the stomach and intestines to the rectum. The nervous system: brain, spinal cord, nerves.

But where was the immune system? It was not to be found all in one place, or with all its parts connected together. It was so important to our well-being that it was dispersed throughout the body, near every organ, every limb. It was housed in the lymph nodes, some of which we call *swollen glands* when our immune system fights against a bad cold or an infection.

The immune system is ultimately made up of cells called *lymphocytes*. Everything that happens in our immune system comes from these cells, travelling in the blood to every part of the body. When I cut my finger, letting bacteria enter my body, the lymphocytes trigger my body's defensive reaction. They signal other cells to begin producing the billions of antibodies that are carried in the blood stream to the infected areas to attack the bacteria. The lymphocytes can trigger a second kind of reaction, our *cellular defense*. While antibodies are the chief protection against bacteria, viruses and parasites work to infect us in a different way. They get inside healthy cells. When the lymphocytes determine we need protection against contaminated cells, they signal the need for the production of *killer lymphocytes*. These *T-cells* then leave the lymph nodes and are carried by the blood stream to attack the troubled cells. It is the killer lymphocytes that stop viruses, attack cancer cells, and reject transplanted organs.[8]

THE TRANSPLANT SURGEON'S BATTLE AGAINST THE IMMUNE SYSTEM

Transplanters have tried many ways to defeat the immune system. British Nobel Prize winner Sir Peter Medawar showed that the immune system was causing the rejection. He also showed that there was a way to defeat the system in laboratory animals, although it didn't work in humans. He transplanted cells from a donor into a mouse fetus before it was born. After birth, the mouse recognized a graft from the donor as *self*, not foreign. The same technique failed in humans because a human fetus and a newborn child have more mature immune systems than a mouse, less susceptible to being taught to accept foreign tissue.[9]

In 1990 surgery researchers at the University of Pennsylvania learned how to trick the immune system of rats into accepting transplanted cells. They were able to cure diabetic rats by transplanting insulin-producing cells into the rat's *thymus*, an organ above the heart that trains immune system cells to tell the difference between the animal's own tissue and alien tissue. The whole process was carried out without the use of powerful and often toxic anti-rejection drugs. Some scientists consider this rat experiment a potential breakthrough in transplant biology, but whether it will work in humans, or even in animals larger than rats is likely to remain unknown for many years.[10]

In the 1950s and 1960s some transplant surgeons tried bombarding the entire body with X-rays, *total body irradiation.* Experiments in Paris, Boston and elsewhere were mostly unsuccessful. In Boston, 12 cases were treated with whole body radiation. Only one patient survived, and his kidney came from his living twin, albeit non-identical.[11]

Surgeons next attempted to defeat the immune system with a new drug, Imuran (azathioprine), first approved for human use in 1961, and still used today. When surgeons combined Imuran with another drug, prednisone, and used a kidney from a living donor closely related to the recipient, the transplant occasionally worked.[12] The results were still not good, but at least not all the patients died.

Surgeons' greater knowledge of tissue matching, along with the *drug cocktails,* as Dr. Starzl called the combinations of drugs, produced somewhat better results in the 1960s. Doctors had learned that each person has *tissue types,* just as each person has a *blood type.* But tissue types are much more complex than blood types, and the chance that two people have identical tissue types is remote unless they are identical twins, or close relatives who have inherited nearly the same package of genes from their parents. For thirty years, transplant surgeons like Dr. Starzl have been learning to identify the tissue types of both the donor and the recipient. The better the match, the higher the chance for success of the transplant. The immune system, deadened by the anti-rejection drugs and deceived by the close match to its own tissue types, reacted less vigorously to reject the transplant. And so, the results improved. The next step in the search for anti-rejection drugs was to add another drug to the Imuran and prednisone cocktail. The transplant recipient now got large doses of three drugs.[13]

In the 1970s researchers developed still another new drug, *cyclosporine,* which Dr. Starzl combined with steroids in a new cocktail.[14] The results improved again. Cyclosporine was different from the other drugs in one important way. It could be used in small doses, and the dosage could be decreased as the patient recovered from the transplant. By gaining experience with cyclosporine combined with steroids, doctors also learned better ways to monitor the immune system. There was less guess-work about mixing the drug cocktail, and a better understanding of how to back off on the anti-rejection drugs so that the patient would suffer fewer infections and other complications.[15]

But the side effects of the anti-rejection drugs were often severe, and they remain so in the 1990s. The treatment-of-choice in the 1980s to prevent transplant rejection became a combination of steroids and cyclosporine, and often Imuran. In the high doses researchers used in the 1970s, cyclosporine did help prevent rejection, but the drug itself damaged the new kidney it was intended to protect. It was *nephrotoxic*—poisonous to the kidney.[16, 17]

THE CATCH-22 OF IMMUNOSUPPRESSIVE DRUGS

The surgeons were in a deadly catch-22. They transplanted a new kidney into the patient's body. The kidney started working, helping the patient, perhaps saving his life. But the immune system recognized the transplanted kidney as foreign and began rejecting it. So the surgeons gave cyclosporine and other drugs to minimize the rejection. The drugs did help prevent the rejection. But at the same time the nephrotoxic cyclosporine damaged the new kidney. Cyclosporine in high doses also caused cancerous growths in the patient. Surgeons soon discovered that they could give lower doses of cyclosporine. It was still nephrotoxic, and the kidney function declined, but the patient's new kidney often worked better than his old ones.

But the other side effects were often serious: hot flashes, sweating, numbness or tingling, runny nose, soreness, swelling and redness of gums, constant and uncontrollable shaking of hands and feet, increase of hair growth that was particularly annoying to women. Some doctors believe the immune system weakening drugs have caused, among other problems, kidney failure, lymphoma, osteoporosis, cataracts, gout, hypertension and severe mood swings. With a weakened immune system, even a common cold can become a threat.[18]

Dr. Starzl and his followers have not yet defeated their opponent, the body's immune system, giving the transplanted organ a chance to live without being rejected. The tissue matching and the drugs have helped, but the drugs cause numerous side effects. Some are serious; most are debilitating. The weakened immune system can leave the patient open to attack from other diseases. The drugs often damage the new kidney the surgeons have implanted. They may cause cancer.[19]

Dr. Starzl had set out thirty years ago to do something most scientists believed was impossible—give the patient a new organ. He and the thousands of workers he has inspired and taught have mastered some surgical techniques, and improved the methods of preserving organs awaiting transplant. They have learned much about suppressing the immune system with drugs, and about matching tissues between donor and recipient. But they have not learned much about the *long-term effects* of the anti-rejection drugs.[20] They have not learned how to help most transplant patients return to work, or to survive more than a few years.

Many transplant patients are as sick, or sicker after the transplant as they were before. That may sometimes be true, Dr. Starzl has said. But at least most of them are not *dead*. "I always had the idea that it was more dignified to go down swinging if you knew that there was some dividend [...] other than letting people bleed out in some back room of a hospital." [21] The "dividend" Dr. Starzl had in mind may have been that some of the transplant recipients would live for a while, most of them in the case of a kidney transplant. The surgeon would also get a "dividend." He had done some "successful" transplants—by his own definition if not by the patients' definition. He would be well paid in money and perhaps in the esteem of his colleagues and of some patients. Medical science would get a "dividend" in improved knowledge of surgery, organ preservation and immune system suppression. Perhaps Dr. Starzl or another transplant pioneer would produce the ultimate dividend. Someone might find the silver bullet of anti-rejection techniques, the drug or procedure that would make transplantation routine, that would fulfill the Starzl dream.

But what of the patient? If all went well he could resume a more or less normal life. But he would probably need expensive and potentially debilitating drugs for as long as he lived. A rejection episode could happen at any time, and probably would happen. Another disease might get past his weakened immune system. He would most likely live a *half-life* with the *half-way technology* of transplant.

If all did *not* go well, he might need a second transplant, or a third, or a fourth. Some doctors believe that with each successive "retransplant" the chances for success diminish because the immune system has become even more sensitive to the presence of alien tissue. The drugs might cause severe and disabling side effects. In either case, he probably would not be able to work. He might become dependent on disability payments. He might be alive, but what kind of life?

The kidney patient considering transplant faces a dilemma with no easy answer. There is the *chance* of a successful transplant, with few complications, with minor rejection episodes, with good kidney function, with no severe side effects. It has happened thousands of times. There is also the chance of a failed transplant, failed second and third attempts, severe reactions from the drugs, other diseases sneaking past the weakened immune system, dependency on a lifetime of drugs. Half of all cadaver kidney transplants have failed within five years. Three quarters have failed within ten years.[22]

LIFE AFTER TRANSPLANT

Although the Hippocratic oath tells doctors *first to do no harm*, the history of medicine is filled with tales of *iatrogenic problems*, harm caused by doctors in the name of helping patients. Patients want doctors *to do something*. So doctors try. Doctors want *to do something* to help the ailing patient. They want to intervene. They want to help. They want to treat aggressively.[23] They want to *control* disease. They want to extend life. They want to perform miracles.

The scientific literature of medicine is mostly numbers—graphs, tables of measurements, and commentary analyzing the numbers. There are few individuals, few life stories. Rarely do people appear as persons, as human beings instead of merely subjects of experiments or therapy. But in 1972, the *New England Journal of Medicine* published an article by Dr. Chad Calland, M.D., a physician whose own end-stage renal disease had been treated first with dialysis, then with transplant. In medical literature style, he titled the article *Iatrogenic problems in end-stage renal failure*. By *iatrogenic problem*, Dr. Calland meant harm inflicted on a patient by a medical doctor in attempting treatment.

Perhaps the most famous iatrogenic problem afflicted the first president of the United States. When George Washington had a sore throat and

---

A Physician With Kidney Disease
Describes Life After Transplant

- [After successful transplants, patients] "can now view life from a different perspective, free from machines, tubes, dialysates, supplies, dietary, fluid and travel restrictions, anemia, the mess of cleaning up after a run, and all the shunt or fistula problems that plague the patient on hemodialysis. Nonetheless, patients with transplants continue to share the anxieties of their friends who remain on hemodialysis, and, in addition, they carry the constant burdens of fear of rejection and of the primary complications of immunosuppressive therapy ..."
- "They may also face worse mental depression. Despite a successful graft, their employment, marital, insurance, mortgage and financial situations have not improved ..."

Source: Calland, 1972.

---

pneumonia in 1800, the doctors treated him with the accepted practice of the day, venesection or phlebotomy—blood-letting. They removed 1500 milliliters of Washington's blood. The blood-letting probably didn't help the sore throat and pneumonia, and it may have made his death inevitable. If the doctors had let him alone, his immune system may have fought off the infections. He may have lived a while longer. Some modern doctors have concluded that President Washington was the victim of *iatrogenic medicine*.[24]

Dr. Chad Calland's article about harm done by doctors to kidney patients was published on August 17, 1972. Three days later he died, perhaps the victim of the iatrogenic problems he had described so vividly. When a San Francisco newspaper wrote about him a year before he died, the headline was *"Five Kidneys and Two Years of Hell."* A magazine headlined its story *"The Incredible Ordeal of Chad Calland, MD."* [25, 26, 27]

Dr. Calland's kidney disease had progressed to end-stage. He was treated first with dialysis, then with transplant. He had nearly every conceivable complication of both therapies, and he had many hours on the dialysis machine or in the transplant ward to contemplate the treatments he was getting. The word he used to describe those treatments was *iatro-*

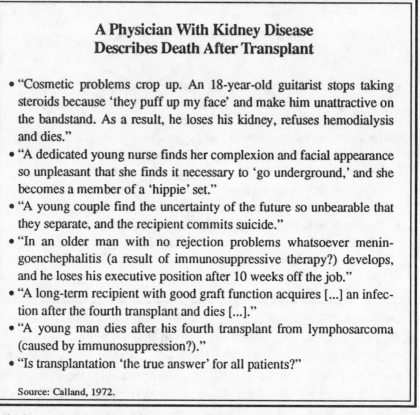

genic; he meant that his fellow doctors had done him *harm* in the name of care. He wanted other doctors to know about it, so he wrote the article for the journal widely read by doctors.

Dr. Calland said he had time to develop close relationships with other patients on dialysis or in the transplant center. He knew forty or fifty patients and some of their families, and although he says he could make no "scientific" observations, he found patterns that he thought could help his fellow doctors care for kidney patients. Although Dr. Calland's article was written nearly two decades ago, many of the practical problems facing dialysis and transplant patients are still present today. The cost of treatment is much less burdensome for the kidney patient because the costs have been spread to all taxpayers by the Medicare End Stage Renal Disease program. The anemia that often weakens dialysis patients can be reduced by the newly approved drug erythropoietin. Cyclosporine has reduced the need for the more toxic anti-rejection drugs. Tissue-matching techniques have helped insure a better match of donor organs, thus less severe rejection. But the problems remain, and Dr. Calland's description of them is the most powerful in the medical literature.

He asks, "Is transplantation 'the true answer' for all patients?" He answers that *neither* dialysis nor transplantation is the "true answer." He recommends that nephrologists and transplant surgeons measure the success of their treatments not only by whether the patient is "alive," but by whether he has a "more nearly 'normal' life, whatever that means to him, and not what it means to the doctor." The transplant surgeon, he writes, makes too little of the "morbidity and mortality of graft rejection," the sickness and death caused by the immune system's attempt to repel the alien organ. The surgeon's work is supported by the statistics he has accumulated on the survival of the transplant and the survival of the patient. But when he reports his statistics, the transplant surgeon "does not mention his patients' fractures, infections, bleeding and other problems."[28]

DR. STARZL MAY BE GETTING READY FOR HIS OWN TRANSPLANT

Dr. Starzl may believe so strongly in organ transplantation that he may be getting ready for his own organ transplant.[29] He has said he lived for days at a time on doughnuts and cheese fries, french fried potatoes drenched in melted cheese, Pittsburgh style. He has been described as a three-pack-a-day cigarette smoker until ten years ago when he saw the first signs of his own heart disease. In the summer of 1990, as he prepared for an international conference on his new wonder drug, FK-506, he felt a severe chest pain as he climbed a flight of stairs in the hospital. Doctors discovered that the main artery supplying blood to his heart was ninety-nine percent blocked, making a heart attack virtually certain. But Dr. Starzl is dedicated to his pursuit of success in what he once saw as the impossible task of organ transplantation. He refused the heart surgery that doctors said he needed to correct the blocked artery. Instead he submitted to a balloon angioplasty, the insertion of a tiny device into the artery to expand it, allowing a better flow of blood to the heart muscle. He continued working on the scientific studies of FK-506 that he would report at the conference in San Francisco. He was risking a heart attack, even a fatal heart attack, but Dr. Starzl has spent his life defying risk. He went to the conference.

After telling the assembled transplant specialists that FK-506 would solve many of the problems of suppressing the immune system, he came back to Pittsburgh where heart surgeons performed bypass surgery, transplanting a vein from his own body to provide an alternate path for blood to his heart.[30] (The rejection problems are different in this kind of graft because the transplanted tissue came from Dr. Starzl's own body, not from an organ donor.)

Dr. Starzl has apparently decided that this new drug, FK-506, is so good at suppressing the immune system, preventing rejection of the transplanted organ, that it will eventually replace other drugs that he has been using for nearly three decades. He made similar comments about his last wonder drug, cyclosporine, which was approved for wide use in the early 1980s. Now, says Dr. Starzl, it is *unethical* to continue treating transplant patients in Pittsburgh with cyclosporine when they could be treated with the unapproved FK-506.

If you had your kidney transplant at the University of Pittsburgh in late 1990, where Dr. Starzl practices, or at the University of California in either Los Angeles or San Francisco, you may have been treated with FK-506. If you had your transplant in Philadelphia, at the University of Pennsylvania, or at any other hospital in the United States, you probably got cyclosporine. Yet Dr. Starzl says it is unethical *not* to use FK-506, and some patients remember the similar conclusion he once reached about cyclosporine. In fact, in the late 1970s, the results from organ transplantation were so poor that Dr. Starzl himself came to the conclusion that transplant might never be a common treatment. That view changed when he started using cyclosporine. Now he thinks it's unethical to use the 1980s wonder drug cyclosporine because the 1990s wonder drug FK-506 is so much better.[31]

Dr. Starzl once "harvested" kidneys from living blood relative donors because of the lower risk of transplant rejection. Now he says it is *unethical* to take a kidney from a healthy donor, transplanting it to a diseased kidney patient relative, because of the risk to the *donor*. He believes that cadaver kidney transplants are so likely to be successful that the risk to the living donor, however small, is not justified.

THE TRANSPLANT CANDIDATE'S DILEMMA

Little wonder that as a transplant candidate I felt confused and afraid. Is transplant a treatment? Or is it an experiment? Is transplant for the benefit of the patient, or is it for the advancement of medical science? Are the transplant surgeons the "heroes," as they often call each other? Or are the patients and their families the true heroes as they face the all-too-frequent horrors of transplant complications? Will transplant someday be as routine as some other surgical procedures? Or will it continue to be a short-term treatment, enormously expensive and risky, occasionally succeeding as a long-term treatment, but failing far more often?[32]

The answer, of course, is that *transplant is both treatment and experiment*. Dr. Starzl and his legions of followers have not yet conquered the immune system. If they do—or, "when they do," as Dr. Starzl would undoubtedly say—the world may be a far better place. Doctors may routinely replace failed organs with new organs. The young Mozart and the little girl in Dr. Starzl's Iowa home town may not be killed by the failure of a single organ system—or by a failed attempt at organ transplant.

Perhaps Dr. Starzl's heroic efforts will someday make organ transplantation more effective than it is today. I hope he stops eating the doughnuts and cheese fries that may have contributed to his own heart disease. I hope he doesn't try to prove the effectiveness of organ transplantation by getting his own heart transplant. The odds are poor.

9

The Third Treatment:
Nutrition—Simple, Low-Cost and
Low-Risk

End-stage renal disease is a death sentence. When the kidneys function at only five or ten percent of normal capacity, the patient usually dies without dialysis or transplantation. Some people don't discover their kidney disease until it is near end-stage; they *must* depend on the high-tech treatments to stay alive. But if you are fortunate enough to have learned about your diseased kidneys while they still have about ten or twenty percent of their capacity, you now have a third treatment alternative—nutritional therapy.

Nobody knows for sure whether nutritional therapy will slow or stop the progression of kidney disease, but some highly respected physicians and scientists who have treated thousands of patients while studying kidney disease have observed that changing the diet, controlling blood pressure and achieving a good balance of blood chemistry constituents like calcium, cholesterol and potassium *may* stop kidney disease from getting worse. And, compared to the risk of dialysis and transplant, nutritional therapy is virtually risk-free. It is simple and natural, without the often-lethal side effects of the high-tech treatments. Many leading nephrologists and researchers in the United States and Europe believe that nutritional therapy *should be tried by all patients with early chronic renal failure.*[1, 2]

WHAT IS NUTRITIONAL TREATMENT FOR KIDNEY DISEASE?

Doctors have known for over a century that dietary treatment improves the symptoms of *chronic uremia*, the poisoning of the body by blood no longer filtered by healthy kidneys. There is little disagreement about that among doctors, maybe none. "The traditional view," wrote prominent Swedish nephrologist Dr. Jonas Bergström, "has been that low protein diet affords symptomatic relief in chronic uremia but does not affect the progression of renal failure." [3] Even though it is a traditional treatment, many nephrologists don't recommend it for their patients nearing end-stage kidney disease. I heard this advice from two prominent nephrologists: "Wait until your kidneys have failed. Do nothing but control your blood pressure until then. When you are near complete kidney failure, then we can treat you with dialysis and perhaps later a transplant." Some nephrologists think this attitude and the resulting advice to patients is *unethical,* even irresponsible. Even if nutritional therapy is not accepted as the treatment-of-choice for *slowing the progression of kidney disease*, it has been accepted for over a hundred years to *reduce the symptoms of the disease.* Some doctors and many patients wonder why some nephrologists ignore this treatment.

The basis of traditional dietary treatment for the symptoms of uremia—*conservative treatment*, physicians call it—is *moderate restriction of protein*, bringing a kidney patient's protein consumption more in line with what the body is believed to need, instead of the vastly excessive amounts most Americans and Europeans actually consume. Traditional moderate protein restriction suggests that the kidney patient cut down the amount of protein he eats to about 40 or 50 grams a day.[4] The average American eats double that amount—about 104 grams a day, two-thirds from animal sources like meat and dairy products. The average European eats somewhat less protein than the average American—about 90 grams a day, half from vegetable sources, like grains and beans; the other half from animal sources.[5]

In third world countries like Bangladesh in Asia, Bolivia in South America, and Zaire in Africa, the average person eats 40 or 50 grams of protein a day, three-fourths or more from vegetable sources. A kidney patient using the moderate protein restriction diet must make a big change in his normal eating patterns. He must learn to eat *less than half* the protein he would normally eat, which means little or no meat, eggs, and dairy products and far more vegetables, fruits and grains. He must eat more like a third world peasant than a rich American or European. But is that restriction a threat to good nutrition? Many scientists have found that it is not, and a major American study of nutrition in China is one of many studies that have found significant health benefits for *everybody* from eating less protein, not just for kidney patients. (More about this study in Chapter 11, Learning About Nutrition.) [6]

Consider the *Recommended Dietary Allowances*, the RDAs that the United States government has published for fifty years. The latest version suggests that adult males should be eating about 56 grams of protein a day—half what Americans actually eat. If the RDAs are right, a kidney patient could cut his daily protein consumption to the 40 or 50 grams that will help protect his body from the effects of damaged kidneys and still be within the government guidelines for normal nutrition for everybody.

There is another kind of diet for kidney patients that many doctors believe provides the far more important benefit of actually *stopping kidney disease from getting worse*. They call it *severe protein restriction*, 25

What Are Amino Acids?

- Living organisms need food to sustain life. The fundamental categories of food—carbohydrate, fat, protein, water, ash, and fiber—provide the energy and the other nutritionally-essential components.
- Proteins contain "amino acids," about 20 natural substances. Nine are believed essential to health and growth, and cannot be manufactured in the body, while the other amino acids are non-essential.
- Foods of animal origin—meat, fish, poultry, dairy products, eggs—contain *all* the essential amino acids. Such foods are called sources of "high biologic value," or "complete proteins."
- Plant foods contain *some*—but not all of, or not enough of—the essential amino acids necessary for good nutrition.
- People who eat mostly vegetable diets must *combine* plant-origin foods to get the "complete protein" their bodies need.

Traditional Cooking Has Known For Thousands Of Years How To Combine Foods To Provide The Essential Amino Acids

Although science only understood the role of amino acids in the 20th century, the ancient cuisines of Asia, the Middle East, and more recently Europe have learned to combine foods in ways that provide "complete protein."

- *grains with legumes* (beans, peas, lentils, chickpeas, peanuts)—rice and beans in China, lentils and rice in India, chickpeas and sesame seeds in the Middle East, pasta e fagioli (pasta and beans) or peas and rice in Italy
- *dairy products with grain*—milk and grain porridge in Europe and the Middle East; in modern American cooking, milk with cereal, pizza with cheese, macaroni and cheese, rice pudding and milk
- *dairy products with legumes*—beans with cheese sauce in Europe, beans with yogurt in the Middle East or lentils with yogurt in India

grams or so a day. Because that amount of protein is less than generally considered necessary for good nutrition, doctors recommend supplementing the severe restriction diet with *amino acids*, or a form of amino acids known as *keto acids*. My own kidney diet is about 25 grams a day of protein, supplemented with about 15 grams a day of *keto acids*, the special form of amino acids that some scientists have observed may contribute to the progression-stopping.

There is serious disagreement among the leaders of the kidney establishment worldwide about severe protein restriction. That's one reason why your nephrologist may not have told you about the third treatment, and is likely to dismiss your questions out of hand when you ask him about what you have read in this book. Many physicians and scientists—especially in Europe—have observed over the last thirty years that severe protein restriction, supplemented with a form of amino acids, can stop the progression of kidney disease, or at least slow it down, without causing malnutrition. Most nephrologists disagree, advising their patients to do nothing about their kidney disease until it gets bad enough to make dialysis or transplant necessary. (That's why I wrote this book: to tell my fellow

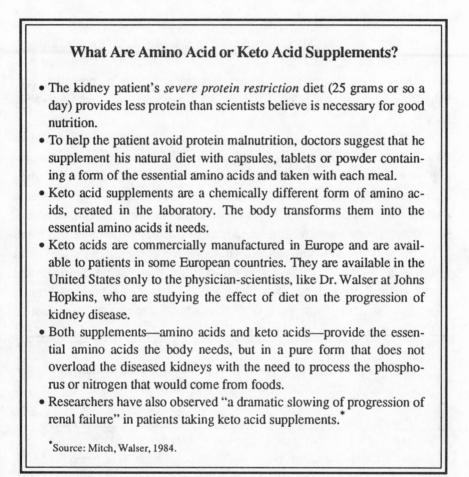

What Are Amino Acid or Keto Acid Supplements?

- The kidney patient's *severe protein restriction* diet (25 grams or so a day) provides less protein than scientists believe is necessary for good nutrition.
- To help the patient avoid protein malnutrition, doctors suggest that he supplement his natural diet with capsules, tablets or powder containing a form of the essential amino acids and taken with each meal.
- Keto acid supplements are a chemically different form of amino acids, created in the laboratory. The body transforms them into the essential amino acids it needs.
- Keto acids are commercially manufactured in Europe and are available to patients in some European countries. They are available in the United States only to the physician-scientists, like Dr. Walser at Johns Hopkins, who are studying the effect of diet on the progression of kidney disease.
- Both supplements—amino acids and keto acids—provide the essential amino acids the body needs, but in a pure form that does not overload the diseased kidneys with the need to process the phosphorus or nitrogen that would come from foods.
- Researchers have also observed "a dramatic slowing of progression of renal failure" in patients taking keto acid supplements.[*]

[*]Source: Mitch, Walser, 1984.

kidney patients about the third treatment, to give you a chance to make your own decision about trying to control your disease, perhaps avoiding dialysis and transplant.)

IS THE THIRD TREATMENT FOR KIDNEY DISEASE REALLY NEW?

Although doctors have recommended the use of nutritional treatment to relieve the symptoms of uremia for over a century, only in the last thirty years have they begun to work on proving that nutritional therapy might actually *stop the progression* of kidney disease. Chronic uremia develops, you will remember, when the diseased kidneys are no longer able to remove toxic substances from the blood. When the kidney patient eats less protein, there is less *nitrogenous waste* in the blood, giving the kidneys less work to do in maintaining a healthy blood chemistry. Reducing protein also reduces phosphorus, another substance doctors suspect may contribute to damaging the diseased kidneys, although nobody knows exactly how.

As early as 1869 British doctors were recommending the use of low protein diets to reduce the effects of uremia.[7] I doubt that scientists working on nutritional therapy in 1990 would quibble with a word of their analysis. Today's doctors would say, however, that the nineteenth century doctors offered no scientific proof of their conclusions. Instead, they presented simply the unproven observations of doctors experienced in treating kidney diseases, assertions without evidence to back them up. When I retrieved some dusty hundred-year-old medical books from the basement stacks of the library, I wondered how much other useful medical knowledge, accumulated from centuries of practical experience, was buried

---

A Nineteenth Century Medical Textbook Recommended Nutritional Therapy for Kidney Disease

- "The diet should be generous and good, but simple. There is I think little doubt that many persons comfortably off, healthy as well as sick, take far more food, especially in the shape of meat, than is required for the perfect performance of the work of their organism or than is conducive to a thoroughly healthy and vigorous state of body."
- "A large proportion of the excess meat taken passes off from the body in the form or urea and other urinary constituents, which it is the special work of the kidney to remove from the blood. It is obviously of the utmost importance to relieve the kidneys of at least this unnecessary and useless work in cases in which they are diseased, when their working power is seriously impaired."
- "The diet should therefore be carefully regulated, so that while the organism is well supplied with the full amount of nutrient materials which it requires, a useless excess which would still further damage the diseased organs is carefully avoided."

Source: Beale, 1869.

---

there. I felt like a medieval monk stumbling across a text from ancient Greece or Rome, rediscovering a simple bit of knowledge that had somehow been lost for over a century. Much of what these nineteenth century doctors asserted in the medical textbooks without scientific evidence was nonsense, I'm sure, but there was practical wisdom there, too, no matter how unscientific.

One scientist who has spent thirty years studying the health-promoting qualities of diet is Dr. James Duke, a botanist for the Department of Agriculture and consultant to the National Cancer Institute. "My favorite sport is finding the science behind the custom, like the gingko seed coincidence. In Japan ginkgoes are eaten with cocktails because they are believed to fight drunkenness. In completely unrelated research, we find that the ginkgo contains compounds that speed up the metabolism of alcohol." How much other wisdom, he wonders, can be found in the customs or the ancient recommendations of medical men? [8]

By the early 1900s more European scientists and physicians were reporting that dietary treatment lessened the symptoms and signs of uremia. In the 1930s, researchers experimented with rats and other laboratory animals to investigate the effects of nutrition on kidney disease. An early scientific paper on the subject, published in 1939, found that nutrition—particularly the amount of protein in the diet—had a crucial role in the course of kidney disease induced in rats. Many other studies in rats have since shown the potential importance of nutritional therapy in kidney dis-

---

The Kidney Establishment Is *Beginning* To Think About Nutritional Therapy

- "The role of diet in the management of chronic renal failure is undergoing a re-evaluation at the moment."
- "It is clear that some diets can relieve the symptoms of even severe uremia, but there is a suggestion both from work in animals and humans that low-protein (which are also low phosphate) diets may be capable of slowing or even stopping the progress of kidney failure, at least in some forms of disease."

Source: Cameron, 1986.

From The Johns Hopkins
Handbook of Nutritional Management

- "There are no contraindications to the use of nutritional therapy in the management of chronic renal failure."
- "Since such treatment may slow or even halt progression of the underlying disease in individual patients, it is worthwhile to try this approach in every patient before accepting dialysis as inevitable."
- "There is no evidence that the conservative management described here induces progressive protein malnutrition or makes eventual dialysis therapy or transplantation more difficult."

Source: Walser, 1984.

---

ease. Studies in dogs, however, have produced conflicting results, convincing the skeptics that controlled trials in humans are necessary to judge the effectiveness of nutritional therapy.[9, 10]

There were attempts during the 1960s and 1970s in both Europe and the United States to introduce low protein diets as routine therapy, but the efforts failed. In the early 1960s two Italian kidney specialists, Dr. C. Giordano and Dr. Sergio Giovannetti, treated uremic patients with severe protein restriction—as little as 6 to 11 grams of protein a day, sometimes supplemented with amino acids. Results were mixed, and protein malnutrition was a frequent result of this severe restriction. Patients also had trouble maintaining such a severely restricted diet.[11] (One small serving of spaghetti with tomato sauce has more than 11 grams of protein. One bagel has more than 11 grams, more than Dr. Giovannetti and Dr. Giordano prescribed for the full day's consumption. You can see how restrictive these diets were, and how difficult to follow.)

About the same time kidney doctors were seeing mixed results from dietary treatment, dialysis was becoming more widely available and the first kidney transplants began to succeed. Doctors concentrated on renal replacement—dialysis and transplant—while dietary treatment stayed in the laboratories of some committed scientists in Europe and the United States, like Dr. Giovannetti at the University of Pisa in Italy and Dr. Walser at Johns Hopkins University in Baltimore. Some doctors now believe that budget pressures caused by increased health care costs in the 1990s and less-than-hoped-for results of renal replacement therapy have caused the new interest in nutritional therapy.[12]

A PIONEER OF THE NEW TREATMENT

Dr. Mackenzie Walser says, "It was a challenge to stand up before a scientific conference of doctors in 1974 to report that nutritional therapy could slow down or stop the progression of kidney disease. Many doctors don't think much of treatments relying on nutrition." Dr. Walser published his first paper on the topic of nutrition and kidney disease in 1975, and he's been working on the problem ever since. Despite the skepticism—and while the kidney establishment was spending billions of dollars on renal replacement therapy—Dr. Walser and a few other scientists (Dr. William Mitch of Emory University, Dr. Sergio Giovannetti and Dr. Giuseppe Maschio of the Universities of Pisa and Verona in Italy, Dr. Norbert Gretz and Dr. M. Strauch of the University of Heidelberg in Germany, Dr. Jonas Bergström of the Huddinge University in Sweden and others) were exploring nutrition and the kidney in both animals and humans. When Dr. Walser suggested that there is a common mechanism underlying progression in all or nearly all kidney disease, and that the process can be treated with diet and drugs, or both, he was relying on evidence he had seen that severe protein restriction plus a form of amino acid supplements slowed progression, or sometimes even stopped it. Some patients on severely-restricted protein diets (20 grams a day or so) supplemented with keto acids (a form of essential amino acids) had a temporary stabilization, or even some improvement in their kidney function.[13]

Dr. Walser has treated hundreds of patients since 1974, exploring nutritional and other factors in the progression of kidney disease. He believes that he and other scientists will soon prove conclusively that restricting protein and phosphorus in the diet, controlling blood pressure, cholesterol and blood fats and other blood chemistry constituents can slow or stop the progression of kidney disease for most people. Although Dr. Walser does not know how to cure kidney disease, he believes he knows how to prevent it from getting worse. He can't yet prove why his treatment works, but he is working to understand the mechanism.

THE KIDNEY ESTABLISHMENT IS SKEPTICAL

Many nephrologists are skeptical of this nutritional therapy because it is not yet proven in a scientifically conclusive way. Dr. Walser himself says it not yet proven. Twentieth century doctors are properly cautious about accepting new theories because they know how much nonsense doctors have proclaimed as science—without proof—before modern scientific methods were applied. Today's medical researchers and doctors want a theory to be proven beyond doubt before they adopt it into the treatment-of-choice category. That's good science and good medicine, good for patients and good for doctors.

I remembered, however, that the tobacco companies insisted for decades that there was no "conclusive scientific evidence" of a connection between cigarette smoking and disease. I also remembered the skepticism of the beef industry when scientists observed in 1990 that the more red meat and animal fat people ate, the more likely they were to develop the common and deadly cancer of the colon.[14] The beef producers association said that neither this study nor any previous studies had conclusively established the link between meat consumption and colon cancer.

Some Early Results From
The Modification Of Diet In Renal Disease Study

Before attempting the controlled study with up to eight hundred patients, the National Institutes of Health scientists tested their methods with a small sample of patients, and made these observations:

- Some patients had a very low GFR even though the creatinine level in their blood was only slightly higher than normal.
- It was hard for kidney patients to follow the low-protein diet.
- There was no evidence of malnutrition in patients on the low-protein diet.
- The level of creatinine in the blood was not a reliable indication of the GFR.
- As blood pressure went up, GFR went down.

Source: Klahr, *N Engl J Med*, 1989.

Maybe the tobacco companies and the beef producers are right; maybe the evidence is *not* conclusive. But if a person chooses to reduce the risk of colon cancer by cutting down on the amount of red meat and animal fat he eats, what's the harm? Except to the beef producers, who will sell less beef. If someone wants to quit smoking cigarettes because of the health risk, what's the harm? Except to the cigarette companies. If a kidney patient wants to try to control his disease by following an "unproven" nutritional treatment, what's the harm? Except to the providers of high technology renal replacement, the kidney business?

There are forces at work in the skepticism of kidney doctors other than the desire for conclusive scientific proof. One is simply that the theory is based on treatment with *nutrition*, and modern scientific medicine has taught doctors to be wary of nutritional treatment. Nutrition has a ring of charlatanism for the ear of modern doctors. "Health foods, vitamins, quacks." Many doctors have little training in nutrition because most medical schools have required little. One physician told me his formal education about nutrition was a single one-hour lecture in medical school; nothing else was required. Some leaders of the medical profession in the 1990s have begun to focus on the fact that doctors are often far more

---

What Do These Early Results Of The Modification Of Diet In Renal Disease Study Mean To You?

They may not mean anything, or they may confirm the theories that restricting protein and phosphorus, and reducing blood pressure may help prevent kidney failure. In any case, no scientists—in the MDRD Study or dozens of others—have found a risk for the patient.

- If creatinine in the blood is a poor measure of kidney function, you may want to ask your doctor to measure your GFR. You could have slightly high creatinine and very low GFR. That may mean that your kidney disease is worse than the doctor expects from looking only at the creatinine level.
- You may have to work hard at following the restricted diet.
- You are unlikely to have problems with malnutrition.
- Your blood pressure should probably be below 140/90 to preserve the kidney function you still have.

interested in *treatment* than in *prevention*, as their whole culture has taught them to behave.[15]

Another force working on kidney doctors is that even simple nutritional treatment requires a patient to make changes in his behavior. Instead of one or two minutes spent writing a prescription, or ordering a test or surgery, the doctor must spend his time convincing the patient *he needs to change his behavior*—teaching him what to do and how to do it. To make conservative nutritional treatment work, the doctor must become a teacher, not just a dispenser of drugs or surgery. His culture and the institutional framework of modern medicine—from training through third-party reimbursement—is out of tune with this role as a teacher. The third party payers—Medicare or insurance companies—usually won't pay for this kind of preventive treatment. So, doctors find themselves without the time, the training or the interest to help their patients work on behavior changes, especially when insurance companies often refuse to pay. Doctors, after all, didn't make the years of extra effort required to achieve a physician's credentials only to practice unreimbursed medicine.

Even if a doctor *does* try to help a patient make behavioral changes, the result is often failure. Doctors say it can be discouraging, even futile work. A dedicated family practitioner who is fighting his own kidney disease, Dr. Murray West of Baltimore, told me he can't even convince many of his patients to take their blood pressure medicines, to say nothing of changing their lifestyles. Dr. Alan Wasserstein, the nephrologist at the University of Pennsylvania who is helping me with my own nutritional therapy, says many of his patients are barely-literate welfare clients from the inner city West Philadelphia neighborhood near the university. They can scarcely understand that they have a disease, he says, without much hope of learning to change their behavior. The National Institutes of Health says that one-third of all end-stage kidney patients live in poverty.[16]

No wonder doctors are skeptical about nutritional treatment. No wonder they prefer to prescribe a drug or surgery, dialysis or transplant. It's so much easier for the doctor, although it may be vastly more difficult and risky for the patient. (The kidney patient often doesn't know how difficult and risky the high-tech treatments are until he has committed himself irrevocably to dialysis or transplant. The books, magazine and newspaper articles, foundation and government publications, radio and television reports available to kidney patients say almost nothing about the risks and outcomes of high-tech renal replacement. The information is all there in the published scientific literature and in the government databases. Some doctors are aware of the risks and outcomes, but patients often don't understand until they are living with the problems of dialysis and transplant. I hope this book will give some kidney patients a chance to learn some facts before they decide on a course of treatment for their disease.)

Still another factor in doctors' skepticism about nutritional treatment is that they hate to be wrong. Doctors—like authors and publishers, businessmen and politicians, popes and saints—have been wrong so often that they are eager to avoid mistakes. Until the nutritional therapy is scientifically proven, Dr. Wasserstein tells me, most nephrologists will continue to ignore it. It's not surprising. Most people hate to be wrong. Who could criticize a kidney specialist for advising dialysis or transplant? They are the "treatments-of-choice." Who could sue a nephrologist for malpractice for having recommended a treatment-of-choice? But, if the nephrologist recommends dietary treatment, and if it fails, the patient—or his medical malpractice lawyer—may well say, "The doctor recommended an unproven treatment." Who can blame a cautious nephrologist for ignoring the conservative treatment rejected by the establishment? (That's another reason I wrote this book. I hope the kidney establishment will start to question its rejection of a simple, inexpensive and low-risk treatment while it pushes the costly and risky high-tech renal replacement therapies that often have less-than-hoped-for outcomes. I hope patients will question their doctors' recommendations of treatments that are *easy for the doctor*—and earn the doctor high fees—while they are *difficult and risky for the patient.*)

A FEW RESEARCHERS CLAIM TO HAVE PROVED THAT NUTRITIONAL THERAPY WORKS.

Some researchers claim to have proved scientifically that nutritional therapy works. In 1989, a team of medical researchers from Australia reported in the *New England Journal of Medicine* on their study of nutritional therapy for kidney disease. They had treated sixty-four patients for eighteen months, finding that the amount of protein in the diet influenced the rate of decline in kidney function. They declared:

> **"We conclude that dietary protein restriction is effective in slowing the rate of progression of chronic renal failure." [17]**

Publication of the study sent a flurry of rumors around the kidney establishment. Was the $50-million federal Modification of Diet in Renal Disease study necessary? Was the dialysis industry threatened?[18] Dr. Walser has criticized this Australian study as poorly designed, poorly carried out, and maybe even unethical because about half the patients in the study received no treatment while their disease proceeded to end-stage. Dr. Walser and other researchers have also criticized the study on technical grounds, claiming that the some of the measurements of kidney function were inaccurate and incomplete.[19, 20]

In early 1991 researchers from the University of Texas reported in the *New England Journal of Medicine* that certain diabetic patients had slowed the progression of their kidney disease by restricting the protein and phosphorus in their diets. The doctors concluded:

> **"We believe that wider use of this treatment is indicated."[21]**

WHY ISN'T NUTRITION MORE WIDELY USED TO TREAT KIDNEY DISEASE?

Dr. Phillip Hall, a leading nephrologist from the Cleveland Clinic Foundation, sums up the accepted establishment view:

> **"Therefore, at present there is no convincing evidence that dietary protein restriction forestalls progressive renal failure in humans. Several studies have shown that patient compliance is difficult [...] Therefore, unless clinically controlled studies now in progress show definite benefit from protein restriction, such diet therapy cannot be recommended." [22]**

Another way to state the argument. "Nutritional therapy may work sometimes for some people. But its value has not been conclusively proven. It is also difficult for patients to follow such a diet. Therefore, we doctors cannot recommend it."

The unstated part of this argument is hard for a layman to understand. "If my kidney disease will get progressively worse, and if there is no treatment for the underlying disease, and if you can't recommend nutritional therapy because it's not scientifically proven, what do you recommend? What can I do? What can you do?"

Some kidney doctors will say, "When your disease is bad enough, when your kidneys stop working, then we can treat you with dialysis or transplant." Some nephrologists have been heard to tell a colleague after a consultation about a patient's newly discovered kidney disease, "Send him back to me when he's vomiting." The kidney specialist was advising the doctor who had first suspected the kidney disease to do nothing until the patient's progressive disease reached the point where uremia was threatening the patient's life, when the patient was desperately ill, vomiting and ready for dialysis. I wondered how a nephrologist could defend this advice when there was another treatment—not scientifically proven, to be sure, but low risk and inexpensive—that might *prevent the kidney disease from getting worse.* I wondered if high-tech medicine had not somehow turned common sense on its head. Advise the patient to let his kidney disease get so bad that there was no possible treatment but the desperate remedies of dialysis and transplant. Ignore conservative nutritional treatment that might stop the kidney disease from getting worse, perhaps eliminating the need for the desperate remedies.[23] Could doctors have become so enamored with the risky and financially rewarding kidney replacement treatments that they could ignore a low-risk treatment that may delay the need for their high-tech dialysis and transplantation treatments?

AN OUTSPOKEN EUROPEAN PIONEER WONDERS WHY DOCTORS DON'T RECOMMEND NUTRITIONAL THERAPY

Doctors and scientists in Italy have been practicing and studying nutritional therapy for kidney disease for three decades. Dr. Sergio Giovannetti, nephrologist, scientist and professor at the University of Pisa, suggests four reasons why nephrologists are so skeptical, why they sometimes start dialysis in patients whose kidney function is still good enough to permit excellent results with dietary treatment. The four reasons he observes: *prejudices, mistakes, greater demands on the physician's time, impact on the physician's income.*

The Doctor's Attitude
Has A Big Impact On The Kidney Patient

- "A very important factor that may increase the percentage of patients willing to try [dietary treatment for kidney disease] is the attitude of the physician."
- "If he is skeptical, the patient will sense this and will refuse even to try, but if the patient realizes that the doctor believes in [dietary treatment] he will be willing to try it."
- "Such an outcome is the natural consequence of satisfactory experience with [dietary treatment] by the doctor himself, but such experience will never take place unless the physician is willing to try [dietary treatment.]"

Source: Giovannetti, 1985.

The *prejudices*, he says, can be seen in some doctors' belief that low-protein diets lead to malnutrition, as in third world countries, and in the often-heard observation that, "My patients have culinary habits quite different from the Italian ones and would never adhere to such dietary restrictions." He argues that both prejudices are unfounded. Third world malnutrition is most often caused by deficiencies in calories, vitamins and protein—plus infectious and parasite diseases—not just protein deficiency alone. About the refusal by some patients to try nutritional treatment, Dr. Giovannetti says that Italian doctors have also had patients who prefer dialysis to dietary restrictions. But if the doctor has a positive attitude about the value of the treatment, he says, the patient is more likely to make an attempt. On the other hand, if the doctor ridicules the treatment as unproven, or, worse, as nutritional quackery, the patient is unlikely to try.

The *mistakes* physicians have made in using dietary therapy, he says, have to do with the choice of which kidney patients may benefit. Some patients will not benefit—particularly those near end-stage uremia with vomiting and anorexia, high blood pressure that has not responded to treatment, severe retention of sodium and water, and those patients who are unable or unwilling to restrict their diets. In other patients, he says, nutritional therapy should be started *early*, when the creatinine level in the

---

Nutritional Treatment
Puts Heavier Demands On The Doctor Than Dialysis

- [Dietary treatment of people with chronic kidney disease] "requires an involvement on the part of the physician which is greater than that connected with dialytic therapy (dialysis)."
- "Dialysis is largely standardized, practically uniform throughout the duration of the life of patients and is often completely entrusted to the nurses or to the patient himself who is instructed by the nurses. Ordinarily, the physician becomes involved only when emergencies arise."
- [Dietary treatment] "requires frequent controls of the patients' conditions and of their compliance that cannot be entrusted to nurses. Changes in the [dietary treatment] are required in accordance with changes in renal function and the difficult decision of when to start replacement of the renal function is the physician's responsibility."
- "All this is well understood and discourages many nephrologists from starting such a 'complicated and involvement-demanding' therapy which is regarded as experimental at best."
- "To start [hemodialysis] or peritoneal dialysis is, in general, much simpler [for the doctor, not the patient] and therefore this is usually done."

Source: Giovannetti, 1985.

---

blood is about 2 mg/dl or less. Professor Maschio of the University of Verona believes conservative treatment is useful for patients very early in their disease, when the creatinine is only slightly above normal.

The *demands on the physician's time*, and the *impact on the physician's income* are troubling, but easy to understand. Doctors are no less human than their patients, subject to the same pressures and weaknesses we all have. Treating a kidney patient with dietary therapy requires more involvement by the doctor, says Dr. Giovannetti, than simply prescribing dialysis, where the treatment is routine, left to the nurses and technicians, requiring the physician's involvement ordinarily only in an emergency. He says, "Everybody knows that the world of dialysis is highly remunerative, especially that of [maintenance hemodialysis], whereas the world of [dietary treatment] is not and this acts by necessity in favor of dialytic therapy if there is a choice."[24] Physicians have families to support, tuitions and mortgages to pay. Is it surprising that some nephrologists choose a treatment method that requires less time and rewards them with greater income? Especially when the treatment has a reputation of being a "miracle of modern medicine, the treatment-of-choice, a life-saving procedure?"

Dr. Giovannetti wants doctors to learn more about nutrition and the kidney, but he concludes that science already knows enough about the potential value of nutritional therapy that doctors should use it more widely. Dietary treatment "already deserves its own place among the various forms of therapy of renal disease with the main purpose to prevent or delay terminal renal failure, and, as such, it should be applied early in the course of the disease and much more extensively." [25]

Dietary Therapy
Can Reduce The Physician's Income

- "Everybody knows that the world of dialysis is highly remunerative, especially that of [maintenance hemodialysis], whereas the world of [dietary treatment] is not and this acts by necessity in favor of dialytic therapy if there is a choice."
- "Travel expenses for meetings, facilities for laboratories, books and medical journals and, finally, gifts of various nature may be easily supported as promotional expenses by the firms making products related to [hemodialysis] and peritoneal dialysis. This is not possible for the firms who make dietary products."
- "Moreover, extra salaries are received in many places by the doctors in charge of dialysis centers and the extra salary is often proportional to the number of patients on dialysis."
- "These are not the least important reasons that explain why some patients are started on [hemodialysis] therapy when their renal function is still good enough to permit a normal life for quite some time with minimal dietary restrictions and, sometimes, even without any."

Source: Giovannetti, 1985.

The Potential Costs of Nutritional Therapy

A patient on a nutritional program may need some or all of these things:
- Frequent clinic visits to teach lifestyle changes; monitor weight, blood pressure, nutritional status
- GFR measurement to find out how well the kidneys are working
- Some form of amino acid supplements to maintain nutritional status
- Vitamin and mineral supplements
- Calcium, potassium supplements
- Blood pressure medication
- Other supplements, fiber, fish oil

I found that living with this program of conservative treatment required some effort and some expense, but the effort was trivial compared to dialysis and transplant. The cost was almost nothing compared to the tens or hundreds of thousands of dollars for dialysis or transplant.

OTHER LEADING EUROPEAN KIDNEY SPECIALISTS DISAGREE—AS DO MOST AMERICAN KIDNEY SPECIALISTS

A few months after Dr. Giovannetti's article was published, two British nephrologists responded that, "The case for low-protein diets in [chronic renal failure] is not established in man." [26] Dr. A. M. El Nahas and Dr. G. A. Coles asked ten questions about dietary treatment which, they claimed, Dr. Giovannetti, Dr. Walser, Dr. Mitch and others had not answered. All of the questions assumed that not enough is known about kidney disease or dietary treatment to make the case for widespread use. For example, they say, some patients live with kidney disease for many years with no treatment at all, perhaps a spontaneous remission of the disease. Other patients seem to improve from *the placebo effect*—results, perhaps, of the attention they get in the clinic and of the patients' own positive attitude, leading to a stable or improved kidney function. In other words, nutritional therapy may not have had anything to do with why the patients were able to stop their disease from getting worse.

Dietary treatment also has risks and costs, say Dr. El Nahas and Dr. Coles. "The most serious hazard of dietary protein restriction is malnutri-

Nephrologists From Many Countries Recommend Nutritional Therapy

- *Italy*—"...the prevention of end stage renal failure is possible in humans as well as in rats [...] and the beginning of [renal] replacement therapy may be delayed and even avoided in some cases. These observations revived the interest in the dietary therapy of chronic renal failure in the last years and this revival is occurring simultaneously with the appearing evidence of the limits of dialysis and transplantation. Only revolutionary improvements in the technologies of replacement of renal function might change the present situation." Dr. Sergio Giovannetti, *Contributions To Nephrology*, 1986.
- *United States*—"The available evidence strongly suggests that, at least in certain groups of patients, appropriate nutritional therapy may have a highly significant effect on the course of renal failure." Dr. Mackenzie Walser, *Lancet*, 1983.
- *United States*—"Nutrition is now a primary tool in treating renal failure." Dr. William E. Mitch and Dr. Saulo Klahr, *Nutrition and the Kidney*, 1988.
- *Germany*—"...the adequate use of a [low-protein diet] can delay the progression of [chronic renal failure] to end-stage renal failure for years, without negatively affecting the patient's condition. This delay also has a considerable economic impact." Dr. Norbert Gretz, *Klin Wochenschr*, 1988.

tion. [...] It would be a great disadvantage if the postponement of dialysis therapy secured by treatment with a low-protein diet was paid for by loss of fitness at the time dialysis is started. [...] If long-term dialysis is postponed by treatment with low-protein diets there will be a considerable cost saving. However, dietary restriction has its price. Firstly, it requires the skills of a renal dietitian. Secondly, dietary restrictions and adjustments require commitment from both patient and family. Exclusion of normal foods is difficult for the family because separate meals may have to be prepared, at extra expense." Finally, they say, supplementation with [amino acids or keto acids] can cost up to £500 per patient per year, about $750 in 1986.[27] I wondered how a scientist could be worried about an expense of $750 a year when he was ready to prescribe dialysis treatments that might cost $30,000 a year.

I asked Dr. El Nahas if he meant to say nutritional therapy was harder for the patient and his family than dialysis or transplant. He replied that he believed no patient should be "burdened" with nutritional therapy unless doctors are more sure of the results. "I think the message from the review article I wrote in the *Lancet* back in 1986 was that no such burden (financial, social, nutritional, etc.) should be put on any renal patient unless we are assured that such therapy would benefit them, and indeed delay the progression of their chronic renal failure and not just artificially bring down serum creatinine levels, which we now know does not reflect what happens to the glomerular filtration rate." [28]

Dr. Giovannetti's answers to the British doctors' ten questions were published a few months later. He agreed that doctors don't know enough about kidney disease to be absolutely sure how and why dietary therapy works, but enough studies have been done to show that it *does lessen the symptoms of uremia, with little or no risk to the patient.* "It is difficult to understand why a low-protein supplemented diet is not to be recommended once its efficacy and safety have been largely proved." [29]

Nephrologists From Many Countries Recommend Nutritional Therapy–Continued

- *Sweden*—"...available clinical data [...] strongly suggest that progression of end-stage renal failure in man may be retarded or halted by [low-protein diet] supplemented with [essential amino acids or keto acids]." Dr. Anders Alvestrand, *Kidney International*, 1983.
- *Australia*—"We conclude that dietary protein restriction is effective in slowing the rate of progression of chronic renal failure." Dr. Benno Ihle, *New England Journal of Medicine*, 1989.
- *Italy*—"We conclude that a moderate dietary restriction of protein and phosphorus is an acceptable and effective regimen for delaying progression of functional deterioration in early renal failure." Dr. Giuseppe Maschio, *Kidney International*, 1982.

I read these studies as a kidney patient, wondering how the physician-scientists could come to such opposite conclusions. I could understand the British doctors' claim that not enough study had been done yet to conclude that nutritional therapy could be widely used to treat kidney disease, but I could also remember the scientists who were saying until the 1980s that there was no conclusive proof that cigarette smoking caused serious health problems. (They may still be saying that in the 1990s, but nobody pays attention.)

I wondered if the nephrologists' objections to nutritional therapy were like the tobacco company claims of the 1960s, 1970s and 1980s? Is nutritional therapy absolutely proven? No; even the pioneers don't claim that. But, so many studies have found that nutritional therapy may stop progression of kidney disease, or at least slow it down. Can the British scientists be serious when they say that nutritional therapy is difficult for a patient and his family? Is it more difficult than dialysis? Is it more difficult than transplant? Is eating less protein worse than plugging yourself into a kidney machine for four out of every 48 hours, drinking no more than three or four glasses of liquid a day, feeling sick most of the time? I wondered how the skeptical nephrologists could defend such a strange idea. Is nutritional therapy really difficult for the patient, I wondered. Or, is it difficult for the nephrologist?

I also wondered about the nephrologists' claim that nutritional treatment has not been proven by a prospective randomized controlled trial, like the government Modification of Diet in Renal Disease study now underway. Is there such a study proving the value of dialysis? Transplant? I couldn't find them in the medical literature, and the nephrologists I asked couldn't tell me about such studies. Yet dialysis and transplant are the "treatments-of-choice" and nutritional treatment is ignored. I hoped this book may prompt some kidney patients to ask their doctors why they were ignoring a treatment that could have such important benefits for the patient, if not for the doctors.

Prominent European nephrologist and scientist, Dr. Jonas Bergström of Sweden, summarized the scientific evidence for and against nutritional treatment:

"**Although each single clinical study which shows that protein restriction may favorably affect the progression of renal failure can be criti-**

cized [...], all these data taken together suggest that there is something to it. [...] In conclusion the challenging concept that the inexorable progression of chronic renal failure can be retarded or stopped by treatment with low protein diet may prove to be of great clinical importance in the future."[30]

IS NUTRITIONAL THERAPY DANGEROUS?

No recent study has found dangerous side effects for patients who follow nutritional therapy. Although not all patients have stopped the progression of their kidney disease, no researchers have found that the therapy has harmed a patient. There is no sudden death as often comes to transplant or dialysis patients. Researchers have not found any significant downside for the patients, any significant risk they incur by following the nutritional therapy.

Another prominent European nephrologist, Dr. Giuseppe Maschio of the University of Verona, has written:

> "We still feel that the scientific ideal [of randomized controlled trials] is less important than routine treatment if this treatment is able to [preserve kidney function] for many years in the large majority of patients, is well accepted by patients, and is not harmful to them." [31]

So why is nutritional therapy not more widely used? It's inexpensive. It's simple and low risk. Is the downside only for the nephrologist? The dialysis clinics? The transplant programs? Is it simply unfamiliar territory for the doctors, something they don't feel comfortable with? How can doctors recommend that patients passively let their disease claim most of their kidney function, waiting for the devastating problems of end-stage renal disease that can be treated only by dialysis or transplant, ignoring a treatment that might have preserved some of the diseased kidneys' ability to function? Can kidney disease be prevented from reaching end-stage? Why don't Medicare and insurance companies pay for this treatment?

These are important questions. I have some clues, but no answers. Each nephrologist has his own answers. The kidney establishment has its answers. The dialysis centers and the transplant programs have their answers. Kidney patients and their families will find their own answers, too, perhaps starting with this book.

10

Deciding What Treatment Is Right For You

S uccessful transplants have restored some kidney patients to nearly normal health, but more than half of kidney transplants from a dead donor, a cadaver, fail within five years, and only about two or three of ten survive for ten years.[1] Some dialysis patients lead active and productive lives without the risks of transplant surgery and anti-rejection drugs, but the average dialysis patient can expect to survive only about five years.[2] Nutritional therapy—if it works for you—is simple and natural, without the risks of either high-tech treatment, but nobody knows for sure why or how it works, or even whether it will work at all.

I felt confused and afraid in the winter of 1989 as I thought about treatment alternatives for my own kidney disease. Two prominent nephrologists had told me there was nothing I could do about my disease except wait for it to get worse. Then I could choose dialysis or transplantation. Leading institutions in the kidney establishment—the National Kidney Foundation and the American Kidney Fund—made the same recommendation. Yet after a morning's work in the medical library I had found a third treatment that the nephrologists and the kidney establishment had chosen not to tell me about. Nutritional therapy offered me the hope of avoiding dialysis and transplant—at least for a while.

As I thought about my own treatment alternatives I wanted to learn how well dialysis and transplant worked as the "treatments-of-choice" that the kidney establishment recommended. I soon discovered that the books for

How The American Kidney Fund Sees Kidney Disease

- "While at present there is no known cure for chronic kidney disease, significant advances in medical research afford today's patient with two major treatment alternatives: *dialysis* and *transplantation.*
- "When chronic kidney failure occurs, you will be referred to a nephrologist (physician specializing in the diagnosis and treatment of kidney disease), who will discuss these treatments with you."
- "In addition, you will also meet other professionals on the staff, each of whom will lend their expertise in providing comprehensive and individualized care. The treatment team includes nurses, technicians, social workers and dietitians. You will be an essential member of this team."
- "It will be your responsibility to comply with the treatment plan and to keep the team informed of any symptoms or problems that may arise."

Source: American Kidney Fund, 1987.

laymen, few as they are, said little or nothing about the *outcome* of dialysis and transplant. By spending an hour or two in a neighborhood library, I could learn more than I would ever care to know about buying cars or computers or microwave ovens, *but I couldn't learn anything there about the life and death risks of high technology treatments for kidney disease.* I would have to dig into the scientific journals and books for facts. I haven't found any non-technical books or articles for laymen that make these facts available, so I have included much statistical information about the *outcomes* of kidney replacement treatments in this book, including extensive excerpts from government databases published in late 1990, which you will find in Appendix 1. (You may want to ask your doctor about some of these facts. Don't be surprised if he doesn't know much about the outcomes of dialysis and transplant, or if he belittles your attempt to learn. Some doctors don't like being questioned closely by their patients, much preferring that the patient simply follow orders. If you or your doctor want to read the original sources for the facts presented here, you will find the citations from the scientific literature in the notes and bibliographies for each chapter. The articles and books are not hard to find in a medical

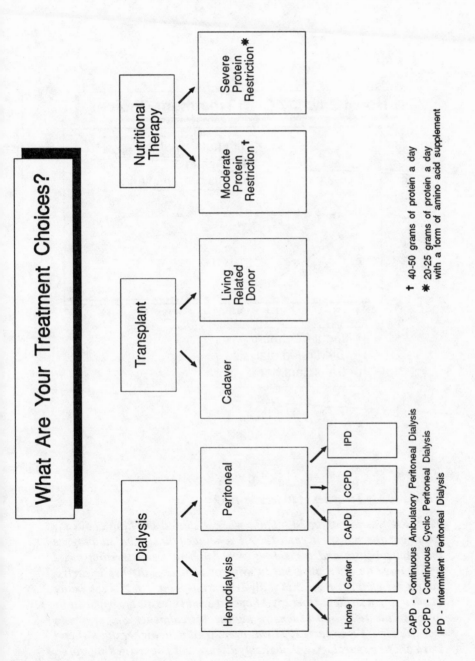

Figure 39 A Kidney Patient's Treatment Choices

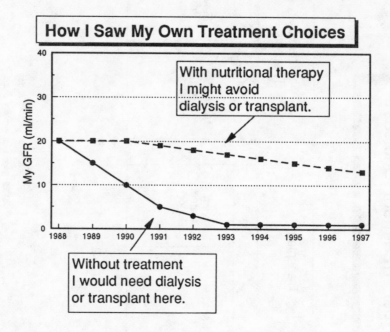

Figure 40 My Treatment Choices In 1989

My GFR was less than 20 ml/min when I started thinking about my treatment alternatives in early 1989. I concluded that if I did nothing, as the nephrologists and the kidney establishment were advising me, I would have no alternative but to wait for end-stage disease to arrive, taking my chances then with dialysis or transplant. I felt much better about trying nutritional therapy. I hoped it would give me the opportunity to avoid the risky and expensive high-tech treatments. So far, it has worked. My GFR in early 1991 was over 20 ml/min, higher than when I started. The nephrologists thought my disease had stopped getting worse.

library. The librarians are often eager to help. If I studied the facts before buying a new car, a computer or a microwave oven, I certainly wanted to know something about dialysis and transplant.)

FOR BETTER QUALITY OF LIFE—DIALYSIS OR TRANSPLANT?

Researchers have been studying the outcome of the renal replacement therapies for twenty years, seeking a better understanding of the effectiveness of dialysis and transplant. Their answer, so far, is that *there is no single best treatment*. Each kidney patient has different health problems, a different life situation and, thus, different needs. I soon learned that, with the help of the physicians and other kidney professionals, I would have to decide which treatment suited me best.

Many studies have compared the quality of life of patients on peritoneal dialysis, hemodialysis and after transplant. (Look back at Chapter 6 for descriptions of the types of dialysis.) A study of about four hundred patients in 1984 found that transplant patients had the best quality of life on nearly all measures.[3, 4] Patients on peritoneal dialysis did better than those on hemodialysis. They were less unhappy with their treatment, had fewer symptoms of uremia, less difficulty with everyday activities, and ranked higher in their own ratings of their health and well being, self esteem and vocational rehabilitation. Over half of peritoneal dialysis patients were in school or working, compared to less than one-third of hemodialysis patients.

A later federal government study of patients in eleven dialysis and transplant centers also found that transplant patients scored highest in quality of life. Home hemodialysis patients were next, followed by peritoneal dialysis patients. Patients who had hemodialysis in a center scored lowest on quality of life. About 45 percent of peritoneal dialysis patients and 43 percent of home hemodialysis patients were able to carry on normal activity with minor symptoms. Only 33 percent of center hemodialysis patients were in this category.[5]

Half the transplant patients described themselves as normal with no complaints and no evidence of disease. About 43 percent of transplant patients said they tired easily, had little energy. Two-thirds of hemodialysis

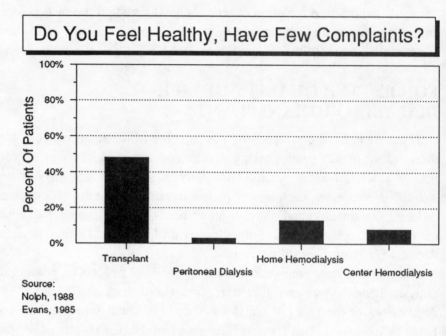

Source:
Nolph, 1988
Evans, 1985

Figure 41 Patients Report Their Health Status

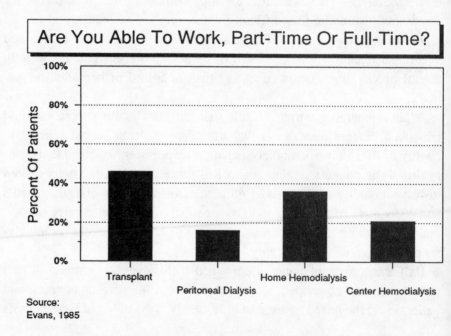

Source:
Evans, 1985

Figure 42 Patients Report Their Work Status

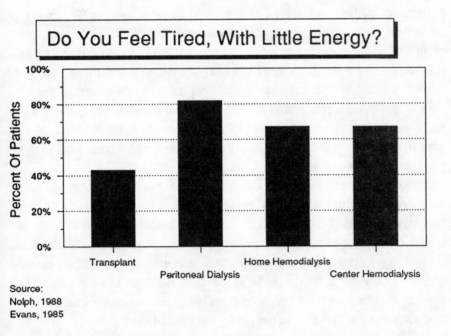

Figure 43 Patients Report Their Energy Level

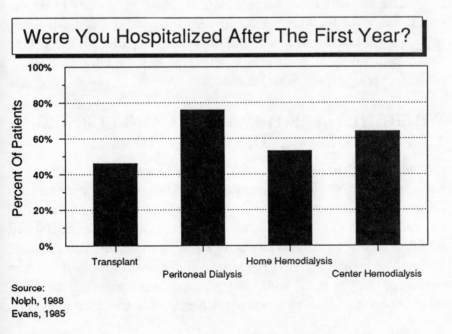

Figure 44 Patients Report Their Need For Hospitalization

patients described themselves as tired and lacking energy; 82 percent of peritoneal dialysis patients saw themselves that way. About half of transplant and home dialysis patients had to be hospitalized after their first year on therapy. Two thirds of in-center dialysis patients and three fourths of peritoneal dialysis patients had been hospitalized. The average hospital stay was about a week. About half of transplant patients were able to work full-time or part-time; 40 percent of home hemodialysis patients, 24 percent of center hemodialysis patients and 16 percent of peritoneal dialysis patients were able to work.

These studies led me to wonder how useful these two treatments really were. A successful transplant seemed to provide the best quality of life— but only about half the transplant recipients described themselves as normal with no complaints and no evidence of disease. That means that about half of successful transplants leave the patient feeling less than normal, unable to continue working. It seemed to me that the "success rate" claimed by the transplant surgeons does not result in similar quality of life results. The patient may be alive, but what kind of life?

Home hemodialysis appears to leave the patient feeling better than in-center dialysis, but is the person who chooses home care rather than in-center care naturally more independent and active, more ready to assume responsibility for his own health? Among all types of dialysis patients, only one of five was able to work full-time, or even part-time. I wondered how effective dialysis really was. It may have kept me alive for a while, but I kept asking myself, what kind of life?

WHERE YOU ARE TREATED MAY INFLUENCE THE DOCTORS' RECOMMENDATIONS

Some researchers have found that *where* you are treated may have an effect on the physicians' recommendations. Many medical treatment facilities are owned by investors seeking to make a profit. That profit motive may influence the treatment they recommend for kidney patients. Harvard scientists studied Medicare records for kidney patients and published the results of their study in 1989. They found physicians at for-profit facilities were more likely to steer their kidney patients toward dialysis at the medical center and away from home dialysis, peritoneal dialysis and transplant.

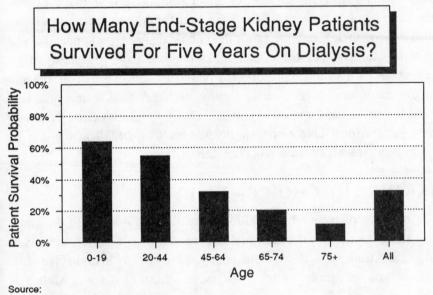

Source:
USRDS 1990 Annual Data Report, E.73

Figure 45 5-Year Survival Of Dialysis Patients

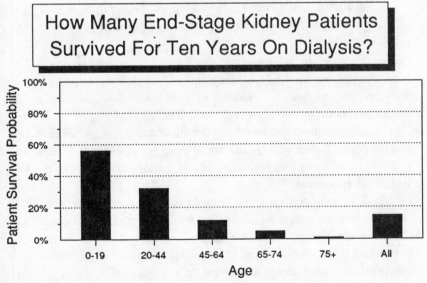

Source:
USRDS 1990 Annual Data Report, E.75

Figure 46 10-Year Survival Of Dialysis Patients

That's hardly surprising because in-center hemodialysis is likely to produce more revenue per year—$30,000 a year for dialysis treatments is not unusual—and therefore more profit than home dialysis, peritoneal dialysis or a transplant. But as a kidney patient, I wondered about the quality of the medical advice I would be getting if I had to be concerned about doctors steering me toward high-revenue treatments rather than a treatment that would be well-suited toward my needs. I was more convinced than ever that a patient must take responsibility for his own health, gathering his own information about treatment alternatives.[6,7]

MAKING THE CHOICE—DIALYSIS

If you have discovered your kidney disease early enough to do something about it, you may decide you do not need the high-tech treatments of dialysis and transplant. If not—that is, if you are already in end-stage renal disease—you will probably have to choose a form of dialysis while you

---

A Physician With Kidney Disease Describes The Dialysis Patient's Discouragement

- "After a number of such visits to the doctor, the patient begins to think that perhaps his very real symptoms of fatigue, dyspnea, muscle weakness and so forth are products of a deranged mind, so that he begins to conceal them because he is ashamed."
- "Eventually, the time comes when the patient complains of nothing, and the doctor is thus wholly unaware of these symptoms, just as he is unaware of the other (marital, financial and social) difficulties that the patient is experiencing."
- "Patients on hemodialysis know these facts better than the physician does, because the patient alone experiences them—often in isolation."
- "Is it any wonder that the patient feels less valuable than any healthy person and doubts the worth of his struggle? Is it necessary to postulate psychiatric disorders to understand the self-evident?"
- "Is dialysis 'the true answer' for all patients?"

Source: Calland, 1972.

decide what to do about transplant, or while you wait for a transplantable kidney to become available for you.

The first choice will likely be the type of dialysis—hemodialysis or peritoneal dialysis. Most doctors believe peritoneal dialysis is best for children with kidney disease while they wait for a transplant. People who live far from a center may also do better on peritoneal dialysis, as will people who feel a strong need for feeling independent and in control of their own treatment. Kidney patients with insulin-dependent diabetes often do better on peritoneal dialysis, as do patients with serious heart disease. Dialysis staffs prefer that patients with AIDS or hepatitis use peritoneal dialysis, minimizing exposure for the staff and other patients. People who want to continue working and traveling or maintaining a variable schedule may do better on peritoneal dialysis. Patients who feel anxiety about the needles used in hemodialysis may prefer peritoneal methods. A more flexible diet is also possible with peritoneal dialysis.

Some circumstances make peritoneal dialysis more difficult, but not impossible. Extreme obesity may interfere with the catheter used to insert and drain the fluid. Back pain or chronic lung disease may be aggravated by the pressure of the fluid in the abdomen. Some patients in nursing homes have successfully received peritoneal dialysis, but the most success has been with patients who can do the procedure themselves. Patients who need the support of a peer group may do better with in-center dialysis.

There are some conditions where peritoneal dialysis may not be appropriate. People with malnutrition, like alcoholics who get enough calories but too little protein, are difficult to treat. High levels of the blood fats triglycerides may be aggravated by peritoneal dialysis. Patients who will be transplanted within a month or two are usually not appropriate for peritoneal dialysis because of the training and practice required to master the technique. People who have poor personal hygiene, or who have trouble taking their medications or keeping clinic appointments will probably have trouble maintaining the schedule of peritoneal fluid exchanges. Peritoneal dialysis may not be appropriate for pregnant women, people with severe bowel disease, and psychotics who are unable to do the procedures reliably.[8]

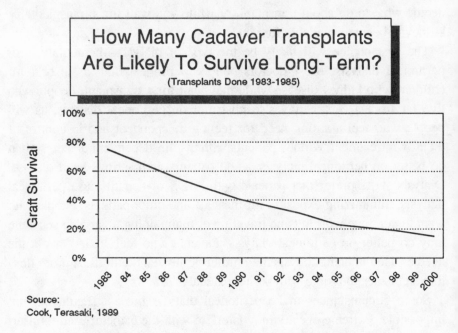

Figure 47 Expected Survival Of Cadaver Transplants

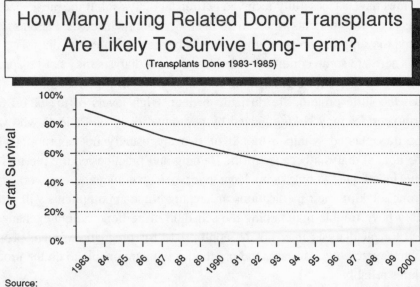

Figure 48 Expected Survival Of LRD Transplants

MAKING THE CHOICE—TRANSPLANTATION

If you choose transplantation and the transplant team considers you a suitable candidate for transplant, you will learn that the chances for long-term success are far greater if you can get a donor kidney that matches your tissue types exactly. If you have a brother or sister whose tissue types and blood type match your own closely, the chances are nine of ten that your new kidney will survive for three years.[9]

If you have no brother or sister who can give you a kidney, or if their blood types or tissue types don't match yours, or if you don't choose to ask someone to give up a kidney for you, you will have to wait for a cadaver kidney to become available. If the kidney is not well-matched to your body, the chances are four of ten that your new kidney will fail within three years. If you have a "regraft," that is, if the surgeons try to replace the failed transplant with a second cadaver kidney, the odds are even worse. About half the regrafts will fail within three years.

Two Prominent Transplant Scientists Comment On The State of Kidney Transplantation

- "If, however, kidney transplantation is meant to provide long-term remission of end-stage renal disease, then the emphasis should be placed on success rates 5, 10 or even 20 years following the transplant."
- "Few patients would be interested in a short-term resolution of the condition, but that is all that has been offered to the recipients of cadaveric donor kidneys up to now."
- "Most of these patients will not have a functioning graft 10 years after the transplantation."
- "Grafts from living related donors fare much better in the long-term, but this approach is not possible for the majority of the patients."

Source: Cook, Terasaki, 1989.

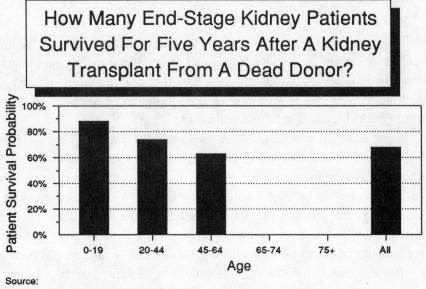

Source:
USRDS 1990 Annual Data Report, E.81

Figure 49 5-Year Patient Survival, Cadaver Transplants

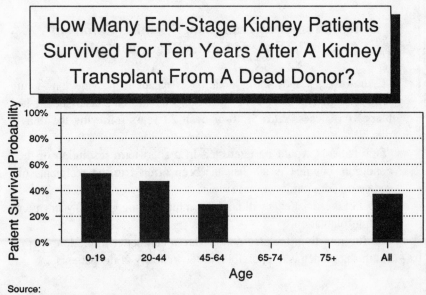

Source:
USRDS 1990 Annual Data Report, E.83

Figure 50 10-Year Patient Survival, Cadaver Transplants

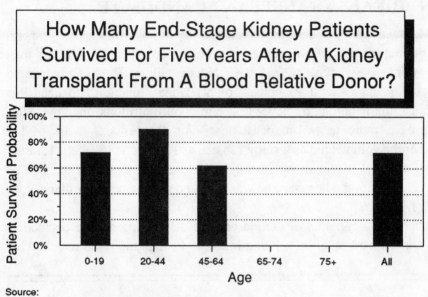

Source:
USRDS 1990 Annual Data Report, E.89

Figure 51 5-Year Patient Survival, LRD Transplants

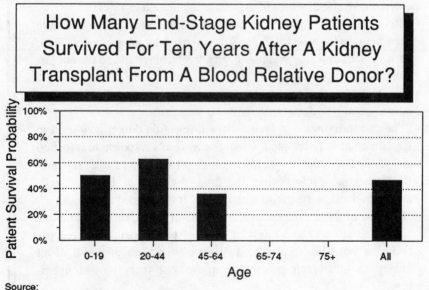

Source:
USRDS 1990 Annual Data Report, E.91

Figure 52 10-Year Patient Survival, LRD Transplants

AN "IDEAL" TRANSPLANT CANDIDATE

I know a kidney patient who lived a nearly normal life for five years on nutritional therapy despite the fact that he started with a GFR of less than 10 ml/min, very close to end-stage kidney failure. He had not started dietary treatment until 95 percent of his kidney function had been lost because the nephrologist never told him about nutritional therapy. After hearing a radio news broadcast describing the research work of Dr. Walser, he volunteered as a study subject, as I had done in 1989. (I started my nutritional treatment with nearly twice the GFR he had at the start of his.) Even with the late start, he was able to delay the need for dialysis for over five years.

Then, the symptoms of uremia became debilitating and he decided to get a kidney transplant. He had a brother whose tissue types matched his

---

How Effective Is Transplantation?

The director of a major laboratory studying anti-rejection drugs commented on the effectiveness of organ transplantation in 1990.

- "More than 80% of cadaveric organs transplanted a decade ago have been completely rejected." (He was referring to *all* transplants from dead persons donating organs—hearts, livers, lungs and so on, not just kidneys.)
- "The rate of graft loss after one year has not improved during the last dozen years."
- "The current immunosuppressants [anti-rejection drugs] now used in the clinic not only cripple the immune system's response to infection and malignant cells, they also cause direct toxicity to vital organs." (For example, cyclosporine, the drug-of-choice in 1991, is well-known to damage the transplanted kidney it is intended to protect.)
- "Because of these inadequacies in our ability to control the immune system specifically and safely, it may not be surprising that our patients are not fully rehabilitated—in one study, less than half of all kidney transplant recipients were employed one year after their operation."

Source: Morris, 1990.

Popular Books About Organ Transplant

"We Have A Donor," by Mark Dowie, St. Martin's Press, New York, 1988. A journalist's book about the people involved in organ transplantations—patients, donors, transplant teams, families. The book offers personal narratives about the transplant experience and explores most of the issues making transplant controversial and dramatic. As I considered the possibility of my own transplant, I learned much.

Many Sleepless Nights; The World Of Organ Transplantation, by Lee Gutkind, W. W. Norton & Company, New York, 1988. The author teaches in the Department of English at the University of Pittsburgh where he had the opportunity to witness the work of Dr. Thomas Starzl and his followers in what some people consider the world's leading transplant center. The author also works as a board member of TRIO, Transplant Recipients International Organization, and has lectured widely on the human dimensions of organ transplantation. The book is a readable, even fascinating description of the realities of transplant as they dominate the lives of patients, donors, families and transplant specialists. The author works hard to present the problems and opportunities from the point of view of each character in the transplant drama, including the deep conflicts of interest between patient, donor and surgeon.

---

own closely, and who was willing to give a kidney. In January, 1990 the transplant surgeons removed a healthy kidney from the brother and transplanted it to the brother with the failed kidneys. I saw him about two months after the operation. He said he was feeling great, was eating about what he wanted—a change for someone who had lived on severe protein restriction for five years—and was preparing to go back to work.

In October, 1990—ten months after his successful transplant—he was hospitalized in an intensive care unit, fighting for his life against rare complications of transplant, perhaps a result of the strong anti-rejection drugs. He was in a coma, not expected to live much longer. His family had almost given up. Surgeons had done eight more abdominal operations since the transplant, removing his spleen, his pancreas and his gall bladder, trying to correct the complications. He was near death.

Then, to the surprise of the physicians, he rallied and his condition began to improve. By the end of 1990 he was still desperately ill—perhaps the result of the transplant surgeons' attempt to treat his kidney disease—but there was hope that he would live. A few days after Thanksgiving he went home.

A Popular Book
By A Prominent Transplant Surgeon

Transplant, by William H. Frist, M.D., A Fawcett Crest Book, Ballantine Books, New York, 1990. The author is the Director of the Heart and Heart-Lung Transplant Program at the Vanderbilt University Medical Center. He has performed over 100 heart and heart-lung transplants. He is a recognized authority on transplant who has published and lectured extensively.

- This sometimes gripping narrative, written with the assistance of ghost writer Charles Phillips, captures the breathless life-and-death world of the transplant surgeon, the patient, the donor and the families.
- Dr. Frist believes, as does Dr. Starzl, that organ transplantation could forever change medicine—if only his fellow doctors would supply more transplantable organs by asking dying people or their families to donate organs.
- Sometimes Dr. Frist's enthusiasm leads to statements that are misleading at best. On page five he writes: *"Over the years, heart-transplant care has improved dramatically. With the discovery of new techniques and drugs, ninety percent of all patients now survive."*
- Dr. Frist was describing heart transplants, where the survival rates for patients and transplanted organs are even worse than for kidney transplants.
- As I had learned in frightening detail, this transplant surgeon's claim that "ninety percent of all patients now survive" may satisfy the surgeon whose patient has somehow escaped the operating table alive. But it may not satisfy the sometimes mutilated, drugged and half-dead patient who may die a few months or years later.

He had been a nearly ideal candidate for a kidney transplant. He was in his early forties, not too old, and his health was generally good, except for his serious kidney disease. His brother's kidney was a close match for his own blood and tissue types. The odds were good, even excellent—probably seven out of ten—that the kidney would survive for five years.[10] But even though all the indications were that the transplant would be successful, his life was threatened within a few months of the transplant operation.

His experience confirmed for me the difficulty of organ transplantation, the desperation of a high-technology medical procedure that is not yet well-understood. Because he and his transplanted kidney survived until January 1991, the people who keep statistics on kidney transplants included his case among "successful" transplants. That is, "He had one-year graft survival. The transplanted kidney didn't fail; it was some other internal organs that failed, perhaps damaged by the anti-rejection drugs. But the transplant was successful." I'm not sure that he and his family will consider it successful if the transplanted kidney fails in a year or two, even though the statistics would call it a "successful transplant."

A NEPHROLOGIST WHO HAS LIVED FOR 24 YEARS ON DIALYSIS NOW CHOOSES TRANSPLANT

A very different case is that of Dr. Peter Lundin of Brooklyn, a practicing nephrologist who has been on dialysis since his second year of college 24 years ago, and who served as president of the American Association of Kidney Patients in 1990.[11] He not only graduated from college and medical school as a dialysis patient, but also completed residency training and has specialized in treating kidney disease for all those 24 years. He has now chosen to seek his own transplant. He has a sister whose blood and tissue types match his own, and who is willing to donate a kidney, but he has chosen not to accept it. Instead, he is waiting for a well-matched kidney from a dead person, a cadaver donor.

This very well informed patient is not only a kidney specialist but also a patient activist in a national self-help and lobbying group for dialysis and transplant patients. He has now judged for himself that the current state-

A NEPHROLOGIST WHO HAS LIVED
FOR 24 YEARS ON DIALYSIS
HAS DECIDED TO GET A TRANSPLANT

- "There was fear implanted in me of transplants in those early days. It really seemed like a game of Russian roulette. More fear was implanted because of many healthy friends on dialysis who sought a transplant and died from rejection, infections, and steroid complications."
- "What has changed in my perspective of transplantation? I think cyclosporine with its blemishes and faults has been a big breakthrough in that it has markedly reduced the number of steroid complications. There is now a much better understanding of the immune system."
- "When I studied transplant immunology [...] it seemed to me that the understanding of the immune system was very sketchy. Now it seems to have improved and is taking off by leaps and bounds, and the kidneys are working better."
- "Another thing that stimulates me to seek a transplant is the limitations of hemodialysis. Even though dialysis allowed me to achieve my goals, I have spent 24 years with considerable denial—dietary restrictions and travel restrictions."
- "I have chosen, even though I do have two sisters who could provide a living related kidney, to go on the cadaveric transplant list. [...] I have always been concerned about how it would alter our relationship, especially if rejection would lead to loss of a kidney from one of [the sisters]. Also, how would I react if they later came down with some illness, even if that illness was totally unrelated to the fact that they had donated a kidney? Would I be able to live with that?"
- "At the present time I feel that waiting for a well-matched cadaveric donor is the best compromise."

Source: Lundin, 1990.

of-the-art of transplantation and anti-rejection drug treatment is far enough advanced that he is willing to try it out on his own body. He is not simply a patient listening to a doctor's advice, but a nephrologist who has watched the outcome of dialysis in his own case, and in hundreds of his patients' cases. He has also observed transplant over the last 24 years, watching the science develop. He is truly well-informed, and he has now chosen to abandon his 24 years of successful dialysis to seek a transplant.

As you consult with your nephrologist and the other kidney professionals, you may not hear many facts about the *risks and outcome* of dialysis and transplant. You may hear instead about the greatly improved "one-year survival rates" that preoccupy the transplant teams, and the new machines, methods and drugs that the dialysis advocates promote. You will judge for yourself, as Dr. Lundin judged for himself. You will probably talk to other kidney patients, people who have had transplants, people who have been on dialysis. You will consult with your family. Then you will make a choice. It won't be easy.

11
Learning About Nutrition

I f you understand good nutrition, I suggest you skip this chapter and go on to Chapter 12 where you will find some specialized techniques that kidney patients have learned. If you're not so sure about nutrition, you may want to spend a few minutes with this chapter.

Somehow I lived through my first fifty years without learning that food was making me sick. I ate whatever I wanted, until my body refused to go on. At 6 feet 3 inches and 255 pounds, I was 75 pounds overweight. My blood pressure was 230/115. My body was saturated with fluid, puffy and swollen. My lungs were so congested with water that I had to sleep sitting up. The neighborhood doctor had been treating me with penicillin, saying I had bronchitis, while I really was in a serious episode of congestive heart failure. Eventually the combination of troubles was so bad I needed emergency hospitalization, intravenous diuretics and a few days of drying the excess fluid out of my system. The hospital dietitian told me my diet was making me sick. I started to pay attention.

Although I didn't focus on it then, my diet was outrageously excessive. As I was preparing this chapter, I tried to remember what I had been eating on a typical day before I started learning about food. Looking back now, I wonder how I survived as long as I did. I often ate over five thousand calories a day, double or triple what I needed. More than half of my calories came from fat, at least twice as much as I needed. I was eating five times the sodium I needed; three or four times the protein, four times the cholesterol. No wonder I was 75 pounds overweight, with clogged arteries, heart disease, high blood pressure and kidney disease.

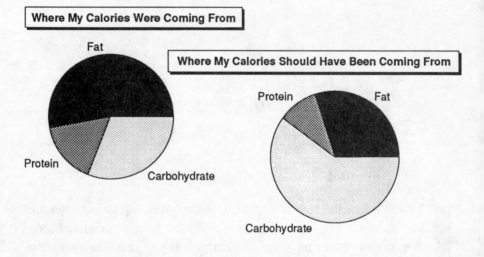

Figure 53 A Nutritional Illiterate (before and after)

The excess calories and fat were making me overweight. The fat and cholesterol were clogging my arteries. The salt was causing my body to retain fluid, raising my blood pressure. The high blood pressure was damaging my kidneys and my heart. My food was making me sick; it was as simple as that. (My sedentary life style and high pressure job contributed to my poor health, but it was the food that was causing the most trouble, and that would be easiest to correct.)

WHY WAS MY DIET SO POOR?

Like some other people under fifty, I considered myself indestructible. I had rarely missed a day of work; had never been hospitalized since childhood when a surgeon removed my ruptured appendix. I was overweight and under-exercised; I didn't have the energy I once had. But I was mostly okay. I had been eating the same diet for fifty years, as well as I could remember, and it worked. Why worry about it?

I had a vague *New York Times* kind of knowledge about nutrition, nothing more. Despite the vigorous efforts of our oldest son, David, I was a nutritional illiterate. David had started learning about nutrition as a hobby while he was in college. He practiced good eating and he tried to teach the family, but we didn't pay attention. He wanted me to learn that the food causing my obesity was probably also aggravating my high blood pressure and causing other health problems.

When my body let me know it would no longer tolerate my eating habits and lifestyle, I started, with David's help, to correct my nutritional ignorance. I had always liked to cook, and to eat good food, and I loved good restaurants, particularly the ones offering ethnic cuisines, so studying food was fun.

BECOMING A NUTRITIONAL LITERATE

A wonderful book helped me start my nutritional education, *The Nutrition Debate; Sorting Out Some Answers*, by Joan Dye Gussow and Paul R. Thomas, professors at Columbia University.[1] They understand that the average consumer hears so much conflicting advice from the "nutrition experts"—the respectable scientists, not just the health food nuts and quacks—that he has little practical guidance. The book collects facts and opinions, science and polemics from dozens of sources—ranging from nutrition scholars like Jean Mayer and D. Mark Hegsted to a General Mills advertisement and a Gary Larson *Far Side* cartoon. It's a marvelous book for somebody who wants to learn about nutrition, the kind of book you can dip into at random, finding a delectable morsel on nearly every page.

RDAs: DOES ANYBODY REALLY KNOW?

After reading their book, I had a clue about why the nutrition debate is so confused. *Nobody really knows for sure what we should be eating.* Lots of people claim to know, and, yes, we have had official federal government *Recommended Dietary Allowances* for fifty years, but informed and unbiased people question what the RDAs mean, how useful they are, or even whether we should have them at all.

The purpose of the original Recommended Dietary Allowances in 1941 was stark. President Roosevelt was preparing the nation for war. He foresaw the day when Americans at war wouldn't have enough food to eat, or, at least not what they had become accustomed to. He prodded the scientists to define minimums that would keep Americans healthy despite wartime deprivation. The result of Roosevelt's prodding was a two-page document called "Recommended Dietary Allowances" for calories and eight nutrients, and a day's menu to meet the requirements—at a cost of 32¢ a day per person at 1941 prices.

Roosevelt had wanted the RDAs for a practical political purpose—helping to prepare the nation for war. By the mid-1980s, however, the RDAs had become vastly more complicated and political. The list of nutrients was up to thirty, individualized for seventeen different groups of people by age and sex. That results in 500 different recommendations. The RDA for vitamin C for a 12-year-old girl, for example, is different from the RDA for a 72-year old man. Some thoughtful nutrition scientists, like D. Mark Hegsted of Harvard, doubt that science has enough information to make recommendations as specific as that. He says, "80-90 percent of the recommendations are really guesstimates."[2]

Dr. Hegsted and others have argued for a new approach, and the topic was high on the federal agenda in 1990 with a battle raging among all the special interests threatened by changes in eating habits. (Egg producers, beef ranchers, hamburger chains, food processing companies and others could be hurt seriously if Americans started to favor mostly unprocessed fresh vegetables, grain and fruits. Imagine the economic change if Americans started to eat mostly vegetarian diets.)

Dr. Hegsted believes that the first principle in establishing dietary standards is, "If it ain't broke, don't fix it." That is, we should know what we're doing before we recommend major changes in the American diet. He thinks that recommendations should be realistic about what food is available and what our habits are now. "Our major concern," he writes, "should be the dietary practices which are relevant to the chronic diseases—not changes in intake of essential nutrients."[3] We should try to do something about the *chronic long-term illnesses that our diet may cause*. For example, if a high-fat, high-cholesterol diet contributes to artery-clogging *atherosclerosis*, which in turn causes heart disease, let's work on learning to eat less fat and less cholesterol, instead of waiting until our clogged arteries need replacing with heart surgery.

What I learned from the Gussow-Thomas book was that science is not even sure yet what nutritional issues to worry about, and the details of nutrition science are probably not as important as we might believe after

Why Don't Some People Know That Diet Causes Disease?

A public health professional wonders why some Americans don't pay much attention to their eating habits—until they get heart disease, or another chronic disease.

- "Why is the food/health connection so vague in the public's mind? Researchers know the magnitude of the association. Health professionals understand it. Yet the public is confused about heart-healthy dietary habits, the diet/cancer connection, and even about what constitutes a good diet."
- "Why does medical school education not include more nutrition courses? As recently as 1983 and 1984, first-year medical students at Harvard organized a campaign to have a nutrition course added to the curriculum."
- "Is the confusion due in part to disagreement by the experts on the definition of a good diet?"
- "What would it take to enable the public to connect food intake with health outcome? How can we break the 'junk food' habits of the American public?"
- "We must acknowledge that food choices come not from government pamphlets or recommendations of dietitians, but from a multi-billion dollar food marketing industry."

Source: Crawford, 1988.

the battering we take from the news media and advertisers. The authors asked one hundred public health experts what parts of our daily lives were truly important to our health. They listed thirty-nine items—only nine involving nutrition. (The most important items were smoking, drug abuse, seat belts, drunk driving, and so on.) We are what we eat, says the ancient proverb, and that's true. But we are not *only* what we eat. Other parts of our lives are important to our health.[4]

WHY THE CONFUSION ABOUT NUTRITION?

Consider *cholesterol.* Not many Americans in the 1990s can spend more than a few hours without being exposed to a warning about cholesterol-laden foods. Package labels, advertising, restaurant menus, news reports, magazine features constantly proclaim the dangers of cholesterol. The message is clear: cholesterol clogs arteries, and clogged arteries lead to heart disease. Many scientists and some doctors are firmly committed to recommending low-fat, low-cholesterol diets to help reduce the risk of heart disease. But they have been puzzled for years by the observation that while lowering cholesterol reduces heart disease, it does not seem to reduce death rates among people on cholesterol-lowering regimes. The puzzle is this: if lowering cholesterol reduces heart disease and heart disease is a significant cause of death, why doesn't lowered cholesterol produce lower overall death rates? Nobody knows for sure, but some clues have begun to appear.

The Surgeon General's Report on Nutrition and Health, 1988

- For the first time, government experts on public health presented the scientific evidence *that diet is linked to chronic disease.*
- The evidence proves, they say, that a diet promoting good health can also prevent many chronic diseases.
- That sounded to me like common sense. But then I remembered that the scientific controversy over nutrition has been raging for decades. I remembered that the culture of modern medicine has taught many doctors to be skeptical of connections between diet and disease. And I remembered the enormous economic interests at stake—from beef and egg farmers to fast food chains and supermarkets. Millions of people make their living by selling us foods that provide what the Surgeon General's Report called poor nutrition.
- The Surgeon General reached these scientific conclusions:
- Among the ten leading causes of death in the United States, five are related to poor diet—heart disease, some cancers, strokes, diabetes, atherosclerosis (clogged arteries).
- Three of the top ten are related to excessive alcohol—accidents (especially automobile accidents), suicide, chronic liver disease.
- One—chronic obstructive lung disease—is related to smoking.
- The tenth is pneumonia and influenza.

Sources: McGinnis and Nestle, 1989. Surgeon General's Report, 1988.

Some researchers have found that lowering cholesterol may result in higher levels of aggressiveness and an increased risk of death from accidents and suicides. One scientist, Dr. Stephen M. Weiss, the chief of the behavior medicine section at the National Heart, Lung and Blood Institute says that lowering cholesterol protects against cardiovascular disease, but "we're also seeing a fairly consistent finding of accidents, suicides and homicides in a small number of people on the cholesterol-lowering regimen. If lowering cholesterol changes people's moods, it may adversely affect the quality of life for certain subgroups of the population. The questions are: Can we identify these people, and if so, can we establish a routine for them?" The *New York Times* quoted Dr. Thomas Chalmers of

---

The Surgeon General's Recommendations, 1988

Despite the scientific and commercial bickering, the report says most people can benefit from this advice:

- *Fats and cholesterol*—Eat less fat (especially *saturated* fat; anything that's solid at room temperature, like butter, margarine, animal fat.) Most oils—olive oil, corn oil, safflower oil and so on—are *unsaturated,* liquid at room temperature. Eat low-fat foods—vegetables, fruits, whole grains, fish, poultry, lean meat, low-fat dairy products.
- *Weight control*—Get to near the desirable weight for your age and build. Balance the calories you take in (energy) with the calories you burn (energy expenditure) in your normal daily life. Limit foods high in calories, fats, sugars. Minimize alcohol. Increase the amount of calories you burn through regular exercise; a brisk half-hour walk three times a week may be as useful as more vigorous exercise.
- *Complex carbohydrates and fiber*—Eat more vegetables, whole grains and cereals, fruits.
- *Sodium*—Avoid high-salt foods (most packaged foods—canned, frozen, boxed—are high in sodium.) Use less salt in cooking and at the table.
- *Alcohol*—Moderation in drinking (no more than two drinks a day.) No alcohol when driving, operating machinery, taking other medications, while pregnant.

Source: McGinnis and Nestle, 1989. Surgeon General's Report, 1988.

Scientists Suspect Some Foods Promote Health, Prevent Disease

Nutrition scientists have clues that some foods can enhance health, but they say they don't know enough yet to be sure, and that any food in excessive quantities can be toxic.

- *Garlic*—The Japanese government has issued nine patents for pain-killers based on garlic. The National Cancer Institute is studying the use of a garlic preparation to stimulate the body's immune system, perhaps retarding cancer. The Department of Agriculture is studying evidence that garlic may reduce blood clots. Loma Linda University is researching the use of garlic to control high blood pressure.
- *Citrus fruits*—The National Cancer Institute is studying evidence that citrus fruits can be used in treating some cancers. The high concentration of vitamin C may fight some viruses, lower cholesterol, and reduce clogging of the arteries.
- *Carrots*—The National Cancer Institute is studying evidence that the high levels of beta carotene in carrots may be useful against cancers caused by smoking, also against colon cancer and heart disease.
- *Broccoli, cauliflower, cabbage, brussels sprouts*—The National Cancer Institute says much evidence shows these vegetables (members of the mustard family) can help the immune system fight cancers of the colon, stomach, lung, prostate and esophagus.

Source: O'Neill, 1990.

the Harvard School of Public Health in September, 1990 saying that scientists lack data about all the potential adverse effects of lowering cholesterol. "If we want to use cholesterol lowering as a prescription for the entire population, it's important to know what we're doing besides lowering cholesterol." In other words, is it dangerous for some people to reduce cholesterol? Nobody knows for sure.[5]

Three weeks later, Dr. Chalmers was quoted by the same newspaper as saying that a new study had "changed my mind" about cholesterol. The ten-year study of 838 patients provided the first evidence that lowering cholesterol levels saves lives in patients whose hearts are functioning normally. "This is the smoking pistol," said Dr. Antonio Gotto, a former president of the American Heart Association. "I think this is really a land-mark study." The consensus of scientists and doctors surveyed by the newspaper was that this long-term study demonstrated once and for all that lowering cholesterol saves lives.[6]

There are other puzzles about cholesterol and heart disease that are poorly understood. The French have the lowest incidence of heart disease in Europe, but they eat more fat than people in other European countries. Some researchers think the French taste for garlic may help protect them from heart disease, or perhaps olive oil. There is some evidence that both these natural foods may have cholesterol-lowering effects. A study of about five thousand Italian men and women between, aged twenty to fifty-nine, found that people who ate more butter had much higher blood pressure and cholesterol. People who ate more olive oil and vegetable oil had lower blood pressure and cholesterol. The *Journal of the American Medical Association* thought the study was important, probably identifying butter as increasing the risk factors for heart disease, and olive or vegetable oils as decreasing the risks.[7]

A 1987 report on a study of six thousand patients in Britain found that too little *linoleic acid* was more important as a cause of heart disease than too much saturated fat.[8] (American marketing executives have not yet learned to popularize the value of *linoleic acid* which is found in fish, wheatgerm, soybeans, avocados, nuts and so on. Some scientists have observed that it helps break down cholesterol and fatty deposits. Imagine the packaged frozen dinner made with soybeans and fish that proudly proclaims "high in linoleic acid.") Does anybody really know what kind of fats are best, or how much we should be eating?

COFFEE, SALT, POTASSIUM AND FIBER

Consider *coffee*. A study of 1,130 graduates of a major medical school found several years ago that coffee drinkers had two or three times the risk of heart disease as those who did not drink coffee. In 1990, however, a new study of 45,589 men aged 45 to 75 found that drinking coffee does *not* make men more likely to develop heart disease. Some earlier studies had also found no link between coffee drinking and heart disease, while some studies did find a link. The president of the American Heart Associa-

---

Why Do The TV Commercials Boast "High In Fiber?"

It's not easy to pass more than a few minutes in front of a television screen without being urged to buy a packaged food that is "high in fiber." *The New England Journal of Medicine* tried to sort out "fiber fact from fiber fiction" in 1990.

- Unprocessed plant foods contain fiber. Hundreds of generations of humans ate coarse foods, not altered by processing, high in natural fiber.
- Modern scientists, particularly Dr. Dennis Burkitt and Dr. Hugh Trowell, observed from their work as medical missionaries in Africa that the patients they treated did not have the "Western diseases"— heart disease, high blood pressure, diabetes, constipation, hemorrhoids, appendicitis, cancer of the intestines, hiatal hernia.
- Dr. Burkitt and Dr. Trowell concluded that their African patients did not have the "Western diseases" because the African diet contained *fiber* that Western food processing had removed.
- Dr. Trowell tried to teach the western world that the bigger and more frequent the bowel movements (because of the fiber), the less the number of visits to the hospital.
- "Thus, we [...] conclude that dietary fiber probably has a role in the nutritional prevention of human disease."

Source: Connor, 1990.

---

tion, Dr. Francois Abbud, said about the new 1990 study: "It is carefully done, and on the basis of this study I feel more confident telling patients that as a public health measure I would not advise them to stop drinking coffee." Does coffee make people more likely to have heart disease? That depends on *which study* we read, and *when* we read it. Does anybody really know the answer? [9]

Consider *salt*, sodium. The common wisdom is that we eat too much salt, aggravating our high blood pressure. But, is that true? The Japanese eat more salt than people in most industrialized countries, and some studies have found that Japan has the highest rates of high blood pressure— hypertension—in the world. In 1986 the World Health Organization found that Japan also had the lowest rate of heart disease in the world. That same

Early Results From The World's
Largest Study Of Diet And Health

American and Chinese scientists published in 1990 the first results of a major study exploring dietary causes of disease. They studied 6,500 people in China, because they could identify people who live in the same way, in the same place, and eat the same foods nearly every day of their entire lives, not usually the case in the United States. Some of their findings:

- *Obesity*—*What* people eat has more to do with obesity than *how much* they eat. The Chinese eat twenty percent more calories than Americans, but Americans are twenty-five percent fatter. Chinese eat twice the carbohydrates, but only one-third the fat Americans eat.
- *Protein*—Eating too much protein, especially animal protein, may cause chronic disease. Seventy percent of Americans' protein comes from animals; only seven percent for the Chinese. Chinese who eat the most animal protein have the highest rates of the "Western diseases"—heart disease, cancer, diabetes.
- *Cancer*—Rich diets promote rapid growth in children, but may also promote cancer. Girls who eat diets high in calories, protein, fat and calcium start menstruating three to six years earlier than Chinese and have higher rates of cancer of the breast and reproductive organs.
- *Osteoporosis*—Calcium from dairy products may not be needed to prevent this bone-weakening disease. Most Chinese eat no dairy products, getting their calcium from vegetables, but only half the calcium that Americans eat. Although life expectancy in China is only about five years less than in the United States (about seventy years compared to seventy-five years for Americans), osteoporosis is uncommon in China.

Sources: Campbell, 1990; Brody, 1990.

year six specialists in heart disease reviewed more than 250 studies made over the ten previous years about the health effects of salt. They found that salt might *perhaps* exert a small influence on blood pressure, but that the effect was minor compared to being overweight or drinking too much alcohol. (Heavy doses of medication—the doctor called them "industrial-strength doses"—kept my blood pressure at controlled but high levels for several years. Then, I lost 75 pounds. With one-third the drugs, my blood pressure came down to more nearly normal levels.)

For the last forty years, scientists have been seeing evidence that *potassium* is an important element in human nutrition. For the million plus years of human life on earth as hunter-gatherers, the available foods were high in potassium and low in sodium. Today, our diets are exactly the reverse—low in potassium and high in sodium. Our bodies are naturally inclined to conserve sodium, which was scarce, and get rid of potassium, which was plentiful during those million plus years.

There is much evidence that the lack of potassium causes disease. People on very low potassium diets have more heart disease than people who take in more potassium. Blacks in the southeastern United States, for example, eat a very low potassium diet and have the highest rate of stroke of any ethnic or geographic group in the country. They also have 18 times more of the kind of end-stage renal disease caused by high blood pressure than whites do. People in Scotland have much more heart disease than people of southern England, France, or Italy where people eat more potassium. Farmers in one part of northern Japan who eat eight or ten potassium rich apples a day (because the apple orchards are there) suffer far fewer strokes than farmers in a neighboring area (with no apple orchards) who eat more rice, but fewer apples.[10]

Nobody knows for sure if all this is simply coincidence. But the human body spent a million plus years becoming accustomed to a high potassium diet. When we skimp on potassium, we may be asking our body to do without enough of something it needs (potassium) and loading up with something it needs less (sodium). (Fruits, vegetables, grains and seeds are all natural sources high in potassium and low in sodium.)

"It's high in fiber" is a phrase we can not escape in the 1990s, but nobody is really sure yet how best to include *fiber* in the diet. Most experts believe fiber is important. Dr. Hugh Trowell, a British physician who worked in Africa for many years, says he taught Nathan Pritikin—the 1970s and 1980s low-fat, low-salt, high-carbohydrate, high-fiber, exercise promoter—that fiber was important. Dr. Trowell has been advocating since the 1930s the diet he observed while working with the African peasant Kikuyu people—high-fiber, high-carbohydrate, low-fat. "The Kikuyu did not get coronaries, diabetes, or high blood pressure. I recommended this type of diet and much physical exercise." [11] Pritikin may have been the man who taught America about diet and exercise to prevent disease, but Dr. Trowell wants us to remember that he helped teach Pritikin. He has also tried to teach the world that the "western diseases" and the "diseases of civilization" are probably caused by our lifestyle—poor diet and too little exercise.

Many doctors are still skeptical about the connection between diet and chronic disease. When I asked a nephrologist in 1988 about my intention to try the low-fat, high-fiber, high-carbohydrate diet recommended by Pritikin and by the Surgeon General's report, he scoffed at me. "It won't hurt," he said, "but you will probably be wasting your time and money." [12]

BLOOD PRESSURE AND POISON ARROWS

In 1990, researchers claimed to have found a hormone in the body that plays a major role in the development of high blood pressure. Their discovery was important because, in the vast majority of persons with high blood pressure, the cause is unknown. The researchers found the hormone after an eight-year search. They had processed hundreds of gallons of blood from people with high blood pressure, looking for a substance common to the blood of all people with hypertension.

When they presented the results of their research to an American Heart Association conference, the researchers said they were astounded to find that every human they studied had tiny quantities of the substance *ouabain* in the blood, and two out of three people with high blood pressure had elevated levels. The reason for the scientists' astonishment is that ouabain is identical to a substance from plants that South American Indians used as a poison on the tips of their arrows and that doctors used to treat patients with heart conditions. Ouabain is derived from the *ouabaio* tree and is related to the *digitalis* family of drugs for heart disease. Dr. John Hamlyn, a physiologist from the University of Maryland, said that until 1990 scientists had no idea that the deadly poison ouabain was present in the body, or that elevated levels of the poison contributed to high blood pressure. The researchers guessed that the poison may slow down the mechanism by which the body regulates levels of sodium, potassium and calcium. They

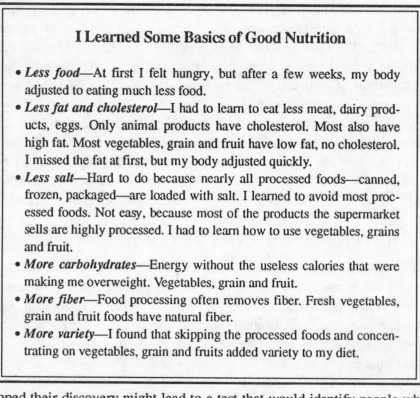

I Learned Some Basics of Good Nutrition

- *Less food*—At first I felt hungry, but after a few weeks, my body adjusted to eating much less food.
- *Less fat and cholesterol*—I had to learn to eat less meat, dairy products, eggs. Only animal products have cholesterol. Most also have high fat. Most vegetables, grain and fruit have low fat, no cholesterol. I missed the fat at first, but my body adjusted quickly.
- *Less salt*—Hard to do because nearly all processed foods—canned, frozen, packaged—are loaded with salt. I learned to avoid most processed foods. Not easy, because most of the products the supermarket sells are highly processed. I had to learn how to use vegetables, grains and fruit.
- *More carbohydrates*—Energy without the useless calories that were making me overweight. Vegetables, grain and fruit.
- *More fiber*—Food processing often removes fiber. Fresh vegetables, grain and fruit foods have natural fiber.
- *More variety*—I found that skipping the processed foods and concentrating on vegetables, grain and fruits added variety to my diet.

hoped their discovery might lead to a test that would identify people who might benefit from reducing their salt intake.[13]

SO, WHAT'S IMPORTANT IN NUTRITION?

Like people with heart disease, high blood pressure, diabetes and other chronic diseases, people with kidney disease must pay closer attention to their diets than people with normal kidneys, but some of the basics are the same. I learned that I could assure good nutrition for myself and my family by remembering one simple sentence.

Eat a variety of mostly fresh and unprocessed foods—mostly vegetables, grain and fruit, not many animal products—and no more at one meal than will fit on one plate.

I found that following this simple formula probably gives me an ample supply of energy, protein, fiber, vitamins and minerals. It also limits the parts of the diet that may contribute to sickness and disease—fat, choles-

A Wise Scientist Sums Up a Life Studying Nutrition

- "I am confident we will bring the major chronic diseases under better control. We will probably debate the factors influencing the accomplishment."
- " But all of the evidence—whether one looks at heart disease, cancer, stroke, hypertension, diabetes or obesity—supports the conclusion that Americans should be advised to reduce their consumption of fat and cholesterol, modify the composition of their dietary fat, reduce their consumption of salt and sugar, and increase their consumption of fruits and vegetables and whole grain cereals."
- "No one has produced evidence that such changes are detrimental or that the current American diet has advantages over this type of diet."
- "Americans have started to modify their diet in these directions, and heart disease and hypertension have decreased markedly."
- "We do not discount the effect of treatment, but nutrition now offers the primary hope for further resolution of these most important public health problems."

Source: Hegsted, 1985.

terol, salt, and sugar. Because of my kidney disease I also need to limit my protein and phosphorus, and other chronic diseases also require some special attention.

There's no magic in this formula, simply the expression of the fact that over the last one-and-a-half million years the human body has adapted to a wide variety of foods that were available and convenient and that helped promote growth and survival. Enormous variations in diets have been successful through history. Eskimos can eat fish, meat and blubber, almost no vegetables. Chinese peasants can eat rice and some vegetables, almost no meat or fish. The Masai in Africa can eat mostly milk and blood. The Toda in India can eat only vegetables and grain, no meat. All can thrive; the human body is remarkably adaptable.[14, 15]

One clue to healthy nutrition is that the human body has evolved over hundreds of centuries by using what food was available. During most of the time our species has inhabited the earth, our ancestors were *hunter-gatherers*, living on meat and fish, vegetables, nuts, roots and fruits. They

---

Good Nutrition For My Kidney Disease

As a kidney patient, I needed the same good nutrition as everybody else, but I also needed to limit the *protein* and *phosphorus* I was eating to give my weakened kidneys less work to do.

- *Less protein*—I learned to limit animal food—meat, fish, eggs, dairy. That reduced protein and phosphorus simultaneously. My low-protein diet is also a low-phosphorus diet.
- *Less phosphorus*—Some vegetables (peas and beans) and some whole grains (wheat, rye, oats) have significant phosphorus as well as protein. Rice and corn have less protein and less phosphorus.

---

ate little grain and almost no dairy products.[16] Their meat and fish came from whatever wild game their hunting produced; the rest, from the food-gathering done mostly by the women and children. The game they hunted—lean and low-fat wild animals—contained only about five percent fat compared to the thirty or forty percent fat of modern domestic food animals, and the fifty or sixty percent fat of processed foods like hamburgers and sausage. Salt was hard to find, as was the honey that provided some sweetness. Processed foods, like refined sugar, were, of course, unavailable. Some people still live the hunter-gatherer life, like the ¡Kung San people of the Kalahari desert in Africa.

Grain and dairy products became important in our diet only recently in evolutionary terms, in the last ten thousand years when people learned to cultivate plants and raise domestic animals for food. Instead of *hunting* wild animals for meat, or wandering through fields and woods *gathering* roots, nuts, fruit and vegetables in the wild, they could sow seeds and reap grain, raise chicken, pigs, cows for meat, eggs and milk.

Only in the last one hundred years have we learned to make the highly-processed foods that we now buy in the supermarket, the high-calorie, high-fat, high-sugar, high-salt, low-fiber, low-potassium foods that our ancestors didn't have and that some people think our bodies are not adapted for. Two thirds of the deaths in the United States each year are caused by cardiovascular disease (heart attack, stroke, high blood pressure), kidney disease and cancer. Some scientists—like Dr. Trowell who has been trying for over fifty years to teach us that our diet and sedentary lifestyle causes disease—believe that our new highly-processed, fast food nutrition is one reason why the "Western diseases, the diseases of civilization" are the biggest killers of the twentieth century.[17] Other scientists and many doctors disagree. Some doctors don't care, perhaps because their culture has taught them to ignore the connection between diet and disease. Nobody knows for sure.

There is little argument in the 1990s on the basics. Eat less food, but a wide variety. Less fat, especially saturated fat, less sugar, less salt. Eat more fresh *unprocessed* foods, vegetables, whole grains, fruit. I found that eating less protein and less phosphorus may have helped stop my kidney disease from getting worse.

While the scientists continue to study nutrition, the rest of us will continue to make the daily choices that can help us feel better, look better, maybe even live healthier and longer lives. People with kidney disease may even be able to avoid dialysis and transplant, at least for a while.

12
Living With A
"Kidney-Friendly Diet"

C omputer people coined the word "user-friendly" to describe computers that were designed for *computer users*—not computer engineers. The idea was that good design could make computers easy to use, the way well-designed cars are easy to drive. We need not be auto mechanics to use an automobile.

A "kidney-friendly" diet makes things easier for weakened, damaged kidneys. When the kidneys aren't working well, give them less work to do. Keep the blood pressure down, keep the cholesterol in balance, minimize the protein and phosphorus kidneys have to deal with. The result—if all goes well—is kidney disease that stops getting worse, or at least gets worse slowly, postponing the need for the desperate high-tech half-way remedies of dialysis and transplant, or perhaps avoiding them entirely.

SOME SECRETS OF A HEALTHY DIET

I learned that people who have successfully adapted to a healthy diet have discovered four secrets:

- #1 Some foods are simply *unhealthy*, perhaps *dangerous*.
- #2 Some people—particularly overweight people—not only eat unhealthy foods, but *they eat too much of everything*. Their portions are simply too big.
- #3 Some of us eat the *same foods* day by day, week by week. There is little variety in our menus.
- #4 Some people get too little *physical exercise*, maybe none.

After being seventy-five pounds overweight for twenty years, I finally learned these four secrets, and began to do something about them. Within six months, I had lost fifty pounds; within a year, seventy-five pounds. My blood pressure was more nearly normal, with one-third the medications I had been taking for four years. My cholesterol was down by forty percent, almost normal. My kidney disease had been nearly stable for two years. I don't know for sure whether my new eating habits caused all these improvements in my health, but the lifestyle changes certainly produced changes in my physical condition that could be measured by scales, blood pressure machines and blood tests.

SECRET # 1: DANGEROUS FOODS

Some foods are downright dangerous. They can make us obese, raise our cholesterol and blood pressure, damage the heart, kidneys and other organs. The most dangerous foods for nearly everybody are foods high in fat, sugar, salt, and cholesterol. For kidney patients, high-protein and high-phosphorus foods can also be dangerous. A problem in identifying dangerous foods is that *nobody seems to think they are dangerous.* Dangerous foods are everywhere. Buy your kids something to munch on at a ball game—cheese fries, hot dog. Stop at a fast-food place for a quick meal—hamburger, french fries, milkshake. Stop for a carryout dinner on the way home from work—fried chicken, mashed potatoes and gravy. Go to a neighborhood diner or family restaurant for a light dinner—bowl of chili, french fries, chocolate cake. Pick up a few things at the supermarket—sandwich meat and sliced cheese, potato chips, ice cream and chocolate syrup.

Some Dangerous Foods In My Life—
High-Fat, High-Cholesterol, High-Salt

- Eggs, processed meats (like sandwich meats, hot dogs, sausages) cheese, butter
- Fast food—hamburgers, french fries, fried chicken, pizza
- Desserts—ice cream, baked goods

Some Foods Could Also Be Dangerous For My Kidneys—*High-Protein and High-Phosphorus*

- Meat, fish, poultry, dairy products, eggs
- *Whole* grains—breads, cereals, pasta
- Peas, beans, lentils, nuts, seeds
- Soy sauce, salt

I had to learn to limit my consumption of all these foods if I wanted to avoid dialysis and transplant.

All these foods can be dangerous for everybody because of their high fat, high salt, high calorie content—but if everybody eats them, how dangerous can they really be? Common sense says that if most Americans eat these foods, they must be okay. But Americans are more overweight than people in many other countries.

The fact is that *dangerous foods can cause disease.* I put the first secret to work for me by identifying the dangerous foods in my diet. I ate so much of so many of them that I had to try to eliminate them from my life. Other people have simply cut down on the amounts, rather than eliminating them entirely. I had no alternative.

SECRET #2: EATING TOO MUCH

I would have an eight ounce hamburger for lunch, or a twelve ounce steak at dinner. I would finish a full plate of spaghetti and meat balls. I would have a sandwich piled high with corned beef or salami. My portions were just too big, but common sense was leading me in the wrong direction again. Most restaurants serve large portions, because, a friend told me, the cost of the food is not the biggest item in a restaurant meal and bigger portions somehow make customers feel they get their money's worth.

I eventually learned that my portions of everything were probably about double or triple what my body could handle. So the solution, once I established a new behavior pattern, was to eat about half what I once ate. At home, I took smaller servings. In a restaurant, I learned a useful technique. As soon as the food was served—like a big plate of pasta—I would divide the serving into two equal portions. When I finished eating half, I would stop, asking the waiter to wrap up the second half so that I could take it home. It was hard at first, but as my body adjusted, I found that I didn't want more food. I reached a more nearly natural weight, and my body automatically adjusted to eating less food.

SECRET #3: RATHER THAN EATING THE SAME-BAD-OLD-MEALS, EAT THE SAME-GOOD-NEW-MEALS

When I took the time to think about what I was eating, I learned that there were really very few different foods in my normal diet. Because many of them were on the dangerous list, and because I was eating far too much of everything, I needed to find a few new meals that could become the mainstay of my diet.

I was eating the All-American Breakfast every day—eggs, bacon, potatoes, toast, butter, coffee with cream. Fat, cholesterol, too many calories. What I needed was something new—cereal, fruit. Oatmeal was a good choice, or almost any cereal. My lunches were usually a cup of soup, a hamburger and some french fries. Fat, cholesterol, calories. A salad was a far better choice. My dinners were beef, chicken, occasionally fish, with perhaps salad and potatoes, rarely vegetables. I needed to learn to eat vegetables and pasta instead of meat and potatoes.

I eventually found some new meals that satisfied me as much as the old ones did, without the health-poisoning effects of the high-calorie, high-fat, and because of my weakened kidneys, the high-protein and high-phosphorus regimen I had followed for fifty years. (You will find in Chapter 13 some suggestions on cooking what have become my favorite foods, and some ideas about eating when you're away from home in Chapter 14.) I still eat only a few basic meals—and many people I know do the same—but now I am eating "the good-new-meals, not the bad-old-meals." The results for me have been dramatic.

SECRET #4: EVEN A LITTLE EXERCISE CAN WORK WONDERS

I was too busy to exercise. I worked twelve or fourteen hour days, often six or even seven days a week. Most meals were business events, except on the weekends. The most exercise I had was running through an airport to catch a plane, sometimes feeling chest pains as I rushed ahead carrying my garment bag. It was a wonder I wasn't dead long before fifty.

When my diseases finally called a halt to my lifestyle, I learned that a half-hour walk every day or two—just a brisk walk, not the running or jogging that seemed too strenuous to me—was enough to give me some of the benefits of exercise. It had to be a *brisk* walk, not a leisurely stroll, so that it would get my heart beating faster and all my other body systems working hard; but jogging, running or weight-lifting wasn't necessary for me, no matter how desirable it might be for others. My weight came down, my pulse rate came down, by blood pressure came down, and my kidney disease stopped getting worse. I don't know for sure what connection existed, if any, between my exercise and all my diseases. But I felt better after a brisk half-hour walk, and when I missed the walk for a couple of days, I felt worse. I suspected there might be a connection.

MAKING LIFESTYLE CHANGES IS NOT EASY

I don't mean to imply that changing the diet and exercise habits of a lifetime is easy. Far from it. Relapses are common. I love to eat scrambled eggs and a toasted bagel while I read the morning paper. Poison for somebody with kidney disease, but I relapse too often. Not often enough, so far, to have gained weight, but my cholesterol goes up after just a breakfast or two like that.

I love good bread, any kind from Italian and French bread to Middle Eastern bread or Indian chapati. Poison for a kidney patient because of the protein and phosphorus content of whole grains. I have to struggle not to eat too much bread.

Somehow, I have had an easier time with meat and dairy products. I occasionally get an overwhelming urge for a hot dog from a street vendor, but that's half fat anyway, not very high in protein. I haven't eaten beef for several years, even before I began working on my life-style changes. I got

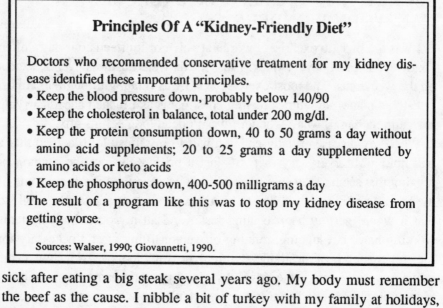

Principles Of A "Kidney-Friendly Diet"

Doctors who recommended conservative treatment for my kidney disease identified these important principles.
- Keep the blood pressure down, probably below 140/90
- Keep the cholesterol in balance, total under 200 mg/dl.
- Keep the protein consumption down, 40 to 50 grams a day without amino acid supplements; 20 to 25 grams a day supplemented by amino acids or keto acids
- Keep the phosphorus down, 400-500 milligrams a day

The result of a program like this was to stop my kidney disease from getting worse.

Sources: Walser, 1990; Giovannetti, 1990.

sick after eating a big steak several years ago. My body must remember the beef as the cause. I nibble a bit of turkey with my family at holidays, but just a nibble. (I do have some turkey stuffing with gravy, however, although probably about half what I once ate.)

Dairy products haven't been a problem for me either, which is surprising because I loved milk and cheese. I could drink a quart of milk with some chocolate chip cookies in a few minutes, or eat a quarter-pound or more of good cheese. The protein and phosphorus content of milk is so high—to say nothing of the fat in whole milk and the salt in cheese—that the damage to my kidneys was probably great. I never drink milk anymore, or eat ice cream or cheese. I do use a bit of grated cheese on pasta, not enough to increase the protein much, just to add some flavor. Somehow the absence of dairy products hasn't been hard for me.

My real deprivation on this kidney-friendly diet is bread and eggs. I haven't quite made it yet to the level of protein and phosphorus consumption that the kidney researchers think is necessary to prolong the life of my kidneys. I get close, and I'm trying hard. It's not easy, but it's far better for me than dialysis or transplant. It may be better for some other kidney patients, too.

13
Cooking For Someone
With Kidney Disease

Most nephrologists and dietitians think that protein-restricted diets are very difficult for kidney patients, maybe too difficult to try. How the kidney professionals can prefer the *extremely difficult dialysis and transplant* to the *mildly difficult* nutritional treatment is beyond me. Would a kidney patient prefer plugging himself into a dialysis machine for four hours out of every two days for the rest of his much-shortened life span? Or, would he prefer altering his diet a bit to prevent the disease from getting worse? Would he prefer the all-too-likely horrors of transplant rejection to a new lifestyle of low-protein, low-phosphorus nutrition? It doesn't make any sense to me, but that's what many kidney professionals tell a patient. Could it be *their own lifestyles* they are protecting, and not the patient's?

Getting my protein consumption down to 20 or 25 grams a day isn't easy, and I work hard trying to sustain it month after month. I don't always succeed. But getting to 40 grams a day, and edging closer to 20 or 25 grams is not nearly so difficult as the kidney professionals seem to believe. And it's nothing compared to a foreshortened life on dialysis or with a transplant. Once I had the basics under some control—avoiding dangerous foods, eating less, finding "the-good-new-meals" to replace "the-bad-old-meals," exercising—I found that the protein and phosphorus restriction followed along quite naturally. Some kidney professionals probably don't know how simple and natural the whole process is. Perhaps they should *try* it before they dismiss it as "too difficult," or a "compliance problem." (Meaning, "The patient won't follow my orders.") While most nephrologists and dietitians believe dietary treatment is too difficult, the director of the federal Modification of Diet In Renal Disease Study, Dr. Saulo Klahr, told me in early 1991 that with some help, patients in the final phase of the study were learning to live comfortably with the low-protein diets. Other researchers reported similar results.[1]

In any case, I found that the kidney-friendly diet was practical. Even my family ate almost the same diet I did, although they ate a bit more protein. In fact, if you like to cook, as I do, you may love the new world of *vegetable cooking* and *ethnic cooking* that opens up to you, perhaps for the first time. There was some grumbling around our house when we first started trying to eat better, but now my wife, two sons and two daughters are enthusiastic fans of what they consider very good cooking.

AM I REALLY GOING TO BE A VEGETARIAN?

I remember the first serious vegetarian I ever knew. She was a professional dietitian who had a weight problem of her own. She started working on the food and sedentary lifestyle habits that were making her obese. She started taking a brisk half-hour walk every day and cutting down on the amount of fats and refined sugars in her diet. She worked on eating less of everything. She tried to eat more complex carbohydrates, and less proteins, fat and sugars. She lost some weight, but not enough. She was determined not to be one of the few obese dietitians in the world, so she decided to adopt a *vegetarian diet*, even a *vegan* diet, no animal foods of any kind, including eggs and dairy products. She ate only foods of vegetable origin. When I became aware of her rigid vegan diet, I can remember how shocked I was. "You mean you eat nothing but vegetables? *Nothing at all but vegetables?*" The idea was so alien to me that I considered her a nut case, a freak.

Like many Americans of my generation, I grew up believing that "vegetables" were the mushy, overcooked boiled cauliflower and broccoli that my family served with the roast beef, mashed potatoes and gravy. Vegetables were disgusting. I later learned that nobody in my family knew how to cook vegetables. Certainly I didn't. No wonder they were so disgusting. As I watched the obese dietitian shed her excess weight on her vegetarian, really *vegan* diet, I was getting a demonstration of the power of good nutrition plus modest exercise. When she became a slim and svelte vegetarian dietitian, I could see there was something to it.

When I started learning to control my kidney disease, I remembered her experience. I also began noticing how many people there are in the world who eat mostly, or even exclusively vegetable foods—in Asia and Europe, certainly, but even in the United States. I started to learn how to cook vegetables in other ways than simply boiling them to mush, as my mother had done. Am I a vegetarian? Yes. Am I a nut case? Certainly some people may call me that, probably some nephrologists. But if I can *control my kidney disease*, if I can eat delicious "good-new-meals" based on grains and vegetables, if I can stay out of the dialysis center and the transplant ward while I learn to enjoy a whole new world of good food, I'm proud to be called a "nut case vegetarian." In fact, if the *New York Times* has it right, I may even be fashionable.

HOW CAN I BUILD A MEAL AROUND VEGETABLES?

My family was skeptical when I began to cook vegetarian meals on the weekends. They were looking for the turkey or chicken or fish. (Roast beef and steak had disappeared from our house long ago.) In my search for some "good-new-meals," and with the help of some of the excellent cook books you will find listed in Appendix 4, I began to find some great menus.

We have always liked Italian food around our house. It's delicious, and easy to cook with a little practice. A satisfying meal for kidney patients and non-kidney patients is the classic pasta and salad—spaghetti with tomato sauce plus a good mixed salad. If the portions are not too large, kidney patients will stay near their low protein target.

No cooking could be easier than a fresh tomato sauce, pasta and a salad. Chop an onion and some garlic, maybe a hot chili pepper if you like spicy food. Sauté them in some olive oil until they soften and the oil is flavored. Add some chopped fresh tomatoes or some chopped canned tomatoes. Bring the mixture to a boil and then reduce the heat and simmer for twenty minutes or so. Meanwhile, cook the spaghetti and make the salad. (You may want to try lettuce other than the iceberg lettuce that is so tasteless. Supermarkets like it because it ships and stores well. It's terrible compared to the other kinds of lettuce you will find in most supermarkets.) Slice very thinly some cucumbers, some scallions (green onions), some radishes, some carrots, some green peppers—some or all, depending on what you happen to have. Mix in some salt and pepper. Sprinkle enough good olive oil over it to coat everything, then some vinegar. (There is a significant difference between the various grades of olive oil. The richly flavored *extra virgin* olive oil is what many Italian cooks like to use for salads.) The result is a delicious and healthful salad.

When the sauce has simmered for a while, add a ladle or two of vegetable broth or hot water with a dissolved bouillon cube and simmer a little longer. Mix the spaghetti or other pasta with the tomato sauce and serve it with the salad. I would be surprised if anyone who likes Italian food realizes that he is eating a "vegetarian" meal. In fact, it's a *vegan* meal. But it's so good and so easy.

As I experimented with vegetable cooking, I learned that some vegetable dishes—prepared with a little care—are so satisfying that even non-kidney patients start to like them. For example, around our house one of the "good-new-meals" is *risotto*, the exquisite Italian dish based on rice cooked very slowly in a flavored liquid, a vegetable or chicken broth. I make the broth from vegetable or chicken bouillon cubes, sometimes from packaged vegetable broth dried ingredients. Adding some other vegetables, like peas, broccoli, summer squash, made a hearty and delicious main dish once I got over the habit of seeing a "joint of meat," as the English would say, in the center of the table. (In most of the world people wouldn't dream of eating a "joint of meat" the way our Northern European forebears taught us to do. Meat as a condiment is much more common in the world than meat as a centerpiece of the meal. Some people think it's much healthier too, to limit the meat. It certainly has been for me.)

WHERE ARE THE 21-DAY MENU PLANS?

Some books on healthful cooking and weight-loss dieting include elaborate plans for weeks of varied menus. I have never understood how anyone can plan meal-by-meal for days and weeks in advance. It makes me think of someone trying to decide on Monday what shirt he will wear on Friday; maybe some people can do it. A much more practical way for me to achieve healthful nutrition was to work on a few dishes that my family and I liked, and that would help me achieve the nutritional goals I had set for myself. It was far more important for me to *set some new patterns* for myself, form some new habits, than to plan things to the last detail. After learning to avoid the dangerous foods and limit portion-sizes, I had to find a few of the "good-new-meals." I found some that were appealing to me and to my family. Some may be appealing to you, too. You may want to try some of the excellent cookbooks listed in Appendix 4, experimenting until you find some "good-new-meals" that suit you. As I browsed the bookstores and libraries for cookbooks, I was amazed at the creativity that has gone into vegetable cooking, particularly in ethnic cuisines. The food section of your newspaper is also an excellent source, and I suspect you will be surprised how many vegetable and grain recipes you will find in the newspapers. It seems that not only kidney patients are interested in healthful nutrition. Maybe the ancient cuisines of Asia and the Middle East have something to teach us and the Europeans.

SOME RECIPES THAT HAVE HELPED ME

One of the happiest parts of my participation in the study at Johns Hopkins University School of Medicine was meeting and working with the other kidney patients. (More about this in Chapter 15.) My fellow patients were eager to share their tips on how to live with a kidney-friendly diet. Dr. Murray West of Baltimore, a physician trying to control his own kidney disease, taught me about *risotto*, a dish I had never cooked, never even eaten until my most recent trip to Italy. (My family and I visited with Professor Giovannetti and his staff at the University of Pisa and Professor Maschio and his staff at the University of Verona.) Dr. West shares some of his recipes in Appendix 5. Sandra Watt and Edith Kahn are also working to control their kidney disease. Gary and Dianne Dulin know more than anybody about low-protein cooking. I am not sure I would have learned as much as I have about living with kidney disease had I not had the help of people like Sandra, Edith, Dianne, Gary and

Murray. I hope you enjoy their tips as much as my family and I have enjoyed them.

14

Eating When You Are
Away From Home

You can find something to eat in *any* restaurant, no matter how bad, but it takes practice. Eating at the home of friends or relatives is trickier, but still manageable once you learn some new techniques. The most important one that I learned was that people don't care if your eating habits seem a bit unusual. Many people in the 1990s are acting on their new knowledge that food causes disease, not only the people we once called the "health nuts" who nibbled sunflower seeds and granola. Even people on low-protein diets are not unusual.

"Nobody wants protein," said a restaurant consultant quoted by the *New York Times* in 1990. "The best-educated, most affluent people in America are willing to pay top-dollar to eat a third-world diet." A travel consultant specializing in health spas said, "They used to pay to starve. Now the typical spa-goer wants plenty to eat, but only vegetables and rice, maybe some pasta or cereal." The newspaper headlined the story: "The New Nutrition: Protein On the Side; Meat is now out of favor." [1] Not only can a low protein diet help you control your kidney disease, but in the 1990s, it is even fashionable.

FINDING GOOD FOODS IN RESTAURANTS

The typical American restaurant—from the cheapest greasy spoon to the most exclusive expense-account place—is a storehouse of poor nutrition. The neighborhood luncheonette specializes in greasy hamburgers, and fat-laden lemon meringue pie with whipped cream. The chic French restaurant serves veal in cream sauce followed by *mousse chocolate*. Too much calories and fat for everybody; too much protein for kidney patients.

Fast food restaurants are even worse. Even the corporate management of McDonald's has apparently realized in the 1990s that the food sold at the neighborhood McDonald's is so nutritionally poor that changes are necessary. As they had decided to do away with wasteful plastic packaging, McDonald's has started ever so slowly to change its menu. Potatoes are fried in vegetable oil, not beef fat. Salads and low-fat milk shakes are available. There is even a low-fat hamburger. Nutrition information is posted in the store, no matter how inconspicuously. I wonder, though, how many customers know that nearly half the calories in many McDonald's meals come from fat. (Next time you are in a McDonald's, try an experiment. Count the customers in the store. Then count the number of *over-*

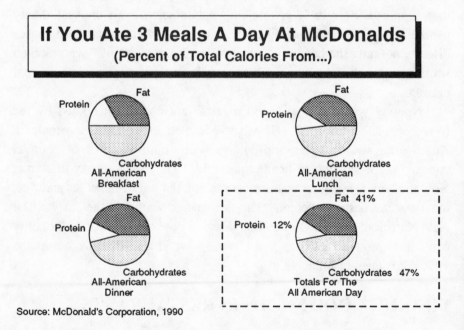

If You Ate 3 Meals A Day At McDonalds
(Percent of Total Calories From...)

Fat
Protein

Carbohydrates
All-American
Breakfast

Fat
Protein

Carbohydrates
All-American
Lunch

Fat
Protein

Carbohydrates
All-American
Dinner

Fat 41%
Protein 12%

Carbohydrates 47%
Totals For The
All American Day

Source: McDonald's Corporation, 1990

Figure 54 Three Meals A Day At McDonald's

weight customers. Could there be a connection between the high-fat Mc-Donald's food and the over-weight customers?)

IF YOU HAVE A CHOICE, ETHNIC IS USUALLY BEST

The world's oldest traditional cuisines—Oriental, Indian and Middle Eastern are the ones I'm most familiar with—are much more likely to offer good nutritional choices than American or northern European cooking. The reasons are fascinating, the subject of some excellent books. People in China, India and the Middle East often depended more on grains and vegetables for their food than on animal foods. Poor people in Europe also fed themselves mostly with grains and vegetables, but rich Europeans ate much more meat. The lord of the manor ate a roast pig; the serfs ate a porridge or gruel made of coarse grain, or coarse black bread. Meat-eating became a symbol of wealth in Europe.[2] Americans are still influenced by

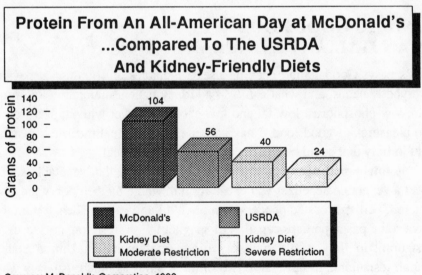

Sources: McDonald's Corporation, 1990
USRDA, Dr. Mackenzie Walser, 1990

Figure 55 Protein From A Day At McDonald's

this medieval European tradition when they ask, "What shall we have for dinner tonight? How about hamburgers or steak?" Can you hear an American answering, "How about peas and rice?" (If the *New York Times* is right, the newly-fashionable eating habits may be changing this centuries-old custom.)

The most popular ethnic cuisines in the United States are Italian, Mexican and Chinese.[3] People in the northeastern states have made Italian cooking the favorite; in the Southwest, Mexican; and in the rest of the country, Chinese. All these traditional cuisines depend heavily on vegetables and grains. Italians use much pasta and rice; Mexicans use rice, beans and corn; Chinese use rice and vegetables. Chinese, Mexican and sometimes Italian cuisines use meat more as a condiment, a flavoring, than as a main element of a meal. Although they have been adapted for American tastes, all three traditional cuisines include some principles of good nutrition, although there is plenty of unhealthy ethnic food, too, especially when the ethnic dishes are adapted to American tastes, like sweet and sour pork or sausage sandwiches.

FINDING GOOD FOOD IN AN ITALIAN RESTAURANT

It's easy. Good Italian cooking uses vegetables and grains, just what everybody needs, and what can help a kidney patient maintain a low-protein, low-phosphorus, low-fat and low-cholesterol diet without sacrificing the pleasures of good food. I have often eaten a typical meal in a restaurant in Italy that could be a perfect kidney patient's meal.

You might start with a cup of minestrone soup, Italian vegetable soup. Next a vegetable appetizer you chose from the table by the door when you entered, perhaps roasted peppers with olive oil and garlic. Then you might have some pasta, perhaps capellini or spaghetti with fresh tomato sauce. A restaurant in Italy would routinely serve small portions. United States Italian restaurants usually serve two or three times as much. An easy way to deal with this problem is the *cut-it-in-half method*. As soon as the dish is served, divide it in half (or in thirds, if it is an enormous portion.) Then eat the smaller portion, asking the waiter to wrap up the rest to take out.

Italians often eat their salad after the meal, a custom we usually follow around our house, too. A simple *insalata mista*, a mixed salad of lettuce (good lettuce, not the iceberg lettuce that looks good in the supermarket, but sometimes tastes like cardboard), radishes, carrots, cucumbers, all sliced very thin, with a dressing of simply olive oil, vinegar, salt and pepper (not the dreadful concoction sold in bottles in the United States under the name "Italian Dressing.")

If you keep the portion sizes small, and if you don't eat bread, you will have eaten a low-protein, low-phosphorus, low-fat, low-cholesterol Italian meal. And you wouldn't have eaten much differently from anybody else in the restaurant in Italy. You can find a similar meal in any Italian restaurant in the United States.

Another elegant and delicious dish in Italian cuisine is *risotto*, now the chic dinner of spa-goers and New Yorkers eating third-world diets. It's great for kidney patients, too, provided the portion sizes are small. (See Chapter 13 for some advice on making *risotto* at home.) *Risotto* is simply good rice simmered slowly so that the cooking liquid is absorbed slowly, flavoring the rice and giving it a more interesting consistency than the library-paste mass of what Americans often call "boiled rice." No wonder we grow up not liking rice. Italian cooks often add vegetables like green or yellow summer squash, broccoli or spinach to the *risotto*. Not many Italian restaurants in the United States serve this dish of northern Italy; most Italian restaurants in the United States are run in the tradition of southern Italian cooking—Naples and Sicily, mostly, where pasta is the staple, not rice. If you see it on a menu, try this very unusual dish. It may become one of "the good-new-meals" around your house as it did around ours.

I still struggle to stay away from the good Italian bread and the butter served by every Italian restaurant in the United States. The bread adds too much protein and phosphorus; the butter, too much fat. But with attention to my portion sizes and my menu choices, I can enjoy wonderful meals in an Italian restaurant in the United States or Italy, despite my kidney-friendly diet.

GOOD FOOD IN A CHINESE RESTAURANT

Traditional Chinese cooking uses mostly vegetables and grain; meat, fish and poultry are condiments, flavorings. Try an experiment next time you are in a restaurant owned and run by recent immigrants from China, Hong Kong or Taiwan. Try this in a small Chinese restaurant after the lunch or dinner rush has ended, when the kitchen staff sits down to eat its own meal. Watch what the cooks and helpers eat. Whenever I have done this experiment, I see the Chinese eating noodles or rice and vegetables, rarely any meat, and certainly not the "sweet and sour pork" that the Americans have been ordering from the Americanized menu. (I haven't seen "sweet and sour pork" on restaurant menus in Hong Kong or Beijing. That dish and all the other Americanized Chinese foods are purely commercial adaptations to the American hunger for meat, the symbol of affluence we learned from our European ancestors. Only now are we learning that our meat and fat eating habits are contributing to our "western diseases.")

In Hong Kong or China, the dishes served by restaurants are based almost exclusively on grains and vegetables. Rice is served with every meal. Noodles are common, like stir-fried noodles with vegetables, something you will see as "Vegetable Lo Mein" on most Chinese restaurant menus in the United States. (If it's not on the menu, ask the waiter to have it made for you. Every Chinese cook knows how to make it, and has the ingredients in his kitchen.) Vegetables are also stir-fried or sautéed and served with rice. An interesting dish is Buddha's Delight, a variety of vegetables stir-fried in a light sauce and served over rice or noodles. I need to use the *cut-it-in-half* method in many Chinese restaurants in the United States. I also need to watch out for tofu, the high protein stuff made from beans. Soy sauce is also high in protein and salt, and is used in nearly every Chinese dish. Adding more at the table is not a good idea for me.

EVEN SOME MEXICAN FOOD IS OKAY

Mexican restaurants are harder to handle than Italian and Chinese because some of the staples of Mexican cooking are high in protein and fat. For example, the "refried beans" served in every Mexican restaurant are made with lard—saturated animal fat—and the beans themselves have a high protein content. I have them on my list of dangerous foods, dangerous not only for kidney patients, but maybe for everybody because of the fat content. Another Mexican food staple is cheese, which seems to find its way into most dishes.

Here's another restaurant experiment. Go to a Mexican restaurant with some other people. Everybody orders something different from the "Mexican Specialties" portion of the menu. When the meals arrive, see if you can tell the difference between them. In my experience in Mexican restaurants in the United States, I can never tell the difference. In fact, I decided at the start of my nutritional therapy that I would steer clear of Mexican restaurants, because of all the beans, cheese, sour cream, hamburger and chicken. But a fellow patient, Dr. Murray West and his wife Therese O'Malley, taught our kidney patients' support group members how to eat at least some Mexican food. They brought to a group meeting all the ingredients for low-protein, low-fat tacos. We all liked it, and we learned how to order something in a Mexican restaurant. Just tell the waiter to leave out the hamburger and the sour cream. You may find some other things too, as long as you watch the portion sizes, and avoid the dangerous foods. Murray and Therese even spent a 2 week vacation in Mexico.

SOME OTHER ETHNIC CUISINES ARE FASCINATING

I learned many years ago that I could often find the best ethnic cooking in very small and inexpensive restaurants tucked away in the corners of ethnic neighborhoods. (In fact, I think some people have discovered a universal law of restaurant dining: The bigger the restaurant, the worse the food. A corollary: The more expensive the restaurant, the worse the food. These laws are not always true, but often enough to make them a useful tool for choosing restaurants.)

The best ethnic restaurants I've ever found in the United States are run by recent immigrants. Sometimes these small restaurants are in the old urban ethnic neighborhoods, like the Italian neighborhoods in New York, Boston, Philadelphia and Baltimore, for example, or Chinatown in New York and Philadelphia. Sometimes, they are in a suburban strip mall, or occasionally even next to a fast food store on a highway. No matter where they are located, they are almost always small, and the owner or his wife does the cooking, or at least supervises the cooks who are often also recent immigrants. (In fact, the law about size is always true, in my experience, with ethnic restaurants. The bigger it is, the worse it is. Perhaps that happens when the owner becomes a manager instead of a head cook.)

Of course, not all small ethnic restaurants are good. Some are dreadful, dirty, and heaven knows what goes on in the kitchen. Sometimes local newspapers or regional magazines review the small restaurants, or publish guides to low-cost or ethnic restaurants, but I have usually found the best ones simply by trial and error. The prices are always reasonable, sometimes very inexpensive, so the cost of a mistake is not high. When I find a good one, I go there often with my family. Sometimes they like the food; sometimes they don't, but whenever my daughters say something like, "We don't like Lebanese food," I suggest that they may be "culture-bound," a label they don't like. The suggestion usually motivates them to try something new. Often they like it.

MIDDLE EASTERN CUISINE

I have never travelled in the Middle East or Greece, so my experience with the cuisines of the eastern Mediterranean comes exclusively from ethnic restaurants in the United States and Europe. I suppose someone who really knows the authentic Middle Eastern cooking (as I know something of the cooking of China, Italy and Mexico, plus France, Belgium, Germany, Austria, Switzerland and Great Britain) would be surprised at my comments. But for kidney patients, the Middle Eastern cuisines have some delights.

A Lebanese or Greek restaurant, for example, has a delicious dish called *baba ghanoush*, a sort of paté of roasted eggplant, garlic, olive oil and spices. Not many Americans grow up eating eggplant or baba ghanoush, so it's something I had to try. The rice rolled in grape leaves or cabbage leaves is tasty and well within the limits of a protein-restricted diet. Vegetable soup and Lebanese salad are also good.

Another staple of this cuisine is not so "kidney friendly"—the paté of chick peas, sesame seeds, olive oil and spices known as *hummus*. It's great nutrition for my family, and they love it, but not so good for me because of the high protein content of the chickpeas and the sesame seeds. Some other vegetarian items on the menu are also on my dangerous list because of the use of chick peas and sesame seeds. The Middle Eastern pita bread is delicious, but I have to be careful not to eat too much because of the protein content. (You may want to try a cup of Turkish coffee after dinner, a deliciously strong brew with a character different from European espresso.)

VIETNAMESE COOKING IS VERY DIFFERENT FROM CHINESE COOKING, WITH SOME DELIGHTFUL SURPRISES

I was too old for military service in Viet Nam and our children were too young, so the horrors of that war are not as immediate for me as they may be for other kidney patients. Going to a Vietnamese neighborhood in Philadelphia or New York doesn't bring back unpleasant memories. Instead, it gives me and my family the chance to enjoy a traditional Asian cuisine that is as different from Chinese cooking as Italian is from English.

The best Vietnamese restaurants I know are small and very inexpensive; most of the customers are orientals. When you are looking over the menu, glance around the room and try the McDonald's experiment. Count the number of customers. Then count the number of *overweight* customers. I don't think I have ever seen an obese person in a Vietnamese restaurant, certainly not an oriental, and I can't remember any overweight Americans either. Could there be a connection? (As I wrote this I tried to remember whether I had ever seen an overweight oriental anywhere—in American Chinatowns or in the Far East. I can't remember any.)

As you look around the restaurant, you will probably see the Vietnamese customers eating with chop sticks from what looks like a large bowl of soup. There are endless variations of this dish that is often called *Phô*. It's a broth based on beef, pork, fish or shell fish with noodles and often vegetables, with generous quantities of the herb I know as *cilantro*. In Viet Nam, I have been told, people eat some variation of Phô two or three times a day. Some versions are very spicy, but there is always a bottle of hot chili sauce on the table to spice it even more. The bowl of Phô is served with a plate of fresh bean sprouts, a wedge of lime, fresh spearmint leaves and a few tiny peppers that look like miniature jalopenas.

The Vietnamese—and the experienced Americans—put some cold fresh bean sprouts into the steaming bowl of soup, squeeze in some lime juice and put the lime twist in the bowl, then add some leaves of fresh mint on the top. A lover of spicy food, like me, adds a tiny pepper and a splash or two of the hot chili sauce. A kidney patient can eat Phô if he skips the meat or fish and doesn't eat all the noodles. It's unlike anything I ever ate before. The combination of steaming hot soup, cold bean sprouts, fresh mint, lime and pepper is very unusual. It sounds bizarre, but my family loves it.

Vietnamese cooking has perhaps adopted some techniques from the French colonial rulers who controlled Indochina for many decades. You will see on the menu appetizers such as "Vietnamese Crêpe," a sort of omelette that a Vietnamese cook may have learned from a Frenchman. Too many eggs for a kidney patient.

There is another appetizer that my family loves—*Nem Nuong*, a dish that a kidney patient can sample, with a little discretion. It's some very small meat balls (not good for a kidney patient) served with a plate of lettuce, thinly sliced carrot, radish and cucumbers, and a dish of special sauce. There are also a few pieces of "rice paper," a wafer thin pancake, thin as a piece of paper, made from rice and steamed for a minute or two to heat and soften it as an Italian cook would boil pasta. The traditional Vietnamese way is to put a piece of rice paper on the plate, add a meat ball or two, add some lettuce, radish, carrot and cucumber, then roll it all up and dip it in the special sauce. A kidney patient can modify the dish slightly by just skipping the meat balls, but enjoying the unusual combination of vegetables, rice paper and sauce. I find it delicious, and my family loves it with the meatballs or without.

INDIAN FOOD HAS SOME GREAT SURPRISES

Although I have never travelled in India, I have sampled what I have been told is good Indian cooking in London and in the United States. The big and expensive rule holds true for Indian restaurants, in my experience; the smaller and less expensive, the better the food. Best of all is the place where the owner is a recent immigrant from India and is still in the kitchen cooking the way thousands of years of Indian cuisine have taught him to cook.

To speak of "Indian cooking," an Indian would probably tell me, is as ridiculous as speaking of "European cooking." (There's not much in common between a dinner in a restaurant specializing in "English" cooking and an authentic Italian restaurant in Florence or Venice. So maybe what I think of as Indian cooking is simply a small sample of what I would find when I visit India. In any case, it is delicious, and with a little care can fit in to a "kidney-friendly" diet.)

The religious beliefs of many people in India teach them not to eat meat. (Their tradition may be the opposite of the European tradition that prosperous people should be eating mostly meat.) A natural result is that Indians have learned to use vegetables and grains, creating interesting and nutritious foods, some of which a kidney patient can use. There are some Indian vegetarian foods on the danger list, though, and you will spot them quickly on the menu. Lentils and peas are staples of Indian cooking, providing much of the protein—too much for a kidney patient. I have to merely sample those dishes. Yogurt is often used; also too much protein for a kidney patient. But there are dozens of dishes based on vegetables with a variety of sauces, like the curries with many spices Americans don't usually encounter. These dishes are often based on potatoes, cabbage, eggplant, and squash, all excellent choices for a kidney patient, provided the portion size is not excessive. The many varieties of Indian bread are delicious, great for dipping in the sauce, but it's easy for me to eat too much bread (because of the protein content.) The rice and chutneys served with the meal are often perfect for a kidney diet.

EATING AT SOMEONE ELSE'S HOME

Some people think eating at the home of a friend or relative is harder than eating in a restaurant, but for some reason it has never been hard for me. There is always *something* to eat, unless the person cooking for you is completely committed to bad food. If they serve you pizza, for example, and only pizza, it will be tough. You'll have to eat very little, or take off all the cheese and non-vegetable toppings, and even then you must limit the amount of pizza crust you eat.

If they serve you, say, hamburgers and potato salad, you can eat some potato salad, maybe half the hamburger roll, but not much more. You'll have to skip the ice cream they serve for dessert. If it's a formal dinner party, with a big prime rib roast, chances are there will be some potatoes, vegetables and salad to go along with it. I try to remember that it's not only healthy for a kidney patient, but for everybody, it seems, to eat less meat. Now in the 1990s, it's even fashionable. Your friends and relatives may tease you about your bizarre eating habits—until, that is, they find out that you're doing it to save your life from a terminal disease. Then they may admire your skill and determination. If they're like some of my friends and relatives, they may even start eating a better diet themselves when they see how much excess weight you lost. They may even call you "skinny." That was music to my ears.

15
A Support Group
Can Make The Difference

By now you may have decided that you want to try *controlling your kidney disease*, with the chance to avoid the need for dialysis and transplant. If so, you may have asked your doctor about the medical research reported in this book. The conversation may have been difficult.

If your doctor is from the "patients-should-follow-orders" school of doctoring, he may have scoffed at your questions. "Where did you learn about nutritional treatment—from the *Readers' Digest*? The book is by a *patient*? What does he know about kidney disease? I've been studying it for twenty years in thousands of patients."

Or, he may have given you a more thoughtful answer. "I'm happy that the author had such good results from nutritional therapy. Some people have hobbled on crutches to the cathedral at Lourdes and come skipping away after a miraculous cure. The author's experience doesn't prove anything to anybody—except that something in his own case caused his kidney disease to stabilize for a while. It my take a nosedive any day. He may even be dead by now, for all I know. Furthermore, nobody can say for sure *why* his disease stabilized. It may be completely unrelated to the nutritional treatment. I've seen it happen dozens of times."

If he is more respectful of you and more candid, he may have even told you some other reasons why he doesn't want to get involved with conservative treatment for your kidney disease. "I don't know much about nutritional treatment. I wouldn't know how to advise you. You would also need help from a dietitian who knows about nutritional treatment for kidney disease, and we don't have a dietitian here who knows about anything but dialysis and transplant. Your insurance company probably wouldn't pay for my services, or the dietitian's services, even if we had one. I would have to argue with the insurance company, or with you, to get paid. If the treatment didn't work out as you hope, you might even sue me for malpractice, for trying a treatment the nephrology profession considers 'unproven.' Even the scientists advocating nutritional therapy say they haven't proven their case yet. The director of the big government study has already said he doesn't think nutritional treatment will ever be practical because it's too hard for patients to follow. So, if you want to try this, you'll have to find another doctor, as the author of the book did."

IF YOU WANT TO TRY NUTRITIONAL THERAPY ANYWAY

If your doctor has given you any of these answers—from the disrespectful "follow-my-orders" to the more thoughtful and candid answers, you may face a dilemma. People with kidney disease need a helpful kidney doctor they can respect and work with, but if he scoffs at a treatment you want to try, the chances are you will fail. You may not have the knowledge or confidence to succeed. You may have to find a doctor who is willing to try to help you, and not in a grudgingly skeptical way.

You will find in Appendix 2 the names and addresses of some physicians-scientists from several cities in the United States and Europe who have experience with nutritional treatment for chronic kidney disease. They may be willing to help you, or to refer you to others who can. Your insurance company may listen to your requests for reimbursement, particularly if you can talk to someone other than a clerk, and if you show them this book and its extensive medical references. Your employer's personnel department may be able to help you with the insurance company. Many companies have come to realize that some doctors are not always interested in preventing or controlling disease. Some are more eager to treat illness than they are to promote health. Some employers have begun active programs to *prevent disease and promote health* among their employees, realizing that money spent on preventing disease is likely to be far better spent than on trying to treat disease when it is far advanced.

I worked hard to find a doctor who would help me with nutritional therapy. You may have to do the same, because if you and the doctor are not on the same team—that is, if he scoffs at your attempts to *control* your disease—your chances of success may be slim. I doubt that I could have come as far as I have with my own treatment without doctors that were sympathetic and helpful.

AFTER YOU HAVE FOUND A HELPFUL DOCTOR ...

If you have some good experience with a "support group," the rest of this chapter will be old news for you. Our family learned about support groups in our attempts to deal with the mental illness of one of our sons. Other people have learned from groups organized to help victims of alcoholism, gambling addiction, divorce, cancer, diabetes and so on. Support groups have worked for our family; in fact, I'm not sure how we would have survived the first years of living with mental illness if we had not been in a support group.

Your doctor may not think much of support groups. He may not have much experience with them; he may consider them amateurish and a waste of his professional time; he may even feel threatened by the prospect of his patients getting organized and discussing the care he is providing. In any case, be prepared to hear your doctor scoff when you ask about a support group, even if he is a helpful doctor you have located after a diligent search. His scorn of support groups doesn't make him a "bad doctor;" it simply means that you will have to take more responsibility and help bring him along. My experience tells me that a successful support group soon convinces the doctor of its value.

WHAT IS A SUPPORT GROUP?

When a suicide attempt brought our son Marc's mental illness to a critical stage in 1983, our family learned about support groups for the first time. The private mental hospital in Philadelphia where Marc was confined for five months organized a family support group for relatives of mentally ill patients. The group was led by a psychiatric social worker with long experience in dealing with mentally ill people and their relatives.[1] About a dozen mothers and fathers, sisters and brothers attended the two hour sessions.

Mental illness is devastating to a family. The mentally ill person suffers terribly, perhaps from delusions, often from depression. His behavior is often bizarre, destructive and even cruel to family members. His actions can cause great harm to the family, to say nothing of the thousands or even hundreds of thousands of dollars of often uninsured expenses for doctors and mental hospitals. (Most insurance policies strictly limit the spending on mental illness, and the price of a month in a private mental hospital in the mid 1980s was over $12,000.)

The worst part, by far, is the *guilt* that the family members feel for having caused, or at least not having *prevented* the mental illness. "What did I do to make Marc like this? What did I *fail* to do that would have prevented this?" And the *loss* of a healthy son or brother, transformed into a pathetic mental patient who never seemed to get well. My wife had the toughest job of dealing with guilt. Her work was not made any easier by the psychiatrist advising us who apparently believed that the mother's behavior toward the infant and young child is the principal cause of mental illness. My wife is a trained psychiatric social worker with the M.S.W. degree from New York University and the A.C.S.W. certification. She should have known better than to listen to the psychiatrist about the mother's causing mental illness. But the feelings of guilt and loss were very real, for her and for the rest of the family. Our daughter Susan felt both the loss and the guilt. "Marc had been a big brother to me. Suddenly he was gone, replaced by a mentally ill person I didn't even know." We needed the support group.

"I REALIZED THAT I WAS NOT ALONE"

At the end of the first session, one parent thanked the leader and the other group members. "I am so happy to learn that other people have the same experiences with mental illness that our family does. We were feeling very alone." I have participated in other support groups since then, including one for kidney patients at Johns Hopkins. I have never attended a meeting where a new group member did *not* say, "I am so relieved that I am not alone with this problem." Perhaps that's the most important function of a support group: people with a common life problem coming together to share information and emotions, to be helpers of others and receivers of help, to take constructive action toward shared goals, to develop a collective willpower and belief—in short, to be a *group* facing a common problem, not an isolated individual.[2,3]

COMMON EXPERIENCES AND NEEDS

You may have personal experience with support groups, or you may just know of them: Alcoholics Anonymous, Gamblers Anonymous, Al-Anon (for family members of alcoholics), Parents Without Partners, Overeaters Anonymous. The groups work when members share a common experience. Alcoholics can often understand and help other alcoholics; gamblers, other gamblers. "Many persons come into Al-Anon thinking that they alone have suffered these 'unique' experiences," writes an expert on support groups.[4] When they realize that their "unique" problem is universal and when they realize they have found a safe place to talk about their own feelings and the ways they have developed to handle the problems, the benefits become obvious and the support group begins to work.

Our informal kidney patients' support group at Johns Hopkins met every three months for the first year. Then, a desire for more frequent meetings arose spontaneously; we decided on monthly meetings, with some people coming to Baltimore from as far as Washington, Philadelphia and even New York. The group was working.

MUTUAL HELP AND SUPPORT

Everybody in our mental illness support group had a mentally ill relative; everybody in our kidney patient support group has kidney disease, or is a family member of the kidney patient. Each person is a member of a group that meets regularly to help one another. Each individual *gives help* and *receives help*. It may even be that the helper gets the most benefit from the process.[5] Some experienced group leaders look for ways to turn *recipients* of help into *givers* of help because they have observed some positive benefits. The giver of help often feels good about helping others, feels a sense of equality with those he helps. The helper often learns while he is helping, as good teachers learn from their students; good managers, from their employees. Often the helper feels social and personal approval from the people he helps. The act of helping others can be a powerful tool.

Kidney patients learning to control their disease with nutritional therapy spend much energy learning how to live on 25 grams of protein a day—less protein than a single Big Mac at McDonald's. It takes some knowledge and ingenuity to eat so little protein, so the support group members share their know-how. At one meeting, a discussion of eating in ethnic restaurants ended with the conclusion that a kidney patient could find something to eat in most ethnic restaurants except one—Mexican. At the next meeting, Dr. Murray West and his wife Therese O'Malley, brought "kidney patient tacos" to the group meeting, complete with everything but the hamburger and grated cheese, and including a nutritional analysis. Murray and Therese were *helping* the rest of us learn to eat some Mexican food. It was the *helper principle* at work.

COLLECTIVE WILL POWER AND BELIEF

Everybody in our kidney patient support group is trying to control his kidney disease with nutrition and other lifestyle changes, like losing excess weight, keeping the blood pressure down with diet, exercise and maybe drugs. It's not easy to *unlearn* the habits of a lifetime. I often ate far more than the one hundred grams of protein the average American consumes in the 1990s, damaging my diseased kidneys. Now I must somehow find the will power and belief to eat one-fifth as much protein. The group has helped me. I can look to the other group members to validate my feelings and attitudes.[6] When Murray West or Sandra Watt, Edith Kahn, or Gary and Dianne Dulin share their cooking tips or recipe ideas, I not only learn some new information, but I sense that this process actually works. They help me in my efforts to help myself.

THE IMPORTANCE OF INFORMATION

We started the support group at Johns Hopkins with the help of Dr. Walser and his team, particularly an experienced renal dietitian, Lynne Ward, the co-author of some of Dr. Walser's research. The purpose was to share information about nutrition, cooking, eating out—in short, living with the nutritional treatment. The first few meetings were informal and unstructured, but Dr. Walser and Ms. Ward were there to provide information, answer our questions. As we became more experienced, we began a newsletter, *The Third Treatment;* my daughter Susan was the editor. Group members began preparing specific contributions for the meetings and newsletter. We were working toward a better understanding of our common problem, trying to control our kidney disease.

In our mental illness group we learned that there is often a biochemical cause of mental illness, not just the mother's inadequate mothering. We learned some ways to cope with our feelings of guilt and loss. We even tried to understand that we were not responsible for causing the mental illness. We learned techniques for dealing with delusions and depression. We learned about books to read, lectures to attend, television shows to watch, other self-help groups to join. We were sharing information.

CONSTRUCTIVE ACTION TOWARD SHARED GOALS

Kidney patients want to live as normally as they can without risking transplant or dialysis. Relatives of mentally ill people want to protect themselves from the erratic behavior of their relative and be a positive influence on his attempt to deal with his mental illness. The members of each group were engaging in activities that could help them avoid being passive toward their illness. They were also working to develop a greater sense of personal responsibility for their own health, and perhaps enhanced self-esteem from having made a difference, to themselves and others. Support groups are oriented to action: share a recipe, a cooking or shopping tip; contribute to a newsletter; present some information on a topic other group members care about. Some experts have called support group members "emotional activists." They are working toward being more aware of themselves and others, of feeling and expressing their emotions, helping others and thus themselves.

SOME SCIENTIFIC EVIDENCE
THAT SUPPORT GROUPS WORK

People who have good experience with support groups know how helpful they can be, but now there is some scientific evidence that they may do more than make people feel better.[7] A psychiatrist treating eighty skin cancer patients at the UCLA medical school organized a support group for half of the patients, but did nothing special for the other half. (It was a *controlled trial*, the kind of study nephrologists say is needed for nutritional treatment; half the patients treated, the other half not.) The support groups met weekly for an hour and a half for six weeks, learning about dealing with exposure to sun light, about loneliness, fear and depression. They used the techniques of support groups to help each other through the emotional and physical crisis of cancer.

After the six weeks of support group sessions ended, the psychiatrist could find little difference between the treated and untreated patients. But six months later there were big differences that could be measured in the laboratory. Two thirds of the support group patients had stronger immune systems than before their work with the support groups. They had 25 percent more of the natural "killer cells" that the body throws into the battle against cancer. Only one of the untreated patients had a similar increase. The support group patients had also improved in other ways compared to the untreated patients. They were more vigorous, less depressed. They were better able to handle their feelings about cancer by consulting a friend or a doctor, or by simply "taking one day at a time." The patients who were *not* in the support groups were more passive, more resigned, more interested in preparing themselves for "the worst" while concealing their distress from people close to them.

Other studies have found similar results. A psychiatrist at Stanford University found that women with advanced breast cancer who participated in a support group while they received medical treatment *lived twice as long* as women who received *only* the medical treatment.[8] A psychologist at the University of Iowa found that even the *spouses* of cancer patients had stronger immune systems if they felt they had strong support systems in their lives. Even the spouses had more killer cells than those who felt more isolated.[9] A psychologist at Stanford found that *monkeys* benefit from support groups. He put a monkey in a stressful situation, with bright lights and loud noises. His body reacted by increasing the level of a hormone that helps prepare for quick action, but suppresses the immune system. The monkey's body may have been getting ready to defend itself against outside attack, but it may have also been weakening its defense against disease. When the psychologist put five other monkeys in the cage, there was no increase in the hormone. Could it be that the "support group" was helping the monkey's body be ready to fight disease?

Do studies like these prove that a support group can help people fight cancer or other diseases? No, say some researchers, but it certainly can't hurt and it may help. Some physician-scientists think the findings are significant enough that *all* cancer patients, and even those at high risk for cancer, should be encouraged to join support groups.[10]

FINDING A SUPPORT GROUP, OR STARTING ONE

If you have found a helpful doctor, and if you are undertaking nutritional therapy, you may want to find a support group. You may have to start one yourself. The American Association of Kidney Patients (AAKP), founded by kidney patients to help kidney patients, has local groups in 26 cities. Their focus is on helping patients who are already on dialysis or who have already had a transplant. Like the National Kidney Foundation and the American Kidney Fund, they don't do much, if anything, about nutritional treatment for kidney disease. It wouldn't be surprising if none of them know much about it. The AAKP publishes a twice yearly magazine, *Renalife*, and a quarterly newspaper, *The Bulletin;* they also organize an annual convention. When I called asking about nutritional treatment to prevent kidney failure, they told me that they didn't have any information about that, but they were very willing to share the information they did have about patients on dialysis and after transplant. Perhaps someday they will help patients *avoid* kidney failure, not just live with it.

The National Kidney Foundation (NKF) has branches in most major cities and much local activity, including support groups for dialysis patients and publications for kidney patients. I wasn't able to find any NKF material about nutritional therapy to prevent kidney failure. (That's one of the reasons I did the research and wrote this book. Nobody else would tell me about it.) You will find in Appendix 3 the addresses and a brief description of the AAKP, the NKF and some other organizations with special interests in kidney disease. I wasn't able to get any help from any of them because, I suppose, nutritional therapy is so widely ignored in the United States.

I'm not sure I could have achieved as much as I have with my own nutritional therapy without the support group at Johns Hopkins. As the support group was invaluable in learning to live with our son's mental illness, the kidney patient support group has been invaluable in learning to live with kidney disease. If I couldn't find one to join, I would have started one. It's not hard, and the rewards are enormous. Write to me. I'll send you some material that may help you get started. A support group can make the difference.

16
Joy And Sadness

My wife is a social worker who helps supervise the care of newborn infants and their mothers at an inner city teaching hospital in Camden, New Jersey. The hospital is the best-appointed building in town, much better than the public schools, as inner city hospitals often are. It is in the midst of what, by some measures, is the poorest urban ghetto in the country, not far from Independence Hall and the Liberty Bell across the river in Philadelphia.

Some of the infants that my wife tries to help have been born prematurely, sometimes weighing as little as a pound or two. Some have been born to ghetto mothers addicted to crack, cocaine or heroin. The babies often stay for days, weeks or even months in an intensive care unit especially designed, equipped and staffed to care for babies born so prematurely that as recently as ten or twenty years ago they would probably have died soon after birth. Now many such infants survive, beneficiaries of some "miracles of modern medicine." Some leave the hospital to return to their drug-abusing ghetto mothers' households in Camden, leaving behind them hospital bills for tens or even hundreds of thousands of dollars, often to be paid by taxpayers.

When my wife first began to work with these tiny babies, she wondered how much medical care had been devoted to *preventing* premature births, instead of keeping the tiny babies alive *after* birth. She soon learned that many of the underprivileged mothers had *no prenatal care*. Instead of receiving the routine care that might have allowed her to carry the baby to the full term, a ghetto mother often showed up in the emergency room with her baby ready to be born weeks early. My wife wondered if the

money spent on heroic efforts in the infant intensive care unit could have
been better spent on *preventing* the premature birth.

A mile or two away is another hospital in inner city Camden. Across the
street, in a building that looks as if it may have once been a supermarket,
is what the large sign calls the "Regional Artificial Kidney and Transplant
Center." Inside are hemodialysis machines and a transplant program. Like
the intensive care unit for premature babies, this center is especially designed, equipped and staffed to provide other "miracles of modern medicine." There were 1,931 units like this one in the United States in 1989,
one unit for every 129,000 people. In 1981 there had been only 1,143 such
centers, one for every 200,000 people. Most of the new centers were
privately-owned, for-profit dialysis and transplant centers. The kidney
business was a growth industry in the 1980s, mostly paid for by money
that Medicare got from taxpayers and that insurance companies got from
premium-payers.[1]

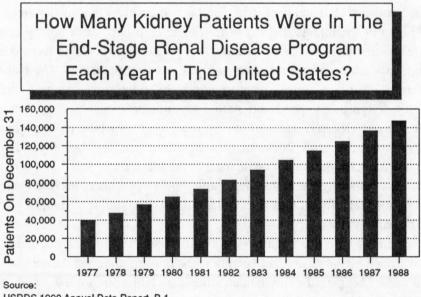

Figure 56 Prevalence Of End-Stage Kidney Disease

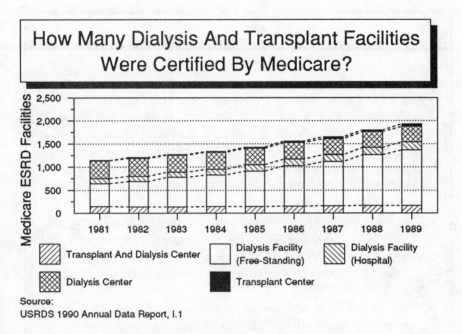

Figure 57 Medicare-Certified ESRD Facilities

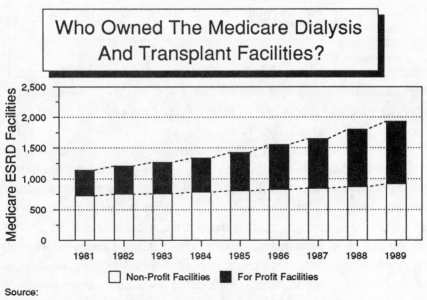

Figure 58 Ownership Of Medicare-Certified ESRD Facilities

A Former Governor Warns About The Cost Of High Technology Medicine

- Richard D. Lamm, former governor of Colorado and now professor of public policy at the University of Denver, has written and lectured extensively on the high cost of high technology medical care.
- "... to impress upon health providers what they are doing when they order marginal services, we should require them to imagine an American worker sentenced to a period of slavery long enough to pay the medical bill for that procedure."
- "Dr. Thomas Starzl recently gave a liver transplant to a 76-year-old woman. It cost $240,000. Dr. Starzl should understand that, with the average U.S. family making $24,000 a year, he has sentenced 100 U.S. families to work all year so that he could transplant a 76-year-old woman."
- "Such actions are cheating our children of resources that they desperately need to build a better life and to revitalize the United States economically."
- "A nation that runs $200 billion deficits and borrows 20¢ from its children out of every dollar it spends must one day demand more accountability from its politicians, from its industries, and from its health providers."

Source: Lamm, 1987.

The artificial kidney and transplant center in inner city Camden, like the nearly two thousand others in the country, is directed and staffed and often owned by people whose livelihoods may depend on *utilization* of the center. If there are not enough kidney patients at the dialysis stations, the director of the program may be judged to be using his resources inefficiently; perhaps his income will be less. If there are not enough transplants done each year, the director may be criticized for not covering the overhead of the transplant program; perhaps his income will also be less. If there are not enough prematurely born infants in the intensive care unit, the hospital administrator may be criticized for not keeping the beds occupied; his income may also be less. I wondered if we must use the armies of medical care workers in the 1990s *simply because they are there?*

A KIDNEY PATIENT LEARNS ABOUT THE MEDICAL CARE SYSTEM

As I read the medical research about my kidney disease and thought about my wife's experience, I began to learn about what the media sometimes call "the health care crisis." I learned that Americans spend far more of our income on medical care than people of other industrialized countries, in some cases twice as much. Yet, by most measures we have about the same rates of sickness and death, sometimes even worse results than the countries that spend far less.[2] I learned that as an average American I worked for the first six weeks of every year in the late 1980s to pay for nothing but medical care. In 1990 Americans spent about $2,500 on doctors, hospitals and drugs for every man, woman and child in the country. By 2000 some experts think the medical bills will be $5,500 per person.[3] Americans were already spending more on medical care than we spent on

---

Transplant Surgeon Dr. Starzl Replies To Governor Lamm

- "The 76-year-old patient whose treatment was decried is coming up to the one-year follow-up mark in excellent condition at home."
- "The enslavement of 100 families, working for one year to pay a $240,000 medical bill, was not required."
- "Surgical fees were written off. The hospital cost of $68,000 has not been paid and may never be."
- "Developments in transplantation and artificial organ technology have changed forever the philosophy by which organ-defined specialties such as nephrology, hepatology, and cardiology are practiced."
- "Until recently, what could be offered victims of vital-organ failure was a rearguard approach designed with diet, medicines, or surgical procedures to extract the last moment of life-supporting function from the failed organ."
- "Now, and for the first time in human history, the breathtaking possibility has emerged of starting over when all else fails, with an organ graft or with a manufactured organ."

Source: Starzl, 1987.

A Potential Transplant Candidate Thinks About The Debate Between Governor Lamm and Dr. Starzl

- Governor Lamm thinks Americans allow doctors and hospitals to spend too much on high technology, life-extending medical care—like Dr. Starzl's $240,000 liver transplant for a 76-year-old woman.
- Dr. Starzl replies that the $68,000 hospital bill was "unpaid" anyway, and the surgeons' fees were "written off."
- I wondered where the hospital got the $68,000 to cover the bills for the woman's liver transplant. The nurses and the operating room staff had to be paid; the electric bill and the drugs had to be paid. *Somebody had to pay the $68,000.*
- I wondered if the *other patients* at that hospital had paid higher hospital bills to make up for the unpaid transplant bill. I wondered if Dr. Starzl knew that *somebody had to pay* the hospital bill.
- Dr. Starzl also didn't specify, in this reply to Governor Lamm's editorial, the *amount* of the "surgical fees that were written off." I wondered if the "write off" may have been subsidized when other taxpayers paid more, or the federal deficit was higher, to make up for the lower income taxes paid by some transplant surgeons.
- I wondered if Dr. Starzl knew that *somebody had to pay for high technology medicine.* I wondered if he knew, as Governor Lamm knew, that all Americans are paying for high technology medicine that we can no longer afford.

food, almost as much as we spent on housing, more than on education or national defense.[4]

Yet I didn't write checks for that $2,500 a year for each member of my family. My medical care was "free." My bills for doctors, drugs and hospitals were "covered." I simply "submitted" the bills to somebody who paid them, my "health insurance company." I had learned to think of my medical care as "free." Maybe that's why I got so much of it. I didn't pay. Somebody else paid.

When I spent a moment thinking about these facts, I understood that, of course, my medical care was *not* free. I paid for everything I got. I may not have been writing checks to doctors, hospitals and pharmacies for more than a token share of my medical bills, *but I was paying nonetheless.* When I bought a new car, Chrysler Corporation used some of the price I paid to pay medical bills for Chrysler employees. Toyota paid less per car for its employees' medical costs. When I paid my telephone bill, or when I bought some new books, the companies would use some of what I paid to cover the medical bills of their employees. Almost one-third of Americans medical bills were paid by city, county, state and federal governments, like the unpaid bills left behind by the "crack moms" and their premature babies at the inner city hospital in Camden.[5] *Somebody had to pay the doctors and hospitals.* My medical care was *not* free, even though I had come to think of it as free. As an American citizen and voter, I had participated in organizing our medical care system in a way that encouraged me to think of medical care as being "free." I was as guilty as anybody of letting myself think of medical care as "free." I had been an entrepreneur. I had provided "free health insurance" for my employees. I had asked my customers to pay more, so that my company would have the money to pay insurance premiums, so that the insurance companies would have the money to pay doctors and hospitals for the medical care that my employees would consider "free." I had contributed to the excessive spending on medical care that some people said America can no longer afford.[6,7]

HOW CAN WE SPEND MORE ON MEDICAL CARE AND BE LESS HEALTHY?

I wondered how Americans could spend so much more on health care than other countries spend, yet not achieve better results measured by life expectancy, infant mortality, and overall sickness and death rates. Where was the money going? *Were we spending money on the wrong things?* Were we asking doctors and hospitals to do with expensive medicine some of what we could do for ourselves with more attention and effort? Could the medical care system expert and former Secretary of Health, Education and Welfare Joseph Califano, Jr. be right when he said this:

"Each of us can do more for our own health than any doctor, any hospital, any machine, or any drug."[8]

Did Secretary Califano mean that the patient was more responsible for his own health than the doctors, the hospitals, the machines, the drugs? Did he mean that Americans could avoid the need for some high technology medicine, prevent some of the chronic diseases that killed most of us? *Did he mean that we don't need as much costly high technology medicine?*

The former governor of Colorado, Richard D. Lamm, has spoken even more bluntly about our excessive demand for medical technology.

"The miracles of medicine have outstripped our ability to pay... Health care is an economic cancer." [9]

I began to realize how my attitudes toward medical care had changed in my lifetime. Some new ideas had penetrated to the marrow of my bones:

- I had come to expect doctors and hospitals to be responsible for my health. *I* was not responsible; *they* were responsible. Doctors knew best. They would do what I needed.

- Doctors and hospitals would treat me *aggressively*. They would *remove* disease from my body with drugs, scalpels, transplants and artificial organs. They would *control* my sickness. They would fix what went wrong with my body. They would prolong my life, cheating death with their "miracles of modern medicine." I would be simply a passive spectator, complying with doctor's orders.

- Someone else would *pay* for these medical miracles, not I. The government would pay, or my insurance company. All this costly treatment was "covered." It was not my financial responsibility, no more than it was my responsibility to preserve my own health. The more medical care I got, and the more expensive it was, the better it was. Medical care was "free." It was my right, my entitlement.

My attitudes were shared perhaps by some other Americans, and by some doctors. Was that a reason why we were spending so much on doctors, hospitals and drugs without a corresponding improvement in the objective measures of our health?

SOME NEW ATTITUDES FOR A KIDNEY PATIENT

America may have a "health care crisis," as some experts say, but for me it was a personal crisis. The doctors had advised me to let my disease get worse, to let it progress until it reached end-stage. Then, they would practice their miracles to rescue me from death. The doctors' attitudes fit in with my attitudes toward medical care. The *doctors* were responsible, not I. They knew what was best. They would treat me aggressively, ripping the disease out of my body with drugs, knives and artificial organs. They would fix what was wrong with my body, and, *somebody else would pay them.* It was the *paradigm* of modern American medicine, the whole constellation of beliefs and institutions surrounding what had come to be considered successful medical treatment.[10, 11]

But there was something wrong here. I began to understand that I had been part of a 20th century perversion of the goals of medical care. Like many Americans, I had asked medicine to do for me—at great cost and with less-than-hoped-for results—some of what I could do for myself. It was the beginning of the sadness and the joy I learned to feel as a kidney patient. The doctors were advising me to do what *they* wanted to do—practice their medical miracles on me at my fellow Americans' expense. They were not doing what *I* wanted them to do—help me control my disease, live with it in as simple and natural a way as I could, avoid the desperate remedies for as long as I could.

I began to see the connections between how the doctors wanted to treat my kidney disease and how some doctors treated people with heart disease. I learned that people with heart disease who live in La Jolla in southern California are three times as likely to have heart bypass surgery as people who live in Palo Alto in northern California. People in some parts of the country are *twenty* times as likely to have heart bypass surgery as people in other parts of the country. Was there that much variation in the *need* for heart bypass surgery? Did people in southern California really need three times as many heart bypass operations as people in northern California? Or, were there other reasons? Some studies have shown that between 20 and 40 percent of all procedures performed on patients are unnecessary; and that 25 to 40 percent of hospitalizations are unnecessary.[12] As a patient, I had demanded some of those unnecessary treatments; the doctors and hospitals had provided them, sometimes even promoted them, perhaps like the extra heart bypass operations in southern California.

On a television news broadcast, I heard Dr. Dean Ornish, a medical school professor at the University of California at San Francisco, discussing his medical research with heart patients and his book on *reversing* heart disease, the disease that kills more Americans than any other disease. He has observed that heart patients can not only *stop their disease from getting worse*, but they can also *reverse the damage*. They can clear out the blocked arteries that may be causing the heart disease. There is no miracle drug or surgery needed—simply some changes in diet and lifestyle. Dr. Ornish teaches his patients to eat a very low fat diet—ten percent of total calories, compared to the thirty percent that the establishment recommends and the nearly fifty percent most Americans really eat. He teaches his patients to take a brisk half-hour walk nearly every day, to stop smoking, and to drink only moderate amounts of alcohol. He teaches them to do a yoga-like meditation twice weekly, concentrating on visualizing a healthy heart. The result of this new diet and lifestyle, Dr. Ornish has observed, is heart disease that gets better without drugs or surgery.[13, 14]

The establishment is skeptical. Dr. Virgil Brown, the new president of the American Heart Association, says Dr. Ornish's studies included too few patients and too many variables to produce valid results. Was it the low-fat diet that produced the improvement; or was it the half-hour walk most days; or was it stopping smoking? We don't know, says Dr. Brown, so we have to do more studies. Also, he says, the program may be too difficult for most heart patients to follow.[15]

The establishment's treatment-of-choice for heart disease has become what the doctors call "the cabbage"—*the coronary artery bypass graft*, the *CABG*. Transplant surgeon Dr. Starzl underwent a CABG in the summer of 1990. Surgeons removed veins from his leg and grafted them to his heart, providing an alternate path for blood to the heart, bypassing the clogged arteries. "This treatment literally and figuratively *bypasses the problem*," says Dr. Ornish. The problem is that the patient's arteries are clogged, not getting enough blood to the heart. When the blood flow is interrupted, the result is often a heart attack and permanent damage, even sudden death. The CABG, says Dr. Ornish, simply *bypasses the problem temporarily*. That is exactly what the operation was designed to do: *bypass the clogged arteries*. If the heart patient doesn't change the *lifestyle* that caused his arteries to become clogged in the first place, the newly transplanted arteries may also become clogged. The surgeons may have solved nothing. If Dr. Ornish is right, transplant surgeon Dr. Starzl's self-described diet of doughnuts and cheese fries may have contributed to his heart disease. The CABG may relieve the symptoms for a while, but may do nothing about the cause of the heart disease, nor about the damage already done.

Modern medicine has turned some things upside down, says Dr. Ornish. The accepted treatment for heart disease is *surgery*, perhaps combined with a lifelong regimen of drugs whose long-term effects are not well-understood. This *aggressive* treatment is considered *normal, routine*. A *conservative* treatment like Dr. Ornish's—sensible diet, moderate exercise, stress-lowering, smoking cessation—is considered *too difficult for patients to follow*. Some doctors accept the complex and radical; they ignore the simple and natural. As a patient, I had encouraged doctors to behave as they do. The result was billions spent on high-tech medicine producing less-than-hoped-for outcomes.

It seemed to me that some heart doctors wanted to treat heart disease in nearly the same way that the kidney doctors wanted to treat my kidney

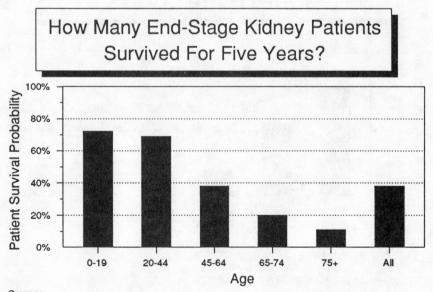

Source:
USRDS 1990 Annual Data Report, E.57

Figure 59 All ESRD Patients, Survival Probability, 5-Year

disease. Let the kidney disease reach end-stage, then treat it with transplant surgery or an artificial organ. Let the heart disease get worse, then treat it with a CABG, heart bypass surgery. Both heart and kidney specialists know about scientifically-supported *conservative treatments* that have been shown to stop the diseases from getting worse, and sometimes even to reverse their harmful effects. But the medical establishment scoffs. I looked again at the government statistics for the survival of the 372,000 Medicare patients who had high technology treatment for their end-stage kidney disease since 1976. I thought the results were poor, no matter what some doctors claimed about "medical miracles."

ANGER MELTS INTO SADNESS

I was angry at first. The doctors knew about simple, low-risk and natural treatments for heart disease and kidney disease. *They knew about them!*

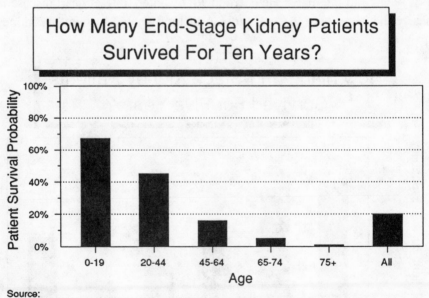

Source:
USRDS 1990 Annual Data Report, E.59

Figure 60 All ESRD Patients, Survival Probability, 10-Year

And they didn't tell me! Instead, they *ignored* them, preferring the high-risk, high-cost, high technology treatments of surgery, drugs and artificial organs. The doctors and hospitals demanded more of our income each year, more than people in any other industrialized country were asked to pay, but the objective measures of Americans' health were no better than those of the Swedes, or Swiss, or Germans. What were we getting for our money? What were we getting for our submission to the risks of high-tech medicine? I felt angry.

Then I heard about the death of Robert DeBragga in 1990. Doctors had diagnosed his terminal cancer twelve years earlier, predicting that he had 36 weeks to live. They prescribed the treatments-of-choice for his cancer—radiation and the use of three different chemotherapy drugs. He agreed to the aggressive treatments, and after a few months was near death. Was it the *cancer* that was killing him, or was it the *cancer treatment*? The answer was not clear. He went to the medical library, as I had done in late 1988. He discovered conservative treatments for his cancer—without the deadly drugs and radiation. He tried the other methods, as I tried the new treatment for kidney disease. His condition improved. He came to believe that *if he had tried the conservative treatments from the beginning*, instead of submitting to the radiation and drug treatments, he might have stopped the cancer. He founded an organization, Project Cure, to teach patients, doctors, bureaucrats and legislators about alternatives to high-tech treatment.[16]

Nearly a decade after his trip to the medical library, Robert DeBragga's cancer turned for the worse. He believed that the radiation and chemotherapy had harmed him, as some kidney patients believe dialysis and transplant harmed them.[17] Nobody can know for sure. He died in 1990, leaving behind a political action movement committed to helping Americans learn that there are alternatives to high technology medicine.[18]

Learning of Robert DeBragga's life and death started melting my anger into sadness. I felt sad that, if he was right, so many other cancer patients were being denied the chance for *conservative treatment* that might have worked, subjecting themselves instead to treatments that Robert DeBragga and some physician-scientists believed caused harm. I felt sad that heart patients were undergoing bypass surgery that some doctors thought would at best only postpone their disease. I felt sad that almost 40,000 kidney patients would be herded to the dialysis machines and the transplant wards every year without ever knowing of a way they might *control* their disease. I felt sad that my attitudes as a patient had encouraged some of the people I had once seen as the miracle workers of modern medicine to become money-eating creatures, wielding scalpels and often-lethal drugs.

THERE WAS JOY, TOO

With my sadness came the joy of learning about the new treatment for my kidney disease. It was there for all to see in the literature of medical science, the work of dedicated physician-scientists around the world, like Dr. Mackenzie Walser, Dr. William Mitch, Dr. Sergio Giovannetti, Dr. Saulo Klahr, Dr. Joel Kopple, Dr. Jonas Bergström, Dr. Norbert Gretz, Dr. Giuseppe Maschio and many others. I had the joy of doing something about my disease, of contributing to my own health, of being more in control of my own life. I had the joy of working with the researchers and other kidney patients in the support group, of helping them succeed—and sometimes fail. I had the joy of plotting a graph of my GFR, the measure of my own kidney function. I could watch it remain stable, sometimes even improve. Most of all, I had the joy of working with my family on this book, trying to put into words and pictures what I had learned, what may help another kidney patient deal with his disease.

A NEW PARADIGM

The old paradigm of medical care has led us to the point where, as Governor Lamm writes:

> **"Health care is clearly entering into a new era: Infinite health needs have run into finite resources. No sector of the economy, no matter how important, can continue to grow at two-and-a-half times the rate of inflation. We are heading rapidly toward an America that has rusting plants, closed factories, staggering trade deficits. Health care cannot continue to operate under the illusion that it can continue with business as usual."** [19]

We can no longer afford to pay for the high technology medical care that too often doesn't help us much anyway. We need to learn new ways. As has so often happened in American history, we need a new book or two, and a "movement." We need Rachel Carson's *Silent Spring*. We need the 1990s equivalent of Earth Day, a start of the environmental movement that helped us all think about protecting our environment. Somewhere in the United States in 1991, I'm sure, somebody is at work right now writing the book that will help Americans think about medical care as Rachel Carson's *Silent Spring* helped us think thirty years ago about the pollution that was fouling our environment.[20] I'm sure that somebody else is at work right now organizing the events and the movement that will dramatize the need for redirecting medical care as Earth Day dramatized the need to protect the environment. These people are at work on one of the great issues of the late 20th century. They are working to help the rest of us lead the American medical care system down the road toward becoming something it is *not*, despite what we call it. We will help our medical care system become a *health care system*.

As the Soviets and East Europeans have learned that communism has converted material and human abundance into scarcity, we will learn that we have transformed some of the medical miracles of our time into arrogant challenges to death, rather than confident enhancements of life. We will learn that it is far better to *prevent* and *control* disease than to *treat* it with heroic and costly medicine that too often leaves patients mutilated and half-dead, like some dialysis and transplant patients. We will learn that we have permitted, perhaps even encouraged our doctors, hospitals, drug companies and the hundreds of thousands of others who are the American medical care industry to spend our money without our consent doing some of the wrong things—like ignoring conservative treatments for kidney and heart disease while promoting dialysis, transplant and bypass surgery. We will learn that patient and doctor are *partners* in attaining good health.

Perhaps Joseph Califano or Richard Lamm will write the book that will become medical care's *Silent Spring*. Perhaps former Surgeon General Dr. C. E. Koop will lead a movement for the new medicine that will rival the environmental movement in its impact on our lives. Or, perhaps it will be the 1990s counterpart of Rachel Carson, a thoughtful and caring person with the vision to see the need for change and the skill and devotion to teach us.

Perhaps it is *you* who will teach Americans about the need to transform *medical care* into *health care*. If so, please let me know about your work. I want to help.

Appendix 1

Facts From The Largest Study Of End-Stage Kidney Disease Ever Made In The United States

As I worked on learning about my kidney disease, I tried to imagine how I might have felt if I had found this book in a neighborhood bookstore on the day after Christmas 1988 when the nephrologist first diagnosed my chronic kidney failure. The doctors' confident descriptions of dialysis and transplant had left me confused and afraid, wanting to know the real facts. I felt like a manager about to hire a new employee, checking the references on the job application; or a home buyer, inspecting the new house for defects. I felt like a baseball or basketball fan studying the box scores in the sports section of the Sunday newspaper to learn how the teams were really doing, or an investor reading the stock tables to find out about the results of his investments. I wanted some *facts* about my kidney disease. I wanted to understand *what really happens* to kidney patients who accept a nephrologist's advice to do nothing about the disease until the kidneys fail, then go on dialysis or get a transplant. Hiring somebody, buying a house, following a sport or checking on an investment were trivial activities compared to the life-and-death matter of choosing a treatment for a terminal disease. Yet I had few facts, certainly less than I had about some trivial things in my life. I wanted more.

I had read about organ transplantation in *Newsweek* a few weeks earlier. The article was headlined, "Interchangeable parts; Transplant surgery is more successful than ever—but organs are in short supply." It quoted the pioneer transplant surgeon Dr. Thomas E. Starzl on the improved results of transplantation in the late 1980s: "We've gone from the unattainable to the routine." The article painted an admiring portrait of the transplant surgeons' work. "The success rate for kidneys is 91 to 96 percent, about the same as it is for corneas, compared with 62 to 65 percent in 1979."[1]

After studying some of the facts, I learned that about one-third of all kidney transplant patients died within five years; two-thirds of cadaver and half of living related transplant recipients died within ten years. That didn't sound to me like the "91 to 96 percent success rate" Newsweek described. The results for transplants from a living blood relative, a living related donor transplant, were better, but not good. About two-thirds of the patients lived for five years; only half, for ten years.[2]

To give you the opportunity to judge for yourself the facts about kidney disease and treatments, I have included in this Appendix extensive excerpts from the most comprehensive study ever done in the United States, perhaps in the world, about *the facts on end-stage kidney disease.* You will find in these pages not the half-truths of some superficial media reports or the sometimes misleading and even self-serving assertions of some advocates of high-technology treatments. Instead, you will find *the facts,* published by the United States government in late 1990. *This is what actually happened to 372,000 kidney patients between 1976 and 1988.* These are not estimates from polls, samples, or studies. These are patient-by-patient descriptions of 372,000 real people who heard a doctor say, "You have end-stage kidney disease."

Your doctor may not know these facts because they were published so recently. You may want to show him this section of the book; it may give him insights into the *actual results,* the *outcome for the patient,* of the treatments he recommends.

These facts are vastly more important than the trivial facts about new houses, new employees, mutual funds or basketball teams that we study every day in our work, in our magazines and newspapers. These are life-and-death-facts for you or for a member of your family. I hope these facts help you to understand, as they helped me.

1. Interchangeable Parts; Transplant surgery is more successful than ever—but organs are in short supply. *Newsweek,* September 12, 1988, p. 61.
2. U.S. Renal Data System, USRDS 1990 Annual Report, The National Institutes of Health, National Institute of Diabetes and Digestive and Kidney Diseases, Bethesda, August, 1990. E.81, E.83, E.89, E.91

UNITED STATES RENAL DATA SYSTEM
1990 ANNUAL DATA REPORT
EXECUTIVE SUMMARY

The United States Renal Data System (USRDS) was created in May 1988 to collect and analyze information on the incidence, prevalence, morbidity, and mortality of end-stage renal disease (ESRD) in the United States. The USRDS is operated by the Coordinating Center (CC) at The Urban Institute, funded by the National Institute of Diabetes and Digestive and Kidney Diseases (NIDDK) of the National Institutes of Health. The Health Care Financing Administration (HCFA) also of the U.S. Department of Health and Human Services participates with NIDDK on the project and supplies expertise and most of the original data to the USRDS.

The USRDS was operational by early 1989, and produced its first annual data report in August 1989. The USRDS entered the implementation phase of the project in May 1990. This USRDS 1990 Annual Data Report is the second volume based on these ESRD data. The annual data reports represent one major vehicle for disseminating information from the US-RDS.

This report addresses extensively the first two goals of the USRDS: 1) to characterize the total renal patient population and describe the distribution of patients by sociodemographic variables across treatment modalities, and 2) to report on the incidence, prevalence, mortality rates, and trends over time of renal disease by primary diagnosis, treatment modality, and other sociodemographic variables. This report makes a modest start toward completion of the third goal, to develop and analyze data on the effect of various modalities of treatment by disease and patient group categories. The fourth goal, to identify problems and opportunities for more focused special studies of renal research issues, is currently being addressed with six special studies requiring new data collection. A report on these six special studies is provided in Chapter XII.

CHANGES SINCE LAST YEAR

This report is larger than last year's report and contains nearly 400 pages of reference tables and 100 pages of text and figures. It contains two entirely new chapters on Transplantation and on Pediatric ESRD, and other chapters have been expanded. The reference tables have been expanded and show more detail by race and by treatment modality. This report represents the largest single compilation of data about ESRD in the United States and possibly in the world. Although many questions are answered here, virtually every table in the report raises new research questions. Future annual data reports will continue to build and expand upon this and the previous report.

The USRDS patient database was updated from HCFA data through March 1990, which allows us to report essentially complete data through December 1988. Institutional data are current through 1989. Over 53,000 new patients (36,000 incident in 1988) and 782,000 additional records have been added to the system since the 1989 report. Because of a delay in receiving hospitalization data, we report hospitalization data only through 1987. Race codes for most purposes have been expanded from white, black, and other to white, black, Asian American, native American, and other.

Our objective in preparing this report has been to present data for the full span of years using consistent definitions, so that valid comparisons can be made across years and among subgroups in the database. We attempt to alert the reader to those cases where changes in the data collection process over the years result in problems in making valid comparisons across years. These warnings appear in the text, in reference table footnotes, and in Chapter XIII, Technical Notes.

Some data reported here differ slightly from data in the 1989 report. The principal reason for changes in data for recent years is delays in receiving data at the HCFA data system. Because of these delays, we do not report data for a given time period until 15 months have elapsed. Even so, some data are still received after 15 months. Differences also may occur because of errors in the date of onset of ESRD which are sometimes corrected at a later date and thus affect data from year to year. Finally, our methods for determining dates such as transplant failure or other modality change are continually being refined, and these refinements will produce small changes in the data from year to year. However, the data in each annual data report represent a consistently defined series of data within which valid comparisons can be made.

The 90-day waiting period for Medicare eligibility causes difficulties in measurement of mortality and survival. The start date for measurement of mortality in this year's report is 90 days following onset of ESRD with a full 365 day followup to day 455 of ESRD (i.e., 12 months, starting at month 3 and ending at month 15). This is in contrast to last year's report for which the followup period was only to day 365 (i.e., 9 months, starting at month 3 and ending at month 12). Mortality analyses based on the full year are both more complete and more comparable to analyses from other research sources. However, since the full year analyses presented in this report start at day 90, they are not perfectly analogous to analyses in the literature that start followup on day 1 (see the discussion in Chapter VI for more detail). Patient mortality for transplant patients is analyzed separately for recipients of living related and cadaver grafts, in contrast to last year when all transplant recipients were analyzed as one group. New aggregate age groups coincide with the definition of pediatric ages, i.e., less than 20 years.

Considerable effort has gone into revising the method of calculating date of graft failure, which leads to different estimates than those generated by HCFA. Reported graft survival is lower than the HCFA estimates by less than one percentage point on average, but larger differences exist for certain subgroups.

CHAPTER I. OVERVIEW

The USRDS is funded and directed by NIDDK of the NIH. Members of the nephrology, transplant, biostatistical, information systems, and epidemiology communities are consulted for advice on specific issues. The USRDS research agenda, reflecting the agenda of NIDDK and the renal community at large, is focused on medical and epidemiological issues central to the causes and effective care of patients with ESRD. The US-RDS Coordinating Center manages and directs a responsive, research-driven information system containing nearly 6 million records for 372,000 Medicare patients who have had ESRD therapy at any time since 1976. The data system contains information on basic demographics of the affected population, diagnoses leading to renal failure, dialysis records (3.4 million), hospital records (1.8 million), transplant information (74,600 transplants and 194,400 transplant followup forms) and details on the 2,181 institutions (14,367 records) providing ESRD services. Besides information collected routinely by HCFA, via its 18 ESRD Networks, the USRDS, in conjunction with these same and other organizations, collects new data on national samples of ESRD patients according to protocols designed by the USRDS. Immediate issues in the current phase of the project include validation of the existing data, further development of a research-oriented data system, extension of the database to non-Medicare populations with ESRD, and the prioritization, design, and implementation of research projects for NIDDK and the kidney community.

CHAPTER II. MAGNITUDE OF THE PROBLEM

The 1988 count of Medicare ESRD patients enrolled at any time during the year (period prevalence) was 172,506. These patients are approximately 93 percent of all ESRD patients in the U.S., an 8.5 percent increase over the 1987 value, and a continuing rate of growth over the last five years of 9.8 percent per year. ESRD patients have from one-fourth to one-fifth the life expectancy of the U.S. general population: at age 40 the expected life of an ESRD patient is 9.3 years compared to 37.4 years for the U.S. general population of the same age. Mortality comparisons with some more common cancers shows lung cancer patients have dramatically shorter life expectancy than do ESRD patients, while prostate cancer patients have longer life expectancy.

In 1988, medical payments for the care of ESRD patients from all sources (Federal, state, and private) were in excess of $5.4 billion per year, a 23 percent increase over the 1987 estimate of $4.4 billion, which was probably low. Federal sources pay approximately 67 percent ($3.7 billion) of this total including contributions to state Medicaid programs. Many other costs are not included in this total, such as the cost of most outpatient drugs, lost production in and out of the labor force, and transfer payments such as disability and social security.

CHAPTER III. CAUSES OF ESRD

The list of causes of ESRD presented in this report has been greatly expanded since the 1989 report. Diabetes mellitus is the leading cause of ESRD accounting for nearly one-third of new ESRD patients in 1988. The newly required reporting of diabetes type has been less beneficial than expected since insulin-dependent diabetes mellitus (IDDM) is seriously over reported, particularly in older patients. It is hoped that in the future, insulin therapy will not be used as the only determinant of diabetes type. Hypertension, the second leading cause of ESRD, is particularly predominant in young black men, though its incidence among white men has shown relatively large increases. More work is planned on the definition by race of hypertension as cause of ESRD.

CHAPTER IV. DEMOGRAPHICS OF ESRD

The number of new patients treated for ESRD per million population is grouped by age, race, gender, and year for the analyses presented in this chapter. Incidence rates are higher in the elderly than in the young population and higher in the black and native American populations than in the white or Asian American populations. Incidence rates are higher among males than among females.

The treated ESRD incidence rate has continued to climb in recent years. On average, the number of patients starting on Medicare-reimbursed ESRD therapy per million population increased at approximately 6 percent per year between 1984 and 1988. When the incidence rates were examined by age for the most recent years (between 1987 and 1988) there was little change for ages less than 19, there was an increase of less than 4 percent for patients of ages 20-44, and as high as 12 percent for patients older than 74. Although the rate of new ESRD cases has increased less in recent years in comparison to the larger increases seen during the early part of the decade, there is little indication that the ESRD treatment program has yet reached stability with regard to reported incidence of new treated cases.

On average, prevalent patients are older now than in the past: the average age of the treated ESRD patient population has increased by 1 year between 1984 and 1988. The average age at onset of ESRD increased by 1.7 years in the same period. The aging of the ESRD population has important implications both for the treatment and for the evaluation of patient outcomes. The types and amount of medical care used by an aging patient population can be expected to change with time. Also, the increase in average age leads to a higher death rate for the recently enrolled ESRD population compared to previous enrollees, which could influence the apparent trends in death rates over recent years.

There are substantial differences in incidence rates among subpopulations with differing ancestry. The incidence rate of treated ESRD is 3 to 4 times higher in the black and native American populations than in the white and Asian American populations. The elevated rate in the black population is found at all ages, except children less than 15 years old. The rate of treated ESRD is increasing twice as fast per year among the native Americans than among other groups. The elevated risk in the black population is especially pronounced for ESRD reported as caused by hypertension, while in the native American population it is especially pronounced for ESRD diagnosed with diabetes. A clearer understanding of the specific determinants of such differences might lead to improved methods for the prevention of ESRD.

The differences in cause of disease by patient ancestry noted above could be partly responsible for differences seen in the average age of newly treated ESRD patients. First ESRD therapy occurs at younger ages in the black and native American populations (average age 57) than in the white (average age 62) or Asian American (average age 58) populations.

There are also differences in incidence rates by gender. In 1988, the percent of the newly treated patient population that was male ranged from 56 percent among white patients to 49 percent among native American patients. The incidence rates of patients with hypertension and of patients with glomerulonephritis as cause of ESRD are higher among males than among females. In the black population, females appear to be at higher risk than males for ESRD caused by diabetes, while the opposite is true in the white population. Incidence rates of ESRD with cystic disease are similar for males and females in the black population, while they are elevated for males relative to females in the white population.

CHAPTER V. METHODS OF TREATMENT

The utilization of treatment modalities is examined among prevalent cases as of the end of each year. Additionally, the modalities used by all patients who started ESRD therapy in 1985 are recorded on a monthly basis over the first three years. Differences among age, sex, and race groups are striking and deserve further investigation. The number of renal transplants performed per year has not shown any increase for the fourth year, while the number of patients awaiting renal transplantation has continued to increase. The lack of available organs has thus created an ever-widening gap between the count of patients on the waiting list and those patients receiving a transplant. The pattern of patients switching treatment modalities during the first year is described for the first time and provides new insights.

CHAPTER VI. MORTALITY

Patient survival among ESRD patients, especially among patients receiving dialysis therapy, is discussed in this chapter. Patterns of mortality by age, race, gender, principal diagnosis, and year of first therapy are examined. Mortality rates for patients receiving hemodialysis and CAPD are compared. Specific causes of death are also examined.

Mortality rates for ESRD patients vary substantially with age, race, and principal diagnosis. Mortality rates are much higher in the elderly patient population than in the younger population. This difference in survival is exaggerated by treatment pattern differences: younger patients are much more likely to receive transplants than are older (over age 64) patients. Among dialysis patients, survival rates are higher on average for black patients than for white patients, although there is no substantial advantage for black patients compared to white patients with glomerulonephritis. Patients with diabetes have substantially higher death rates than do other patients. Patients with ESRD due to hypertension tend to have somewhat elevated death rates. There is no indication of a substantial trend in mortality rates with the year of first ESRD therapy in the results reported in this chapter, although there have been minor fluctuations from year to year.

An analysis of patient survival comparing hemodialysis to CAPD therapy revealed relatively small differences in survival for these two therapies. An analysis of patient survival in the 90-day interval immediately following a switch in dialytic modality showed little change in mortality rates following such a switch.

Cardiac/atherosclerotic cause is the leading cause of death in all age groups. This report examines for the first time race and sex differences in the death rates by causes of death besides those related to the age of patients. The death rates are strikingly lower among the patients having ever received a renal transplant than among dialysis-only patients. For both groups, cardiac causes predominate.

CHAPTER VII. TRANSPLANTATION

Kidney transplantation is for many patients the preferred method of treatment, but as noted in Chapter V, the supply of cadaver donor grafts has not grown for the last four years. Patient survival for recipients of cadaver transplants has improved since at least 1983, with the largest improvements occurring in the period just after 1983. Precise reasons for the improved patient survival are not known, but these results are contemporaneous with the introduction of cyclosporine in 1983.

Graft survival has improved over the 1983-88 period, particularly for cadaver grafts. As was the case for patient survival, the benefits were largest in the immediate post-1983 period. Most improvement has come in the first year following a transplant, but there have also been improvements in the period beyond 1 year post transplant for cadaver donor grafts.

Kaplan-Meier survival estimates show an improved graft survival for both living related and cadaver donor transplants for 0 antigen mismatches (HLA A, B, DR) compared to 5 or 6 mismatches. Black patients have a consistently higher level of mismatched grafts than do whites when compared over the 1983- 88 period. The lower level of mismatches for white recipients is consistent with the observation that most donors are white; therefore white phenotypes are more common in the donor pool. Black patients also have a consistently lower level of graft survival than do white patients both for living related and for cadaver donor transplants.

Access to transplantation was measured by age, sex, and race groups as the percent of the prevalent dialysis patients transplanted in 1984 and 1988. On this basis, for patients in the 20-44 age group, blacks and other races compose a substantially lower percentage of patients transplanted than do white patients, and the disparity between black and white patients increased between 1984 and 1988. For patients in the 45-64 age group, the black-white comparison showed similar results as for the younger age group, and females showed strikingly lower percentages than did males. Possible reasons for these differences need to be further explored.

CHAPTER VIII. HOSPITALIZATION

Hospitalization measures several aspects of ESRD therapy. For transplantation and vascular access or peritoneal catheter placement, the hospital stay is part of the therapy. Hospitalization can also be an indication of the severity of the illness or of the presence of comorbid conditions. In all cases it is a measure of the quality of life of the patient and of the monetary cost of ESRD. This chapter examines trends in hospitalization over time, and examines differences between dialysis and transplant patients and among races and disease groups.

Hospitalization rates of ESRD patients declined markedly for all patient subgroups between the 1980-83 and 1984-87 periods. The decline was greater for transplanted patients than for dialysis-only patients. This trend is consistent with overall trends in hospitalization and with the financial incentives of the diagnosis-related group (DRG) system used by Medicare to pay for inpatient care.

There appears to be a selection of healthier patients for transplantation; patients transplanted in the first three years of ESRD have much lower hospitalization rates before their first transplant while on dialysis than do patients who have only dialysis during their first three years. The hospitalization rate is somewhat higher after the transplantation as compared to the pretransplant period, but it is not as high as that of the dialysis only group.

Blacks treated by dialysis therapy only have lower hospitalization rates than do whites, but blacks who are transplanted have higher hospitalization rates during and after the transplant than do whites. Patients with diabetes and hypertension as causes of ESRD have more hospitalizations than patients with other diseases. Whites have more hospitalizations than blacks for diabetes and hypertension, but race differences are insignificant for other disease groups.

The results for hospitalization by race, and by race and disease group, are consistent with the results for mortality included in this report.

CHAPTER IX. PEDIATRIC ESRD

There were 833 new pediatric (less than 20 years of age at onset) ESRD cases covered by Medicare in 1988. Over half of these were in the 15-19 age group. While whites comprise the majority of patients, blacks are represented in greater proportions among new ESRD patients aged 15-19. Thus, the incidence of ESRD is higher for black children than it is for white children, similar to the differences observed for adult Americans. Asian Americans have a lower incidence rate than do white Americans. For children younger than 15 years old, the incidence rates are similar for blacks and whites, but those for native American children are somewhat higher. Geographical differences for incidence rates in pediatric patients are described by Network area, since the rates are difficult to determine due to small sample sizes in smaller areas (e.g., states).

The distribution of diseases causing ESRD is dramatically different for children compared to adult ESRD patients. In contrast to adults, diabetes and hypertensive ESRD account for a small percent of incident cases over the 1986- 88 period, while glomerulonephritis and congenital diseases account for 38 and 20 percent of all cases, respectively. Along with age of the patient, the disease causing ESRD may influence the primary choice of treatment modality.

Transplantation is the primary choice of treatment modality within all pediatric age groups, followed by peritoneal dialysis in the younger pediatric patients (??10 years old) and hemodialysis in the older pediatric patients. Living related transplants occur approximately as frequently as cadaver transplants in pediatric patients, in contrast to adult ESRD patients for whom cadaver grafts far outnumber living related grafts. Male pediatric patients are 33 percent more likely to receive a cadaver transplant than female pediatric patients. Similarly, white pediatric patients are 18 percent more likely to receive a cadaver transplant than black pediatric patients. Graft survival is higher for living related transplant recipients than for cadaver transplant recipients, although patient survival does not appear different between living related and cadaver transplant recipients. In 1984, transplant patients had higher two-year patient survival rates than did dialysis patients, while the 1987 two-year patient survival rates for transplant and dialysis are comparable.

CHAPTER X. INSTITUTIONS PROVIDING ESRD SERVICES

The wide proliferation of dialysis and transplant units has made renal replacement therapy a readily available service in most areas of the U.S. The number of dialysis units has grown from 987 in 1981 to 1,712 in 1989. This growth rate of 7.1 percent per year, compounded annually, mirrors the growth in ESRD prevalence of 9.8 percent per year in the last five years. The number of transplant centers has grown at an annual rate of 4.3 percent, from 156 to 219, in the 1981-89 period. Dialysis units are widely distributed. As of 1989, there were 317 metropolitan areas and 400 non-metropolitan areas having at least one dialysis unit. Transplant units were located in 104 metropolitan and 3 non-metropolitan areas in 1989.

The distribution of dialysis patients across types of units shows that, as of 1989, just under 53 percent of dialysis patients were being treated in for-profit freestanding units, representing an increase from 39 percent in 1981. Dialysis units in hospitals treated 18.8 percent of patients in 1989, down from 29.2 percent in 1981. The average size of transplant units, as measured by the median number of transplants per year, has been declining since reaching a high of 36 in 1986 to 30 in 1989. The freestanding dialysis units have shown the smallest increases in size over the last 8 years.

CHAPTER XI. INTERNATIONAL COMPARISONS

An international perspective is provided by comparing USRDS findings with those of other ESRD registries for European countries, Canada, Japan, and Australia. The incidence of treated ESRD is highest in the U.S. This finding is related in part to the high incidence of ESRD among the U.S. black population and to the relatively greater acceptance of older patients. Differences in the use of various treatment modalities are striking and are explained partly by specific policies, cultural beliefs, and acceptance of older patients.

CHAPTER XII. USRDS RESEARCH STUDIES

The special data collection and analysis efforts currently being conducted by USRDS and some of those proposed for the future are described in this chapter. Six such "special studies," which require the collection of new, primary data, have been initiated: 1) Measurements of severity of illness and case mix at initiation of renal replacement therapy; 2) Data validation, comparing USRDS data with primary data from original sources; 3) Renal biopsy examined as an indicator of specific renal diagnoses and subsequent outcomes; 4) Erythropoietin (EPO) use and quality of life; 5) Examination of peritonitis episodes in patients treated by CAPD; and 6) Assessing pediatric patient growth (plus development of secondary sexual characteristics in older children), as affected by ESRD treatment modality. More than 30 other studies have been proposed and are under consideration for the future.

"Existing data studies" are analyses that use basic information routinely obtained from HCFA on all Medicare and some non-Medicare ESRD patients. Several such studies can be undertaken each year, depending upon their scope. Twenty existing data studies have been approved by NIDDK since November 1989; eight are nearing completion and have had preliminary results reported.

CHAPTER XIII. TECHNICAL NOTES

This chapter provides extensive documentation of the USRDS database and of the methodologies used in this report. It discusses data quality issues and describes in detail the changes in the data and the methods since the 1989 report. Although HCFA and the USRDS present similar data, there may be slight differences in the actual numbers presented in this report and those found in HCFA publications. As noted above, these differences are largely due to data updates and quality screens applied to the USRDS data. Readers of the nearly 400 pages of reference tables will find this chapter an essential reference.

The USRDS database provides an extraordinarily comprehensive and detailed picture of 93 percent of the ESRD population in the United States. It is a dynamic database. Each year new data are added, data errors are corrected, and methods and definitions are refined. For these reasons, the data reported in this annual volume will vary slightly from year to year, although each report presents an internally consistent series of data, as summarized here.

USRDS 1990 Annual Data Report
Incidence Of Reported ESRD Therapy A.1
Incidence Counts Of Reported ESRD Therapy
By Year, By Age, Race, Sex, and Primary Disease Causing ESRD

.	1977	1978	1979	1980	1981	1982	1983	1984	1985	1986	1987	1988
AGE AT ESRD												
0- 4	28	37	40	61	77	101	99	110	121	116	121	114
5- 9	68	81	95	103	91	100	83	105	87	110	111	89
10-14	209	208	185	205	169	214	198	213	209	196	195	191
15-19	435	420	455	426	438	444	428	399	411	427	454	439
20-24	661	654	641	643	662	712	667	755	772	751	773	807
25-29	886	838	861	908	927	1097	1086	1155	1211	1304	1229	1311
30-34	944	879	974	1149	1223	1349	1371	1457	1481	1654	1590	1722
35-39	977	951	977	1059	1138	1296	1379	1479	1696	1830	1880	2091
40-44	1063	1034	1068	1133	1204	1289	1439	1519	1665	1803	2054	2159
45-49	1265	1199	1338	1315	1373	1455	1649	1725	1916	1984	2152	2393
50-54	1593	1558	1708	1790	1813	2044	2062	2106	2269	2399	2647	2884
55-59	1757	1734	1916	2073	2255	2465	2572	2813	3020	3119	3327	3561
60-64	1722	1665	1960	2209	2389	2768	3132	3418	3813	3920	4355	4533
65-69	2022	1679	1937	2212	2288	2574	3260	3376	3739	4117	4598	4743
70-74	1382	1159	1411	1560	1677	2050	2797	2802	3312	3566	3949	4062
75-79	564	574	795	904	953	1189	1764	1920	2169	2559	2820	3030
80-84	225	171	278	330	350	453	755	772	992	1131	1331	1500
85 plus	31	54	83	99	99	168	250	275	345	408	472	531
	15832	14895	16722	18179	19126	21768	24991	26399	29228	31394	34058	36160
RACE												
White	11020	10229	11277	12363	13155	15223	17085	18139	20047	21532	23132	24357
Black	3977	3838	4509	4771	4949	5859	7060	7407	8156	8619	9513	10045
Asian	33	30	39	58	133	310	316	383	504	508	548	633
Native Amer.	27	37	40	70	131	196	260	263	272	335	343	440
Other	398	393	460	511	409	112	145	134	160	240	367	586
Unknown	377	368	397	406	349	68	125	73	89	160	155	99
	15832	14895	16722	18179	19126	21768	24991	26399	29228	31394	34058	36160
SEX												
Male	9007	8280	9270	10118	10580	12023	13739	14608	15918	17236	18504	19663
Female	6825	6615	7452	8061	8546	9745	11252	11791	13310	14158	15554	16497
	15832	14895	16722	18179	19126	21768	24991	26399	29228	31394	34058	36160
PRIMARY DIAGNOSIS												
Diabetes	1212	1423	1631	2251	3637	5019	5906	7107	8174	9263	10179	11034
Hypertension	1664	1841	2031	2510	3944	5401	5804	6513	7423	7852	8884	9647
Glomeruloneph.	2021	1937	2071	2171	3129	3886	4096	4359	4572	4686	4882	5003
Cystic Kidney	539	514	571	608	835	1011	1052	1063	1153	1204	1227	1196
Other Urologic	920	852	997	1112	1496	1744	1884	1926	2167	2169	2041	1995
Other Cause	286	309	347	424	724	1239	1527	1661	1850	1840	1963	2048
Unknown Cause	1486	1340	1470	1516	1813	1887	1876	1902	2112	2228	2623	2394
Missing Disease	7704	6679	7604	7587	3548	1581	2846	1868	1777	2152	2259	2843
	15832	14895	16722	18179	19126	21768	24991	26399	29228	31394	34058	36160

APPENDIX 1

USRDS 1990 Annual Data Report
Incidence Of Reported ESRD Therapy   A.2
Incidence Rates Per Million Population Of Reported ESRD Therapy
By Year By Age, Race, Sex, and Primary Disease Causing ESRD, Unadjusted

	1977	1978	1979	1980	1981	1982	1983	1984	1985	1986	1987	1988
AGE AT ESRD												
0- 4	2	2	3	4	5	6	6	6	7	6	7	6
5- 9	4	5	6	6	6	6	5	6	5	6	6	5
10-14	11	11	10	11	9	12	11	12	12	12	12	11
15-19	21	20	22	20	21	22	22	21	22	23	25	24
20-24	33	32	31	30	31	33	31	35	37	37	39	42
25-29	50	47	47	46	46	53	51	54	56	59	56	60
30-34	61	55	59	65	65	72	71	74	73	80	75	79
35-39	79	73	72	75	79	83	85	87	96	98	100	109
40-44	95	91	93	97	100	104	110	112	118	126	132	134
45-49	110	106	119	119	125	132	147	150	165	166	174	184
50-54	134	132	146	153	156	178	184	191	207	220	242	259
55-59	159	154	169	178	195	214	223	246	266	277	299	327
60-64	184	176	204	218	230	261	293	314	347	358	400	415
65-69	239	196	223	251	257	285	355	364	396	426	465	475
70-74	225	182	214	228	240	286	383	376	437	465	508	514
75-79	138	138	186	187	192	234	338	358	394	454	488	513
80-84	81	62	100	112	116	146	238	238	298	331	378	415
85 plus	15	24	36	44	42	69	98	105	128	147	165	180
0-19	10	10	11	11	11	12	11	12	12	12	12	12
20-44	59	56	56	58	59	64	65	68	72	76	77	82
45-64	145	140	158	166	176	196	211	225	245	254	276	291
65-74	233	190	219	241	249	285	367	369	415	443	484	492
75 plus	92	88	123	133	136	170	253	264	304	346	380	406
RACE												
White	59	54	59	63	67	77	85	90	99	105	112	117
Black	158	151	174	178	182	212	252	260	283	294	320	333
SEX												
Male	86	78	87	92	95	107	121	127	137	147	156	164
Female	61	59	66	69	72	82	93	97	109	114	125	131
PRIMARY DIAGNOSIS												
Diabetes	6	7	7	10	16	22	25	30	34	38	42	45
Hypertension	8	8	9	11	17	23	25	28	31	33	36	39
Glomeruloneph.	9	9	9	10	14	17	17	18	19	19	20	20
Cystic Kidney	2	2	3	3	4	4	4	4	5	5	5	5
Other Urologic	4	4	5	5	7	8	8	8	9	9	8	8
Other Cause	1	1	2	2	3	5	7	7	8	8	8	8
Unknown Cause	7	6	7	7	8	8	8	8	9	9	11	10
Missing Disease	36	31	35	33	15	7	12	8	7	9	9	12
TOTAL												
	73	68	76	80	83	94	107	112	122	130	140	147

USRDS 1990 Annual Data Report
Prevalence Of Reported ESRD Therapy B.1
December 31 Point Prevalence Counts Of Reported ESRD Therapy
By Year By Age, Race, Sex, and Primary Disease Causing ESRD

	1977	1978	1979	1980	1981	1982	1983	1984	1985	1986	1987	1988
AGE AT ESRD												
0- 4	40	53	61	84	123	175	210	235	267	276	292	298
5- 9	164	194	223	264	263	310	340	389	420	490	536	558
10-14	477	546	598	654	691	771	825	865	872	885	932	973
15-19	1228	1403	1572	1669	1752	1826	1851	1885	2006	2081	2190	2240
20-24	2095	2459	2706	2992	3303	3602	3811	4012	4148	4220	4264	4339
25-29	2714	3229	3756	4289	4732	5278	5774	6198	6638	7118	7484	7797
30-34	2869	3398	4131	4989	5820	6605	7326	8122	8867	9640	10172	10796
35-39	3080	3694	4233	4798	5564	6431	7335	8437	9718	10810	11786	12760
40-44	3251	3890	4467	5059	5596	6379	7318	8088	8889	10054	11217	12538
45-49	3836	4287	4957	5558	6120	6758	7608	8374	9237	9941	11149	12473
50-54	4538	5320	6062	6661	7392	8114	8592	9384	10109	10937	11805	12922
55-59	4647	5504	6519	7539	8347	9412	10162	10964	11731	12535	13341	14126
60-64	4107	4982	5984	6930	8060	9139	10423	11616	12755	13520	14876	16003
65-69	3433	4331	5348	6159	6969	8047	9397	10425	11532	12643	13997	14985
70-74	2051	2736	3469	4262	4924	5734	6995	7921	8791	9934	10864	11676
75-79	782	1206	1684	2117	2576	3115	4029	4805	5533	6277	7115	7793
80-84	269	359	544	713	855	1092	1565	1848	2249	2722	3215	3634
85 plus	51	79	135	195	254	352	488	587	748	872	1111	1295
	39632	47670	56449	64932	73341	83140	94049	104155	114510	124955	136346	147206
RACE												
White	27364	32703	38334	43935	49549	56231	63246	69827	76535	83410	90657	97307
Black	10270	12488	15096	17455	19814	22827	26380	29656	32948	36014	39534	42868
Asian	72	100	139	197	328	591	841	1094	1413	1697	1994	2324
Native Amer.	65	100	135	199	318	480	684	852	982	1142	1287	1494
Other	1077	1278	1531	1769	1857	1665	1570	1508	1477	1521	1691	2044
Unknown	784	1001	1214	1377	1475	1346	1328	1218	1155	1171	1183	1169
	39632	47670	56449	64932	73341	83140	94049	104155	114510	124955	136346	147206
SEX												
Male	21982	26312	31061	35737	40252	45600	51528	57177	62694	68293	74278	80083
Female	17650	21358	25388	29195	33089	37540	42521	46978	51816	56662	62068	67123
	39632	47670	56449	64932	73341	83140	94049	104155	114510	124955	136346	147206
PRIMARY DIAGNOSIS												
Diabetes	2438	3101	3847	4996	7100	9913	12710	16038	19408	22896	26441	29937
Hypertension	4023	5193	6377	7781	10170	13356	16310	19154	22074	24877	27820	30517
Glomeruloneph.	7309	8490	9715	10991	13047	15576	18051	20533	22958	25176	27304	29216
Cystic Kidney	1928	2258	2631	2993	3530	4217	4838	5408	5971	6503	7097	7561
Other Urologic	2833	3324	3889	4453	5286	6236	7176	8014	8938	9571	9990	10362
Other Cause	489	725	968	1246	1774	2670	3608	4540	5482	6349	7162	7953
Unknown Cause	4729	5277	5935	6522	7296	7998	8632	9227	9822	10454	11383	11780
Missing Disease	15883	19302	23087	25950	25138	23174	22724	21241	19857	19129	19149	19880
	39632	47670	56449	64932	73341	83140	94049	104155	114510	124955	136346	147206

USRDS 1990 Annual Data Report
Methods Of Treatment C.1
Living ESRD Patients On December 31
By Treatment Modality By Year

Counts, Percentages

		1980	1981	1982	1983	1984	1985	1986	1987	1988
Transplant	N	7417	9633	12210	15237	18876	23145	28219	32867	36967
	%	11.42%	13.13%	14.68%	16.19%	18.12%	20.21%	22.58%	24.10%	25.11%
Unknown	N	7897	7119	6908	6683	6644	6773	6902	7180	7469
	%	12.16%	9.70%	8.30%	7.10%	6.37%	5.91%	5.52%	5.26%	5.07%
Center Hemo	N	43576	48823	53689	59959	62636	65012	69442	75793	83410
	%	67.10%	66.56%	64.57%	63.74%	60.13%	56.76%	55.56%	55.58%	56.65%
Home Hemo	N	2561	2117	2194	1893	3479	5630	5253	4543	2757
	%	3.94%	2.88%	2.63%	2.01%	3.33%	4.91%	4.20%	3.33%	1.87%
Center Self Hemo	N	454	730	857	1256	1100	1130	1117	1164	1125
	%	0.69%	0.99%	1.03%	1.33%	1.05%	0.98%	0.89%	0.85%	0.76%
CAPD	N	1270	3351	5300	6589	7996	9592	10330	11032	11683
	%	1.95%	4.56%	6.37%	7.00%	7.67%	8.37%	8.26%	8.09%	7.93%
CCPD	N			1	16	135	403	624	770	907
	%			0.00%	0.01%	0.12%	0.35%	0.49%	0.56%	0.61%
Other Peritoneal	N	1221	1473	1928	2045	2265	2086	2260	2304	2328
	%	1.88%	2.00%	2.31%	2.17%	2.17%	1.82%	1.80%	1.68%	1.58%
Unknown Dialysis	N	542	102	58	379	1033	751	821	704	574
	%	0.83%	0.13%	0.06%	0.40%	0.99%	0.65%	0.65%	0.51%	0.38%
TOTAL	N	64938	73348	83145	94057	104164	114522	124968	136357	147220
	%	100.00%	100.00%	100.00%	100.00%	100.00%	100.00%	100.00%	100.00%	100.00%

USRDS 1990 Annual Data Report, Patient Survival E.57
Five Year Survival Probabilities: From Day 91 to Five Years +90 Days For All Patients
By Year Of Incidence By Age, Race, Sex, and Primary Disease Causing ESRD
Using Aggregate Categories, Adjusted for Age, Race, Sex, and Primary Disease

	1977	1978	1979	1980	1981	1982	1983	1984	1985	1986	1987	1988
AGE												
0-19	87.1	81.3	84.4	73.7	84.0	77.0	86.0	71.6	.	.	.	.
20-44	61.0	61.6	62.0	64.7	66.5	66.7	65.8	68.7	.	.	.	.
45-64	39.7	39.9	38.1	40.3	39.9	39.6	38.3	38.0	.	.	.	.
65-74	25.7	22.1	23.2	22.9	22.7	22.3	18.2	20.0	.	.	.	.
75 plus	9.6	10.2	9.5	11.7	10.5	10.6	7.9	10.8	.	.	.	.
RACE												
Black	40.2	40.3	41.0	44.0	42.8	40.6	39.7	40.8	.	.	.	.
Non-Black	37.1	36.8	35.7	37.4	37.3	37.9	36.0	36.9	.	.	.	.
SEX												
Female	39.6	39.1	38.5	39.9	40.9	40.5	38.7	40.0	.	.	.	.
Male	37.4	36.4	36.6	38.6	37.8	37.8	36.3	36.9	.	.	.	.
PRIMARY DIAGNOSIS												
Diabetes	23.3	23.4	23.5	24.2	24.6	23.5	24.6	23.5	.	.	.	.
Hypertension	42.3	41.8	41.3	43.6	41.5	41.3	39.5	41.0	.	.	.	.
Kidney Diseases	51.2	50.1	49.1	50.5	50.8	49.4	49.6	50.1	.	.	.	.
Other	37.6	39.2	37.6	38.9	43.4	44.2	35.9	39.8	.	.	.	.
TOTAL PROBABILITIES												
Total Crude Prob.	44.5	45.5	43.2	43.8	44.6	43.2	38.4	39.2	.	.	.	.
Total Adjusted Prob.	38.4	37.9	37.6	39.3	39.2	39.0	37.3	38.3	.	.	.	.

USRDS 1990 Annual Data Report, Patient Survival E.59
Ten Year Survival Probabilities: From Day 91 to Ten Years +90 Days For All Patients
By Year Of Incidence By Age, Race, Sex, and Primary Disease Causing ESRD
Using Aggregate Categories, Adjusted for Age, Race, Sex, and Primary Disease

	.	1977	1978	1979	1980	1981	1982	1983	1984	1985	1986	1987	1988
AGE													
	0-19	74.7	66.1	67.0	.	.	.	.	.	.	.	.	.
	20-44	45.0	43.7	44.5	.	.	.	.	.	.	.	.	.
	45-64	16.6	15.5	15.8	.	.	.	.	.	.	.	.	.
	65-74	6.2	5.5	4.5	.	.	.	.	.	.	.	.	.
	75 plus	2.3	1.4	0.9	.	.	.	.	.	.	.	.	.
RACE													
	Black	19.9	18.5	19.1	.	.	.	.	.	.	.	.	.
	Non-Black	20.2	19.4	19.2	.	.	.	.	.	.	.	.	.
SEX													
	Female	21.7	20.2	19.9	.	.	.	.	.	.	.	.	.
	Male	19.0	18.4	19.2	.	.	.	.	.	.	.	.	.
PRIMARY DIAGNOSIS													
	Diabetes	10.2	9.0	8.0	.	.	.	.	.	.	.	.	.
	Hypertension	23.1	21.1	20.5	.	.	.	.	.	.	.	.	.
	Kidney Diseases	28.4	27.0	27.8	.	.	.	.	.	.	.	.	.
	Other	20.0	21.3	20.7	.	.	.	.	.	.	.	.	.
TOTAL PROBABILITIES													
	Total Crude Prob.	25.5	26.1	24.9	.	.	.	.	.	.	.	.	.
	Total Adjusted Prob.	20.3	19.3	19.6	.	.	.	.	.	.	.	.	.

USRDS 1990 Annual Data Report, Patient Survival E.73
Five Year Survival Probabilities: From Day 91 to Five Years +90 Days, For Dialysis Patients (Censored At First Transplant)
By Year of Incidence By Age, Race, Sex, and Primary Disease Causing ESRD
Using Aggregate Categories Adjusted for Age, Race, Sex, and Primary Disease

	1977	1978	1979	1980	1981	1982	1983	1984	1985	1986	1987	1988
AGE												
0-19	64.6	66.7	58.8	65.3	68.5	65.4	78.9	64.2	.	.	.	.
20-44	46.7	47.9	48.2	50.0	49.6	51.7	51.4	54.8	.	.	.	.
45-64	35.6	36.1	33.9	35.7	35.0	34.5	32.9	32.1	.	.	.	.
65-74	25.6	22.0	22.9	22.9	22.6	22.1	18.0	19.8	.	.	.	.
75 plus	9.6	10.2	9.5	11.7	10.5	10.6	7.9	10.8	.	.	.	.
RACE												
Black	35.8	36.0	35.8	39.2	38.6	36.4	35.5	36.5	.	.	.	.
Non-Black	31.6	31.5	30.3	31.6	30.6	31.6	29.8	30.5	.	.	.	.
SEX												
Female	35.1	35.0	34.1	35.3	36.0	35.8	34.2	35.0	.	.	.	.
Male	31.6	30.9	30.5	32.4	31.2	31.3	29.7	30.4	.	.	.	.
PRIMARY DIAGNOSIS												
Diabetes	20.2	19.8	17.7	20.0	19.4	17.8	19.4	17.7	.	.	.	.
Hypertension	35.5	36.4	35.9	38.1	35.0	35.5	34.1	35.8	.	.	.	.
Kidney Diseases	44.0	43.5	42.5	43.8	43.5	43.2	43.4	43.6	.	.	.	.
Other	33.1	34.5	32.8	33.8	37.6	39.2	30.3	34.5	.	.	.	.
TOTAL PROBABILITIES												
Total Crude Prob.	38.1	39.2	37.0	37.4	37.5	36.7	32.6	33.2	.	.	.	.
Total Adjusted Prob.	33.2	32.9	32.3	33.7	33.3	33.3	31.7	32.5	.	.	.	.

APPENDIX 1

USRDS 1990 Annual Data Report, Patient Survival E.75
Ten Year Survival Probabilities: From Day 91 to Ten Years +90 Days For Dialysis Patients (Censored At First Transplant)
By Year of Incidence By Age, Race, Sex, and Primary Disease Causing ESRD
Using Aggregate Categories, Adjusted for Age, Race, Sex, and Primary Disease

	.	1977	1978	1979	1980	1981	1982	1983	1984	1985	1986	1987	1988
AGE													
	0-19	56.9	60.8	55.5	.	.	.	.	.	.	.	.	.
	20-44	32.3	31.3	32.1	.	.	.	.	.	.	.	.	.
	45-64	13.7	12.8	12.2	.	.	.	.	.	.	.	.	.
	65-74	6.1	5.5	4.5	.	.	.	.	.	.	.	.	.
	75 plus	2.3	1.3	0.9	.	.	.	.	.	.	.	.	.
RACE													
	Black	16.6	14.5	15.3	.	.	.	.	.	.	.	.	.
	Non-Black	15.6	15.2	14.4	.	.	.	.	.	.	.	.	.
SEX													
	Female	17.8	16.5	15.8	.	.	.	.	.	.	.	.	.
	Male	14.6	14.0	14.4	.	.	.	.	.	.	.	.	.
PRIMARY DIAGNOSIS													
	Diabetes	8.5	7.8	5.5	.	.	.	.	.	.	.	.	.
	Hypertension	17.3	16.6	15.6	.	.	.	.	.	.	.	.	.
	Kidney Diseases	22.3	20.8	21.7	.	.	.	.	.	.	.	.	.
	Other	16.0	17.2	16.0	.	.	.	.	.	.	.	.	.
TOTAL PROBABILITIES													
	Total Crude Prob.	20.0	20.6	19.2	.	.	.	.	.	.	.	.	.
	Total Adjusted Prob.	16.1	15.2	15.1	.	.	.	.	.	.	.	.	.

USRDS 1990 Annual Data Report, Patient Survival E.81
Five Year Survival Probabilities: From Day 1 to Five Years For First Transplant Patients (Cadaveric)
By Year Of First TransplantBy Age, Race, Sex, and Primary Disease Causing ESRD
Using Aggregate Categories Adjusted for Age, Race, Sex, and Primary Disease

	1977	1978	1979	1980	1981	1982	1983	1984	1985	1986	1987	1988
AGE												
0-19	65.1	67.5	60.0	70.4	61.5	59.0	66.3	88.2	.	.	.	.
20-44	69.0	68.0	65.0	65.3	73.8	72.3	72.2	74.4	.	.	.	.
45-64	51.2	43.8	48.3	48.4	56.8	58.6	56.5	62.5	.	.	.	.
RACE												
Black	51.1	42.3	52.6	52.0	64.6	68.1	63.6	68.2	.	.	.	.
Non-Black	62.7	60.3	56.2	57.4	66.0	62.9	63.5	66.9	.	.	.	.
SEX												
Female	66.5	54.5	54.9	52.1	64.4	67.9	64.2	69.6	.	.	.	.
Male	53.5	52.6	55.7	59.8	63.5	62.1	63.1	66.1	.	.	.	.
PRIMARY DIAGNOSIS												
Diabetes	47.9	40.0	38.2	30.7	48.0	48.4	47.4	53.0	.	.	.	.
Hypertension	61.4	59.1	56.3	64.9	73.4	69.6	68.9	71.6	.	.	.	.
Kidney Diseases	65.5	63.2	69.6	72.4	76.0	74.7	73.8	78.3	.	.	.	.
Other	62.9	52.9	60.0	59.3	67.4	68.2	65.0	73.7	.	.	.	.
TOTAL PROBABILITIES												
Total Crude Prob.	62.9	56.7	60.0	60.4	66.1	66.8	64.5	68.1	.	.	.	.
Total Adjusted Prob.	59.5	53.4	55.1	56.3	63.5	65.2	63.6	67.7	.	.	.	.

USRDS 1990 Annual Data Report, Patient Survival   E.83
Ten Year Survival Probabilities: From Day 1 to Ten Years For First Transplant Patients (Cadaveric)
By Year Of First Transplant By Age, Race, Sex, and Primary Disease Causing ESRD
Using Aggregate Categories Adjusted for Age, Race, Sex, and Primary Disease

	1977	1978	1979	1980	1981	1982	1983	1984	1985	1986	1987	1988
AGE												
0-19	63.2	48.4	52.5	.	.	.	.	.	.	.	.	.
20-44	53.0	48.6	46.8	.	.	.	.	.	.	.	.	.
45-64	24.4	16.8	28.6	.	.	.	.	.	.	.	.	.
RACE												
Black	34.5	22.4	31.5	.	.	.	.	.	.	.	.	.
Non-Black	38.1	34.9	38.6	.	.	.	.	.	.	.	.	.
SEX												
Female	39.2	31.3	39.0	.	.	.	.	.	.	.	.	.
Male	38.4	30.8	34.1	.	.	.	.	.	.	.	.	.
PRIMARY DIAGNOSIS												
Diabetes	19.0	10.4	21.0	.	.	.	.	.	.	.	.	.
Hypertension	53.9	39.4	37.0	.	.	.	.	.	.	.	.	.
Kidney Diseases	40.7	41.3	48.3	.	.	.	.	.	.	.	.	.
Other	40.8	34.7	42.1	.	.	.	.	.	.	.	.	.
TOTAL PROBABILITIES												
Total Crude Prob.	42.9	37.2	41.6	.	.	.	.	.	.	.	.	.
Total Adjusted Prob.	38.6	30.8	36.6	.	.	.	.	.	.	.	.	.

USRDS 1990 Annual Data Report, Patient Survival E.89
Five Year Survival Probabilities: From Day 1 to Five Years, For First Transplant Patients (Living Related)
By Year Of First Transplant By Age, Race, Sex, and Primary Disease Causing ESRD
Using Aggregate Categories Adjusted for Age, Race, Sex, and Primary Disease

.	1977	1978	1979	1980	1981	1982	1983	1984	1985	1986	1987	1988
AGE												
0-19	40.5	60.5	52.1	46.2	82.6	84.3	61.3	72.0	.	.	.	.
20-44	81.9	80.8	73.3	81.2	81.3	84.0	83.5	89.6	.	.	.	.
45-64	28.0	60.3	49.5	55.1	66.4	71.8	68.1	62.4	.	.	.	.
RACE												
Black	26.9	52.1	43.8	59.8	64.0	76.3	62.1	59.7	.	.	.	.
Non-Black	58.0	77.0	60.9	66.7	75.8	77.2	79.9	77.6	.	.	.	.
SEX												
Female	49.1	74.0	60.6	64.0	82.9	75.1	78.6	66.1	.	.	.	.
Male	49.2	63.7	56.9	65.0	64.2	78.3	73.2	76.7	.	.	.	.
PRIMARY DIAGNOSIS												
Diabetes	19.5	49.1	26.5	36.5	60.3	62.7	61.7	53.9	.	.	.	.
Hypertension	58.7	76.4	47.9	66.0	81.6	80.2	79.7	72.8	.	.	.	.
Kidney Diseases	53.8	73.0	76.4	84.8	71.2	91.3	82.7	81.6	.	.	.	.
Other	73.1	75.7	86.2	78.9	76.6	77.1	70.1	88.7	.	.	.	.
TOTAL PROBABILITIES												
Total Crude Prob.	66.6	74.8	75.1	72.9	75.5	77.6	75.5	72.3	.	.	.	.
Total Adjusted Prob.	49.6	68.9	59.0	64.6	73.6	75.9	75.0	71.6	.	.	.	.

APPENDIX 1

USRDS 1990 Annual Data Report, Patient Survival E.91
Ten Year Survival Probabilities: From Day 1 to Ten Years For First Transplant Patients (Living Related)
By Year Of First Transplant By Age, Race, Sex, and Primary Disease Causing ESRD
Using Aggregate Categories Adjusted for Age, Race, Sex, and Primary Disease

	1977	1978	1979	1980	1981	1982	1983	1984	1985	1986	1987	1988
AGE												
0-19	34.2	58.3	49.5	.	.	.	.	.	.	.	.	.
20-44	70.8	69.7	62.6	.	.	.	.	.	.	.	.	.
45-64	23.1	38.9	35.7	.	.	.	.	.	.	.	.	.
RACE												
Black	18.0	49.7	40.1	.	.	.	.	.	.	.	.	
Non-Black	50.4	53.6	46.9	.	.	.	.	.	.	.		
SEX												
Female	43.4	49.3	49.7	.	.	.	.	.	.	.	.	
Male	40.8	53.7	44.3	.	.	.	.	.	.	.	.	
PRIMARY DIAGNOSIS												
Diabetes	16.4	25.3	16.8	.	.	.	.	.	.	.	.	
Hypertension	48.1	75.0	43.2	.	.	.	.	.	.	.		
Kidney Diseases	46.6	56.7	58.7	.	.	.	.	.	.	.		
Other	55.5	59.3	74.2	.	.	.	.	.	.	.		
TOTAL PROBABILITIES												
Total Crude Prob.	53.9	58.5	62.7	.	.	.	.	.	.	.	.	
Total Adjusted Prob.	42.4	51.8	47.1	.	.	.	.	.	.		.	

USRDS Annual Data Report 1990, Transplant Outcome G.1
Counts of First Renal Transplants (Cadaveric)
By Year of First Transplant By Age, Race, Primary Disease Causing ESRD and
By Selected Transplant Characteristics

.	1977	1978	1979	1980	1981	1982	1983	1984	1985	1986	1987	1988
AGE												
0- 4	6	8	11	12	12	15	18	31	33	29	37	28
5- 9	3	15	23	16	31	28	25	35	36	45	35	42
10-14	24	42	59	55	53	63	61	70	72	79	84	65
15-19	54	100	109	95	109	119	141	149	150	164	179	146
20-24	85	154	176	174	217	240	243	288	306	341	279	258
25-29	99	192	208	243	250	347	390	424	405	524	506	410
30-34	93	196	243	261	336	447	493	583	574	750	652	617
35-39	83	198	229	241	299	401	524	604	660	782	783	733
40-44	91	184	204	239	287	381	411	513	571	715	789	708
45-49	90	167	206	226	238	341	372	447	559	669	672	675
50-54	74	143	156	188	213	286	326	406	425	579	615	557
55-59	34	93	96	97	117	152	215	271	331	452	486	474
60-64	5	30	39	23	39	61	72	147	180	248	285	332
65-69	2	6	3	15	11	5	27	32	58	100	140	172
BENEFICIARY RACE												
Black	177	324	359	433	488	705	799	924	1050	1231	1241	1187
White	531	1128	1307	1367	1574	2082	2410	2952	3186	4055	4073	3797
Other	35	76	96	85	150	99	109	124	124	191	228	233
SEX												
Male	459	964	1110	1195	1420	1851	2094	2515	2758	3476	3458	3142
Female	284	564	652	690	792	1035	1224	1485	1602	2001	2084	2075
DISEASE GROUP												
Diabetes	45	101	131	160	235	397	489	676	840	1113	1143	1091
Hypertension	55	145	133	182	233	367	442	503	628	753	807	808
Glomeruloneph.	180	373	415	437	527	778	880	1137	1135	1455	1445	1314
Cystic Kidney	25	61	84	84	106	178	217	301	331	437	512	468
Other Urologic	43	104	126	134	139	186	255	259	312	376	352	269
Other Cause	11	39	52	59	72	131	194	256	307	364	351	356
Unknown Cause	86	166	214	203	232	269	312	336	356	420	415	366

APPENDIX 1

USRDS Annual Data Report 1990, Transplant Outcome G.3
Counts of First Renal Transplants (Living Releated) By Year of First Transplant
By Age, Race, Primary Disease Causing ESRD and
By Selected Transplant Characteristics

.	1977	1978	1979	1980	1981	1982	1983	1984	1985	1986	1987	1988
AGE												
0- 4	.	1	4	8	17	32	36	40	41	39	53	40
5- 9	7	10	20	25	21	41	29	42	51	39	50	28
10-14	17	40	46	42	36	60	81	95	82	75	65	71
15-19	29	65	94	69	106	143	148	133	128	137	124	108
20-24	37	87	116	112	153	213	214	187	191	189	175	152
25-29	48	99	133	151	173	263	266	237	271	263	245	221
30-34	37	65	98	111	210	239	268	254	254	262	224	242
35-39	21	44	77	76	107	174	174	176	198	206	195	186
40-44	21	38	47	71	71	125	121	127	140	130	155	118
45-49	12	37	39	47	63	92	98	98	118	106	116	96
50-54	7	19	30	31	50	68	76	76	86	74	88	80
55-59	6	9	14	9	22	46	41	37	50	54	65	45
60-64	1	5	4	.	2	14	12	12	12	19	28	22
65-69	2	1	1	3	2	1	4	2	3	5	13	9
BENEFICIARY RACE												
Black	20	48	82	72	80	175	188	189	196	179	164	163
White	207	439	595	647	862	1280	1335	1288	1383	1380	1385	1206
Other	18	33	46	36	91	56	45	39	46	39	47	49
SEX												
Male	138	297	447	435	624	945	960	938	952	955	923	877
Female	107	223	276	320	409	566	608	578	673	643	673	541
DISEASE GROUP												
Diabetes	11	41	40	73	113	249	270	287	328	361	336	278
Hypertension	13	28	35	35	59	128	114	117	121	116	127	113
Glomeruloneph.	52	122	176	208	279	451	531	477	494	444	469	427
Cystic Kidney	5	9	18	22	28	43	56	64	63	64	68	52
Other Urologic	19	40	40	35	79	108	131	115	137	136	119	88
Other Cause	8	24	41	33	42	92	135	184	164	179	182	158
Unknown Cause	26	61	98	89	115	155	129	132	146	115	117	88
Missing Disease	111	195	275	260	318	285	202	140	172	183	178	214

USRDS Annual Data Report 1990, Transplant Outcome   G.21
Five Year Graft Survival Probabilities
For First Transplants (Living Related) By Year of Transplant
By Age, Race, Sex, and Primary Disease Causing ESRD, Unadjusted

	1977	1978	1979	1980	1981	1982	1983	1984	1985	1986	1987	1988
AGE												
0- 4	.	100	25.00	62.50	76.47	65.63	63.89	75.00	.	.	.	.
5- 9	42.86	80.00	35.00	72.00	76.19	51.22	48.28	69.05	.	.	.	.
10-14	47.06	50.00	50.00	61.90	55.56	58.33	66.67	61.05	.	.	.	.
15-19	48.28	50.77	58.51	62.32	67.92	70.63	71.62	67.67	.	.	.	.
20-24	86.49	66.67	73.28	73.21	69.28	69.95	70.09	70.59	.	.	.	.
25-29	72.92	67.68	66.92	72.85	73.41	69.96	72.56	74.26	.	.	.	.
30-34	64.86	55.38	66.33	73.87	63.81	71.13	72.39	77.17	.	.	.	.
35-39	76.19	52.27	62.34	61.84	57.01	67.82	69.54	74.43	.	.	.	.
40-44	52.38	57.89	61.70	54.93	57.75	61.60	61.16	62.20	.	.	.	.
45-49	50.00	45.95	56.41	55.32	58.73	69.57	67.35	62.24	.	.	.	.
50-54	71.43	52.63	66.67	51.61	60.00	51.47	61.84	59.21	.	.	.	.
55-59	50.00	55.56	57.14	55.56	59.09	63.04	73.17	67.57	.	.	.	.
RACE												
Black	65.00	45.83	45.12	56.94	45.00	55.43	55.32	44.44	.	.	.	.
White	62.80	59.23	65.21	67.85	66.01	68.59	70.79	73.14	.	.	.	.
Other	83.33	57.58	65.22	58.33	74.73	66.07	77.78	84.62	.	.	.	.
SEX												
Male	63.77	55.89	59.73	65.06	64.10	64.76	68.96	69.51	.	.	.	.
Female	65.42	60.54	68.12	68.12	66.75	70.67	69.41	70.42	.	.	.	.
DISEASE GROUP												
Diabetes	63.64	46.34	50.00	60.27	52.21	59.44	59.63	64.46	.	.	.	.
Hypertension	69.23	42.86	45.71	51.43	64.41	60.16	59.65	60.68	.	.	.	.
Glomeruloneph.	61.54	49.18	59.09	67.79	64.87	65.41	71.94	70.23	.	.	.	.
Cystic Kidney	80.00	33.33	50.00	68.18	60.71	74.42	67.86	79.69	.	.	.	.
Other Urologic	63.16	65.00	67.50	62.86	72.15	69.44	75.57	78.26	.	.	.	.
Other Cause	37.50	50.00	51.22	63.64	64.29	64.13	62.96	69.02	.	.	.	.
Unknown Cause	76.92	59.02	65.31	61.80	52.17	74.19	68.22	64.39	.	.	.	.
Missing Disease	63.96	68.21	70.55	71.15	73.58	74.04	80.69	82.14	.	.	.	.
TOTAL PROBABILITY												
Total Crude Prob.	64.49	57.88	62.93	66.36	65.15	66.98	69.13	69.85	.	.	.	.

USRDS Annual Data Report 1990, Transplant Outcome G.25
Ten Year Graft Survival Probabilities For First Transplants (Living Related)
By Year of Transplant By Age, Race, Sex, and Primary Disease Causing ESRD, Unadjusted

		1977	1978	1979	1980	1981	1982	1983	1984	1985	1986	1987	1988
AGE													
	0- 4	.	100	0.00	.		.		.	.		.	.
	5- 9	42.86	80.00	30.00	.		.		.	.		.	.
	10-14	17.65	35.00	34.78	.		.		.	.		.	.
	15-19	37.93	44.62	47.87	.		.		.	.		.	.
	20-24	70.27	56.32	66.38	.		.		.	.		.	.
	25-29	56.25	60.61	56.39	.		.		.	.		.	.
	30-34	48.65	43.08	58.16	.		.		.	.		.	.
	35-39	52.38	50.00	55.84	.		.		.	.		.	.
	40-44	38.10	52.63	53.19	.		.		.	.		.	.
	45-49	25.00	32.43	41.03	.		.		.	.		.	.
	50-54	57.14	42.11	43.33	.		.		.	.		.	.
	55-59	33.33	33.33	42.86	.		.		.	.		.	.
RACE													
	Black	35.00	39.58	32.93	.		.		.	.		.	.
	White	46.86	49.66	54.79	.		.		.	.		.	.
	Other	72.22	51.52	58.70	.		.		.	.		.	.
SEX													
	Male	47.83	48.15	49.22	.		.		.	.		.	.
	Female	47.66	49.78	57.97	.		.		.	.		.	.
DISEASE GROUP													
	Diabetes	36.36	39.02	32.50	.		.		.	.		.	.
	Hypertension	46.15	42.86	31.43	.		.		.	.		.	.
	Glomeruloneph.	42.31	40.98	48.30	.		.		.	.		.	.
	Cystic Kidney	60.00	33.33	33.33	.		.		.	.		.	.
	Other Urologic	52.63	47.50	57.50	.		.		.	.		.	.
	Other Cause	25.00	45.83	43.90	.		.		.	.		.	.
	Unknown Cause	42.31	47.54	51.02	.		.		.	.		.	.
	Missing Disease	53.15	58.46	63.27	.		.		.	.		.	.
TOTAL PROBABILITY													
	Total Crude Prob.	47.76	48.85	52.56	.		.		.	.		.	.

USRDS Annual Data Report 1990, Transplant Outcome G.31
One Year Graft Survival Probabilities For First Transplants (Cadaveric)
By Year of Transplant By Age, Race, Sex, and Primary Disease Causing ESRD, Unadjusted

	1977	1978	1979	1980	1981	1982	1983	1984	1985	1986	1987	1988
AGE												
0- 4	50.00	62.50	36.36	50.00	58.33	40.00	44.44	41.94	30.30	55.17	72.97	60.71
5- 9	33.33	60.00	56.52	43.75	64.52	50.00	64.00	68.57	75.00	60.00	54.29	73.81
10-14	62.50	73.81	57.63	58.18	71.70	60.32	57.38	75.71	79.17	74.68	77.38	72.31
15-19	51.85	53.00	72.48	68.42	66.06	63.87	68.79	73.15	67.33	75.00	75.98	74.66
20-24	63.53	53.90	64.77	62.64	62.67	66.67	68.31	67.71	77.12	73.02	78.14	75.58
25-29	53.54	53.65	60.58	62.96	65.60	65.13	67.69	74.29	77.04	76.34	77.87	77.80
30-34	51.61	51.02	58.02	60.15	63.39	61.74	65.31	73.07	79.44	76.00	76.07	79.42
35-39	62.65	54.55	47.16	61.00	65.22	59.10	62.98	71.36	74.09	74.30	76.37	76.26
40-44	57.14	50.54	49.51	61.51	59.58	59.32	63.75	67.25	78.63	77.20	73.76	77.12
45-49	42.22	43.71	52.43	58.41	61.34	62.46	64.78	68.01	75.31	73.99	75.60	77.93
50-54	56.76	53.15	53.21	54.79	58.22	62.24	62.88	70.94	73.41	79.45	78.70	78.10
55-59	52.94	51.61	54.17	58.76	55.56	57.89	57.67	77.12	69.49	73.67	75.51	77.64
RACE												
Black	51.98	44.75	47.91	55.43	57.99	57.02	58.57	65.04	69.43	70.35	74.46	72.79
White	56.87	54.34	57.38	61.59	63.47	63.26	66.10	72.29	76.77	76.77	76.14	77.90
Other	42.86	51.32	58.33	63.53	61.33	57.58	62.39	79.84	79.84	81.15	81.58	80.26
SEX												
Male	54.47	50.31	53.42	60.50	61.55	61.16	64.23	70.50	76.18	75.29	75.85	76.54
Female	55.99	55.32	59.05	59.86	63.13	62.22	64.05	71.45	73.22	75.81	76.20	77.30
DISEASE GROUP												
Diabetes	44.44	46.53	52.67	50.62	61.70	57.18	57.87	67.90	76.31	71.70	73.40	76.54
Hypertension	58.18	49.66	48.87	58.79	59.23	58.86	63.35	68.79	72.29	74.63	74.47	75.62
Glomeruloneph.	52.22	54.16	51.08	60.18	59.77	62.85	66.14	72.91	77.97	76.98	77.58	77.78
Cystic Kidney	36.00	45.90	42.86	67.86	57.55	63.48	70.51	71.76	72.51	78.49	79.30	80.77
Other Urologic	72.09	58.65	68.25	66.42	66.91	63.44	67.84	71.04	71.79	77.93	74.72	80.67
Other Cause	54.55	58.97	69.23	57.63	69.44	54.20	59.28	71.09	73.29	70.88	74.64	76.69
Unknown Cause	60.47	53.61	57.94	67.00	67.24	69.52	64.42	74.11	76.97	77.86	77.83	71.58
Missing Disease	55.37	51.02	57.66	58.95	62.28	61.21	64.65	69.36	73.39	77.46	76.60	75.41
TOTAL PROBABILITY												
Total Crude Prob.	55.05	52.16	55.51	60.27	62.12	61.54	64.17	70.85	75.09	75.48	75.98	76.84

APPENDIX 1

USRDS Annual Data Report 1990, Transplant Outcome G.43
Five Year Graft Survival Probabilities For First Transplants (Cadaveric)
By Year of Transplant By Age, Race, Sex, and Primary Disease Causing ESRD, Unadjusted

	1977	1978	1979	1980	1981	1982	1983	1984	1985	1986	1987	1988
AGE												
0- 4	33.33	12.50	9.09	25.00	58.33	20.00	27.78	35.48	.	.	.	.
5- 9	0.00	13.33	34.78	31.25	22.58	28.57	44.00	51.43	.	.	.	.
10-14	45.83	47.62	27.12	34.55	33.96	25.40	32.79	42.86	.	.	.	.
15-19	22.22	30.00	56.88	42.11	44.95	31.93	48.23	48.32	.	.	.	.
20-24	44.71	36.36	44.32	44.25	41.01	45.00	46.91	48.26	.	.	.	.
25-29	38.38	39.06	35.10	42.39	40.00	43.52	47.69	49.29	.	.	.	.
30-34	31.18	32.14	37.45	36.40	42.26	41.16	43.41	46.66	.	.	.	.
35-39	38.55	34.85	31.00	37.34	40.13	40.15	39.69	47.85	.	.	.	.
40-44	32.97	25.54	25.98	35.15	42.86	41.73	43.55	46.39	.	.	.	.
45-49	22.22	20.96	33.01	34.96	39.50	38.12	39.52	48.10	.	.	.	.
50-54	36.49	30.77	33.97	35.64	37.09	41.96	42.33	47.54	.	.	.	.
55-59	23.53	35.48	32.29	23.71	26.50	33.55	36.74	53.87	.	.	.	.
RACE												
Black	25.42	23.15	25.35	28.87	31.35	30.78	32.54	36.58	.	.	.	.
White	37.29	33.78	37.11	39.21	41.17	42.89	45.27	50.68	.	.	.	.
Other	20.00	36.84	39.58	37.65	47.33	40.40	47.71	58.87	.	.	.	.
SEX												
Male	33.55	31.22	31.98	36.74	38.87	39.92	41.83	46.52	.	.	.	.
Female	33.80	32.45	39.72	36.81	40.40	39.71	43.06	49.63	.	.	.	.
DISEASE GROUP												
Diabetes	20.00	26.73	25.19	27.50	36.60	33.50	34.15	40.68	.	.	.	.
Hypertension	27.27	26.21	29.32	26.37	33.48	34.06	36.88	41.15	.	.	.	.
Glomeruloneph.	31.67	33.51	32.53	40.05	37.95	40.10	46.25	50.84	.	.	.	.
Cystic Kidney	20.00	22.95	29.76	42.86	36.79	44.94	52.07	56.15	.	.	.	.
Other Urologic	41.86	39.42	47.62	38.06	43.17	41.94	45.10	52.90	.	.	.	.
Other Cause	36.36	35.90	34.62	27.12	33.33	32.06	34.54	48.05	.	.	.	.
Unknown Cause	45.35	33.13	36.45	41.87	40.95	47.21	41.99	43.75	.	.	.	.
Missing Disease	34.56	31.54	37.23	38.02	43.41	43.62	45.37	50.94	.	.	.	.
TOTAL PROBABILITY												
Total Crude Prob.	33.65	31.68	34.85	36.76	39.42	39.85	42.28	47.68	.	.	.	.

USRDS Annual Data Report 1990, Transplant Outcome G.47
Ten Year Graft Survival Probabilities For First Transplants (Cadaveric)
By Year of Transplant By Age, Race, Sex, and Primary Disease Causing ESRD, Unadjusted

		1977	1978	1979	1980	1981	1982	1983	1984	1985	1986	1987	1988
AGE													
	0- 4	33.33	12.50	0.00	.	.	.	.	.	.	.	.	.
	5- 9	0.00	13.33	17.39	.	.	.	.	.	.	.	.	.
	10-14	25.00	30.95	18.64	.	.	.	.	.	.	.	.	.
	15-19	14.81	18.00	36.70	.	.	.	.	.	.	.	.	.
	20-24	32.94	24.68	30.68	.	.	.	.	.	.	.	.	.
	25-29	29.29	25.00	25.48	.	.	.	.	.	.	.	.	.
	30-34	20.43	19.90	25.93	.	.	.	.	.	.	.	.	.
	35-39	24.10	24.75	25.33	.	.	.	.	.	.	.	.	.
	40-44	20.88	18.48	16.18	.	.	.	.	.	.	.	.	.
	45-49	11.11	16.77	23.79	.	.	.	.	.	.	.	.	.
	50-54	21.62	13.29	19.87	.	.	.	.	.	.	.	.	.
	55-59	17.65	16.13	15.63	.	.	.	.	.	.	.	.	.
RACE													
	Black	14.69	11.42	13.37	.	.	.	.	.	.	.	.	.
	White	25.24	22.25	25.94	.	.	.	.	.	.	.	.	.
	Other	11.43	25.00	28.12	.	.	.	.	.	.	.	.	.
SEX													
	Male	22.00	19.19	21.17	.	.	.	.	.	.	.	.	.
	Female	22.18	21.63	27.45	.	.	.	.	.	.	.	.	.
DISEASE GROUP													
	Diabetes	11.11	12.87	12.98	.	.	.	.	.	.	.	.	.
	Hypertension	18.18	14.48	19.55	.	.	.	.	.	.	.	.	.
	Glomeruloneph.	19.44	17.96	23.61	.	.	.	.	.	.	.	.	.
	Cystic Kidney	20.00	16.39	17.86	.	.	.	.	.	.	.	.	.
	Other Urologic	27.91	30.77	34.13	.	.	.	.	.	.	.	.	.
	Other Cause	9.09	17.95	19.23	.	.	.	.	.	.	.	.	.
	Unknown Cause	32.56	21.69	21.03	.	.	.	.	.	.	.	.	.
	Missing Disease	22.82	22.45	26.36	.	.	.	.	.	.	.	.	.
TOTAL PROBABILITY													
	Total Crude Prob.	22.07	20.09	23.50	.	.	.	.	.	.	.	.	.

USRDS Annual Data Report 1990, Institutional Providers 1.1
Counts Of Medicare ESRD Facilities By Year
By Certification Type And Ownership Type

	1981	1982	1983	1984	1985	1986	1987	1988	1989
Certification Type									
TRANSPLANT CENTER	8	17	19	26	30	31	40	44	52
DIALYSIS CENTER	385	385	365	362	354	353	343	334	339
DIALYSIS FACIL HOSPITAL	105	114	112	122	132	143	148	161	174
DIALYSIS FACIL (FREE-STANDING)	497	552	637	688	769	876	961	1099	1199
TRANSPLANT AND DIALYSIS CENTER	148	139	141	143	145	154	158	164	167
	1143	1207	1274	1341	1430	1557	1650	1802	1931
Ownership Type									
INDIVIDUAL-FOR PROFIT	15	16	18	23	30	34	38	42	44
PARTNERSHIP-FOR PROFIT	15	17	20	23	34	44	52	67	75
CORPORATION-FOR PROFIT	307	342	399	433	478	560	617	717	790
OTHER-FOR PROFIT	79	80	80	78	85	92	99	106	109
INDIVIDUAL-NOT-FOR-PROFIT	3	3	3	4	6	7	7	7	7
CORPORATION-NOT-FOR-PROFIT	454	469	476	499	520	541	570	595	635
OTHER-NOT-FOR-PROFIT	112	119	117	120	117	118	111	110	110
STATE-GOV NON-FED	49	52	52	54	52	52	52	52	51
COUNTY-GOV NON-FED	36	34	34	33	33	32	30	31	30
CITY-GOV NON-FED	17	17	18	17	17	15	14	15	15
CITY/COUNTY-GOV NON-FED	5	5	5	5	5	6	6	6	6
HOSPITAL DIST/AUTH GOV NON-FED	31	31	29	31	32	33	31	30	31
OTHER-GOV NON-FED	4	4	5	5	5	4	4	4	7
VETERANS ADMINISTRATION GOV FED	14	17	15	15	15	16	15	15	14
PUBLIC HEALTH SERVICE- GOV FED	2	1	1	1	1	3	4	4	3
OTHER-GOV FED	0	0	0	0	0	0	0	1	1
UNKNOWN-MISSING ON FORM	0	0	2	0	0	0	0	0	3
	1143	1207	1274	1341	1430	1557	1650	1802	1931

Appendix 2

Some Physicians And Scientists Experienced With Nutritional Therapy For Chronic Renal Disease

California

Joel D. Kopple, M.D.[1]
Harbor Medical Center
1124 Carson Street, C-1 Annex
Torrance, California 90502
(213) 212-4101

Shaul G. Massry, M.D.[1]
University of Southern California
Division of Nephrology
2025 Zonal Avenue GNH-4250
Los Angeles, California 90033
(213) 224-5261

District of Columbia

Juan P. Bosch, M.D.[1]
George Washington University
Division of Renal Diseases
2150 Pennsylvania Avenue, N.W.
Washington, D.C. 20037
(202) 994-3859

Florida

C. Craig Tisher, M.D.[1]
University of Florida
Division of Nephrology
Box J224 JHMHC
Gainesville, Florida 32610
(904) 392-3755

Jacques J. Bourgoignie, M.D.[1]
University of Miami
P.O. Box 016960 (R-126)
Miami, Florida 33101
(305) 547-4691

Georgia

William E. Mitch, M.D.[1]
Emory University
218 Glenn Building
69 Butler Street, S.E.
Atlanta, Georgia 30322
(404) 589-3620

Iowa

Lawrence G. Hunsicker, M.D.[1]
University of Iowa Hospitals and Clinics
Internal Medicine
T312 General Hospital
Iowa City, Iowa 52242
(319) 356-4900

Massachusetts

Andrew S. Levey, M.D.[1]
New England Medical Center Hospital/
Massachusetts General Hospital
Division of Nephrology
750 Washington Street
Boston, Massachusetts 02111
(617) 326-7544

J. Michael Lazarus, M.D.[1]
Brigham and Women's Hospital/
Beth Israel Hospital
454 Brookline Avenue Suite 27
Boston, Massachusetts 02115
(617) 732-5950

Maryland

Mackenzie Walser, M.D.[2]
    Johns Hopkins University School of Medicine
    Department of Pharmacology
    725 North Wolfe Street
    Baltimore, Maryland 21205
    (301) 955-3832

Missouri

Saulo Klahr, M.D.[2]
    Washington University School of Medicine
    Renal Division
    600 South Euclid Avenue
    St. Louis, Missouri 63110
    (314) 362-8231

North Carolina

Vardaman Buckalew, M.D.[1]
    Bowman Gray School of Medicine
    Dept. of Medicine/Nephrology
    1940 Beach Street
    Winston-Salem, North Carolina 27103
    (919) 748-6324

Vincent W. Dennis, M.D.[1]
    Duke University School of Medicine
    Division of Nephrology
    P.O. Box 3014
    Durham, North Carolina 27710
    (919) 228-6373

New York

Jerome G. Porush, M.D.[1]
    Brookdale Hospital Medical Center
    568 Rockaway Parkway, 2nd Floor
    Brooklyn, New York 16212
    (718) 240-5607 or (718) 240-5615

Ohio

Lee A. Hebert, M.D.[1]
    Ohio State University
    N210 Means Hall
    1654 Upham Drive
    Columbus, Ohio 43210

    (614) 293-5505

Pennsylvania

Alan G. Wasserstein, M.D.[3]
    University of Pennsylvania Medical Group
    Renal Division
    210 White Building
    3400 Spruce Street
    Philadelphia, Pennsylvania 19104
    (215) 662-2690

Tennessee

Paul E. Teschan, M.D.[1]
    Vanderbilt University Medical Center
    422 Medical Arts Building
    Nashville, Tennessee 37232-1371
    (615) 322-6539

Texas

Meyer Lifschitz, M.D.[1]
    University of Texas Health Science Center
    7703 Floyd Curl Drive
    San Antonio, Texas 78284-7882
    (512) 696-9660 (ext. 4685)

Europe

France

M. Aparicio, M.D.[2]
Service de Nephrologie
Hôpital Pellegrin-Tripode
33076 Bordeaux CEDEX, France
56.79.55.37

Germany

M. Strauch, M.D.[2]
Nephrologische Klinik
Klinikum Mannheim
Postfach 23
6800 Mannheim 1, Germany

N. Gretz, M.D.[2]
Nephrologische Klinik
Klinikum Mannheim
Postfach 23
6800 Mannheim 1, Germany

Italy

G. Barsotti, M.D.[2]
Clinica Medica 1°
University of Pisa
56100 Pisa, Italy

M.G. Gentile, M.D.[2]
Divisione Nefrologica
Ospedale S. Carlo Borromeo
20100 Milano, Italy

Sergio Giovannetti, M.D.[2]
Clinica Medica 1
University of Pisa
56100 Pisa, Italy
(050) 502586

Giuseppe Maschio, M.D.[2]
Division of Nephrology
University of Verona
Ospedale Civile Maggiore
37126 Verona, Italy
(045) 932528

Ester Morelli, M.D.[2]
Clinica Medica 1
University of Pisa
56110 Pisa, Italy

L. Oldrizzi, M.D.[2]
Division of Nephrology
University of Verona
Ospedale Civile Maggiore
37126 Verona, Italy

C. Rugiu, M.D.[2]
Division of Nephrology
University of Verona
Ospedale Civile Maggiore
37126 Verona, Italy

Sweden

Jonas Bergström, M.D.[2]
Department of Renal Medicine
Huddinge University Hospital
S-1486 Huddinge, Sweden

Switzerland

Johan B. Rosman, M.D.[2]
   University Hospital of Basel
   CH-4031 Basel, Switzerland

United Kingdom

G. A. Coles, M.D.[2]
   Cardiff Royal Infirmary
   Newport Road
   Cardiff CF2 1SZ, United Kingdom
   (0222) 492233

A. M. El Nahas, M.D.[2]
   Department of Renal Medicine
   Northern General Hospital
   Herries Road
   Sheffield S5 7AU, United Kingdom
   (0742) 434343

Australia

Benno U. Ihle, M.D.[2]
   Royal Melbourne Hospital
   Victoria 3050, Australia
   347-4052

Sources: 1. Department of Health and Human Services, National Institutes of Health, National Institute of Diabetes and Digestive and Kidney Diseases, Information Handbook for The Modification of Diet in Renal Disease Study (MDRD). Revised January 18, 1990.
2. Published books or studies.
3. Personal communication.

Appendix 3

Directory Of Kidney Disease Related Organizations

American Association of Kidney Patients (AAKP)
Suite 302
1 Davis Boulevard
Tampa, Florida 33606
(813) 251-0725
Erwin Hytner, Executive Director
Kris Robinson, Assistant Director
Publication: *Renalife* (twice yearly magazine), *Bulletin* (quarterly newspaper)
Convention: Annual **Membership Fee:** $15 annually
Local Groups: 26

American Diabetes Association (ADA)
1660 Duke Street
Alexandria, Virginia 22314
(703) 549-1500 or (800) ADA-DISC
Sheila Mylet, Coordinator, Patient Information
Publications: *Diabetes*; *Diabetes Care*; *Diabetes Spectrum*; *Clinical Care*; *Diabetes Forecast*.
Local Groups: 58

American Dietetic Association
216 West Jackson Boulevard
Chicago, Illinois 60606
(312) 899-0040

American Kidney Fund (AKF)
Suite 1010
6110 Executive Boulevard
Rockville, Maryland 20852
(301) 881-3052 or (800) 638-8299
M. Suzanne Popplewell, Information Specialist
Publications: *AKF Nephrology Letter*; *AKF Torchbearer*; *AKF Newsletter* (for Health Professionals); patient and public education brochures.

American Nephrology Nurses' Association (ANNA)
Box 56
North Woodbury Road
Pitman, New Jersey 08071
(609) 589-2187
Ron Brady, Executive Director
Publications: *ANNA Journal*; *ANNA Update* (bimonthly newsletter); *Core Curriculum for Nephrology Nursing*; *Standards of Clinical Practice for Nephrology Nursing*; position statements and clinical monographs.
Local Groups: 4 regions, 62 chapters.

American Society of Nephrology (ASN)
Suite 700
1101 Connecticut Avenue, NW
Washington, DC 20036
(202) 857-1190
Carolyn M. Del Polito, Ph.D.
Publication: *ASN abstract book.*

American Society of Pediatric Nephrology (ASPN)
c/o University of Texas Health Science Center
5323 Harry Hines Boulevard
Dallas, Texas 75234
(214) 688-3438
Billy S. Arant, Jr., M.D., Secretary/Treasurer

American Society of Transplant Physicians
c/o The Wright Organization
716 Lee Street
Des Plaines, Illinois 60016
(312) 824-5700

American Society of Transplant Surgeons
c/o Arnold Diethelm, M.D.
Department of Surgery
UAB Station
Birmingham, Alabama 35294
(205) 934-5200
Arnold Diethelm, M.D., President

International Pediatric Nephrology Association (IPNA)
  Albert Einstein College of Medicine
  1825 Eastchester Road
  Bronx, New York 10461
  (212) 904-2857
  Ira Greifer, M.D., Secretary General
  Publication: *Pediatric Nephrology.*

International Society for Peritoneal Dialysis
  3800 Reservoir Road, NW
  Washington, DC 20007
  (202) 784-3662
  James F. Winchester, M.D., Secretary/Treasurer
  Publication: *Peritoneal Dialysis International.*

National Kidney Foundation, Inc.
  30 East 33rd Street
  New York, New York 10016
  (212) 889-2210 or (800) 622-9010
  John Davis, Executive Director
  Publications: *The Kidney; American Journal of Kidney Diseases;* patient and
public education materials; *CNSW* (newsletter); *CNSW Perspectives; CRN Quar-
terly; CNNT Action Update; Kidney '89.*
  State Groups: 50
  Other Services: Council of Nephrology Nurses and Technicians; Council of
Nephrology Social Workers; Council on Clinical Nephrology; Dialysis and Trans-
plantation; Council on Urology.

North American Transplant Coordinators Organization (NATCO)
  P.O. Box 15384
  Lenexa, Kansas 66215
  (913) 268-9830
  Dede Gish Panjada, Executive Director
  Publications: *NATCO Newsletter;* Patient care brochures.

Polycystic Kidney Research Foundation (PKRF)
  922 Walnut Street
  Kansas City, Missouri 64106
  (816) 421-1869
  Jean G. Bacon, Executive Director

Publications: *Polycystic Kidney Disease?*; *Short History of the PKR Foundation*; *PKR Progress* (quarterly newsletter); *Your Diet and PKD*; *First International Workshop Book.*

Psychonephrology Foundation
c/o Westchester County Medical Center
Valhalla, New York 10595
Norman B. Levy, M.D., President
Publications: *Psychonephrology I: Psychological Factors in Hemodialysis and Transplantation*; *Psychonephrology II: Psychological Problems in Kidney Failure and Their Treatment*; *Psychonephrology III and IV.*

Renal Physicians Association
Suite 500
1101 Vermont Avenue, NW
Washington, DC 20005-3457
(202) 898-1562
M. Eileen Widmer, Executive Director
Publications: Various publications available at no cost to members. A legal resource directory is presently being prepared, for which there will be a cost.

Transplantation Society
c/o New England Deaconess Hospital
185 Pilgrim Road
Boston, Massachusetts 02215
(617) 732-8547
Mary L. Wood
Publications: *Transplantation*; *Transplantation Proceedings.*

United Network for Organ Sharing (UNOS)
1100 Boulders Parkway
Suite 500
Richmond, Virginia 23225
(804) 330-8500
Gene Pierce, Executive Director
Publications: *UNOS Update*; *Transplant Perspective.*

Source:
Department of Health and Human Services, National Institues of Health, National Institute of Diabetes & Digestive & Kidney Diseases, 1989.

Appendix 4

Cookbooks About Many Cuisines

Vegetarian

Atlas, Nava. *American Harest: Regional Recipes For The Vegetarian Kitchen.* New York: Fawcett Columbine, 1987.

Hazelton, Nika. *Nika Hazelton's Way With Vegetables.* New York: M. Evans And Company, Inc., 1976.

Hazen, Janet. *Glories Of The Vegetarian Table.* New York: Addison-Wesley Publishing Company, Inc.,1988.

Sacharoff, Shanta Nimbark. *The Ethnic Vegetarian Kitchen.* San Ramon: 101 Productions, 1984.

Spear, Ruth. *The Classic Vegetable Cookbook.* New York: Harper & Row, Publishers, Inc., 1985.

Thomas, Anna. *The Vegetarian Epicure: Book Two.* New York: Alfred A. Knopf, Inc., 1978.

Italian

Hazan, Marcella. *The Classic Italian Cookbook.* New York: Ballantine Books, 1973.

Hazan, Marcella. *More Classic Italian Cooking.* New York: Ballantine Books, 1978.

Simmons, Marie. *365 Ways To Cook Pasta.* New York: Harper & Row, Publishers, 1988.

Greek

Metaxas, Daphne. *Classic Greek Cooking*. Concord: Nitty Gritty Productions, 1974.

Indian and Middle Eastern

Jaffrey, Madhur. *Indian Cooking*. New York: Barron's Educational Series, Inc.,1982.

Roden, Claudia. *A Book Of Middle Eastern Food*. New York: Vintage Books, 1972.

Chinese and Vietnamese

Lee, Beverly. *The Easy Way To Chinese Cooking*. New York: The New American Library, Inc., 1963.

Lo, Kenneth. *New Chinese Vegetarian Cooking*. New York: Pantheon Books, 1986.

Ngo, Bach, and Zimmerman, Gloria. *The Classic Cuisine Of Vietnam*. New York: Nal Penguin Inc., 1979.

Miscellaneous

Rosso, Julee, and Lukins, Sheila. *The New Basics Cookbook*. New York: Workman Publishing, 1989.

The Gilroy Garlic Festival Association, Inc. *The Garlic Lovers' Cookbook: Volume II*. Berkeley: Celestial Arts, 1985.

Wilson, Jane Weston. *Eating Well When You Just Can't Eat The Way You Used To*. New York: Workman Publishing, 1987.

Appendix 5

Some "Kidney-Friendly" Recipes

I have included a chart and three graphs with each recipe to show the nutritional content of one serving quickly and easily. I found that paying close attention to the nutritional content of my foods at the start of my lifestyle changes helped me develop new cooking and eating habits. They soon became second nature.

Nutrition Information For One Serving		
	Ordinary Ingredients	Low-Protein Ingredients
Calories	294	
Protein	4	
Fat	13	
Phosphorus	61	
Potassium	139	

Protein and fat measurements are in grams; phosphorus and potassium are in milligrams. When the recipe shows the option of low protein ingredients, the nutritional values for the special version are shown under "Low Protein Ingredients."

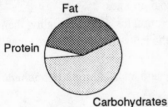

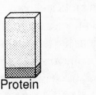 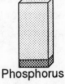

This graph shows how many of the total calories in the recipe come from fat, protein and carbohydrates. Some nutrition experts say that fat should be limited to 30% or less of total daily intake of calories. Some scientists have found that a diet of about 10% of calories from fat may help reverse heart disease.

These graphs show the approximate amount of my daily targets for protein and phosphorus provided by one serving of the recipe. The targets may be different for each person. My targets, illustrated by the graphs, are 24 grams of protein and 500 milligrams of phosphorus per day.

Murray West's
Microwave Risotto

· ·

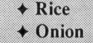

+ Rice
+ Onion

Stove-top risotto in the traditional Italian style takes about 30 or 40 minutes to prepare. Murray West's microwave risotto takes a bit less time, and much less attention. It's almost as good as the traditional dish, and a very appealing meal.

Preparation Time: *5 minutes* **Cooking Time:** *20 minutes*
Servings: *4*

2 tbsp olive oil (extra virgin is best)
2 tbsp butter
1 cup arborio rice (or other rice)
1 onion, chopped
2 ½ cups hot water
3 bouillon cubes (dissolved in the water)

1. In a microwave dish with a cover, heat the olive oil and butter on high for 2 minutes.
2. Add the rice and onion. Cook on high for 4 to 5 minutes.
3. Add the chicken broth and cook on high for 9 minutes. Stir thoroughly, then cook on high for 9 minutes longer. (Stirring at the half-way point assures that the rice, broth and onions are thoroughly mixed.)
4. Remove from the microwave, stir thoroughly and let stand for 4 to 5 minutes to let the rice absorb the flavors.

· ·

	Ordinary Ingredients	Low-Protein Ingredients
Calories	294	
Protein	4	
Fat	13	
Phosphorus	61	
Potassium	139	

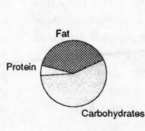

Murray West's
Vegetable Paella

◆ **Sweet Pepper** ◆ **Chili Pepper** ◆ **Red Onion**
◆ **Zucchini** ◆ **Tomato** ◆ **Rice**

Paella is a favorite of Spanish and Portuguese cooking. It usually includes shellfish (lobster, clams, mussels), chicken and sausage, with rice, tomatoes, onions and peppers. Dr. Murray West, of Baltimore, adapted this classic for a low-protein gourmet dinner hearty enough for a complete meal. You can buy arborio rice in a good Italian deli or some supermarkets.

Preparation Time: *10 minutes* **Cooking Time:** *60 minutes*
Servings: *4*

4 tablespoons olive oil (extra virgin is best)
1 red or green pepper, seeded, thinly sliced
1 chili pepper or jalopena pepper, seeded, chopped
1 red onion, thinly sliced
2 cloves garlic, minced
1 zucchini, cut in ½ inch cubes
1½ tsp thyme
2 or 3 tomatoes, or 1 small can tomatoes, chopped, drained
1½ cups rice (arborio rice is best)
3 bouillon cubes dissolved in 3 cups hot water

1. In a large pan with a cover, heat the oil briefly. Sauté the pepper, chili pepper and onion over medium heat for about 15 or 20 minutes until the onions are lightly browned.

2. Add the garlic, zucchini, tomatoes and thyme. Cover and simmer for about 15 minutes.

3. Add the rice and chicken broth. Cover and reduce heat. Simmer, stirring occasionally, until the rice is done, 20 to 25 minutes.

	Ordinary Ingredients	Low-Protein Ingredients
Calories	429	
Protein	8	
Fat	15	
Phosphorus	129	
Potassium	568	

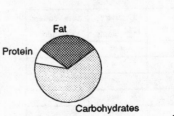

Murray West's
Baked Peppers, Onions and Potatoes

- ✦ **Peppers**
- ✦ **Potatoes**
- ✦ **Onion**

A winter or summer main course that is ready to serve 35 minutes after you start.

Preparation Time: *10 minutes* **Cooking Time:** *25 minutes*
Servings: *4*

5 red or green peppers, seeded, 1-inch cubes
5 potatoes, peeled and quartered
1 medium onion, quartered
1 cup olive oil
pepper to taste

1. Preheat the oven to 425 degrees.
2. Mix all ingredients together in a baking dish, taking care that all the vegetables are covered with the olive oil. Lots of any kind of pepper—black, red, dried chili, fresh chili—adds zest.
3. Bake for about 20 to 25 minutes in the 425 degree oven.

	Ordinary Ingredients	Low-Protein Ingredients
Calories	660	
Protein	4	
Fat	54	
Phosphorus	99	
Potassium	796	

Sandra Watt's
Braised Broccoli

- -

+ **Broccoli**
+ **Oyster sauce**
+ **Ginger**

Preparation Time: *5 minutes* **Cooking Time:** *10 minutes*
Servings: *1*

⅔ cup broccoli, raw, fresh or frozen
1 tbsp peanut oil (or other vegetable oil)
1 tbsp oyster sauce (buy it in an oriental grocery, or some supermarkets)
½ tbsp soy sauce
1 tsp sugar
½ tsp sesame oil (from oriental grocery)
½ cup liquid from blanching the broccoli
2 slices fresh ginger, thinly sliced
1 tsp corn starch

1. Cut the broccoli into bite size pieces. Bring lightly salted water to boil in a saucepan. Drop the broccoli into the boiling water and blanch it for one minute (to seal the flavor). Drain in a colander, but save 1/2 cup of the liquid.
2. Heat the vegetable oil in a wok and stir fry the broccoli and ginger root for 1 minute. Add oyster sauce, soy sauce, sugar, sesame oil and cooking liquid. Let it boil.
3. Mix the corn starch with 1 tbsp cold water and stir into the liquid until it thickens slightly. Toss broccoli in the sauce and serve.

- -

	Ordinary Ingredients	Low-Protein Ingredients
Calories	333	
Protein	5	
Fat	30	
Phosphorus	123	
Potassium	542	

Carbohydrates   Protein

Fat

Protein

Phosphorus

Sandra Watt's
Lo Mein

- ◆ **Lo mein noodles**
- ◆ **Bean sprouts**
- ◆ **Bok choy**
- ◆ **Oyster sauce**

Preparation Time: *5 minutes* **Cooking Time:** *10 minutes*
Servings: *2*

1 package lo mein noodles (2 cups)
¼ cup hot water and bouillon cube
1 tbsp oyster sauce
1 tbsp dry white wine or Chinese rice wine
½ tbsp light soy sauce
1 tbsp vegetable oil
2 cups boy choy stems and leaves, thinly sliced (from most supermarkets, or all oriental groceries)
OR 2 cups shredded cabbage
⅓ cup bean sprouts

1. Drop the lo mein noodles into enough boiling water to cover, cooking for two or three minutes. Then drain and rinse the noodles.
2. Mix the sauce in a small bowl, stirring together the bouillon dissolved in water, oyster sauce, rice wine or dry white wine, soy sauce and sesame oil. Set the sauce aside.
3. Heat a wok (or a skillet) over high heat. Then add the vegetable oil. Stir fry the bok choy or cabbage over high heat for one minute. Remove the stir-fryed vegetables from the wok.
4. Add the sauce, bean sprouts and noodles to the wok. Cook until heated. Then add the bok choy or cabbage and serve.

	Ordinary Ingredients	Low-Protein Ingredients
Calories	510	
Protein	17	
Fat	9	
Phosphorus	229	
Potassium	360	

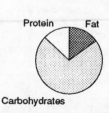

Sandra Watt's
Fried Rice

- ✦ rice
- ✦ peas
- ✦ mushrooms

Preparation Time: *5 minutes*   **Cooking Time:** *15 min-utes*
Servings: *2*

> *1 tbsp peanut (or other oil)*
> *1 egg substitute (optional)*
> *½ onion, diced*
> *2 mushrooms*
> *⅓ cup frozen peas*
> *1 cup cooked rice*
> *2 medium romaine leaves, chopped*
> *⅓ cup bean sprouts*

1. Preheat a wok and add ½ tbsp of oil.
2. Add egg substitute to the hot oil.
3. Lift and tilt the wok to form a thin sheet of egg about 3 to 4 inches wide.
4. Cool without stirring for about 2 minutes until set.
5. Slide the egg sheet onto a cutting board and cut into ¾ inch wide strips. Cut the strips into 2 inch lengths.
6. Return the wok to high heat. Add ½ tbsp oil.
7. Stir fry the onion for 30 seconds.
8. Add mushrooms, beansprouts and peas. Stir fry for 1 minute.
9. Add the rice. Cook and sir for 2 to 3 minutes or until heated.
10. Add romaine and toss slightly.
11. Stir in the egg strips.

	Ordinary Ingredients	Low-Protein Ingredients
Calories	434	
Protein	10	
Fat	14	
Phosphorus	172	
Potassium	462	

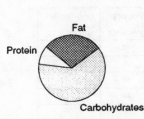

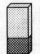

Edith Kahn's
Hungarian Cabbage

- ✦ **Cabbage**
- ✦ **Onion**
- ✦ **Tomatoes**

Preparation Time: *5 minutes* **Cooking Time:** *30 minutes*
Servings: *3*

½ head red cabbage, shredded
1 onion, chopped
1 16-oz can stewed tomatoes
2 tbsp vegetable oil
2 tbsp paprika (more or less to taste)
pepper

1. Sauté the shredded cabbage and chopped onions in the oil until both are soft and the onion is translucent.
2. Add the stewed tomatoes, paprika and pepper.
3. Cover and simmer for 20 minutes.

	Ordinary Ingredients	Low-Protein Ingredients
Calories	160	
Protein	3	
Fat	10	
Phosphorus	87	
Potassium	31	

Fat

Protein

Carbohydrates

Protein

Phosphorus

Edith Kahn's
French Toast

- -

✦ **low protein bread**
✦ **egg substitute**
✦ **milk substitute**

Preparation time: *5 minutes*   **Cooking time:** *5 minutes*
Servings: *1*

1 slice low protein bread
1 tbsp Second Nature egg substitute
½ tsp Farm Rich milk substitute

1. Blend egg and milk substitute.
2. Spray frying pan with Pam and melt small amount of margarine for flavor.
3. Dip the bread in the liquid and brown in the frying pan on both sides.

- -

	Ordinary Ingredients	Low-Protein Ingredients
Calories		117
Protein		2
Fat		4
Phosphorus		4
Potassium		14

Protein — Fat — Carbohydrates

Protein

Phosphorus

Edith Kahn's
Low Protein Cake

- -

> ✦ **cocoa**
> ✦ **low protein flour**

Preparation Time: *10*   **Cooking Time:** *35*
Servings: *8*

> *6 tbsp cocoa*
> *3 cups low protein flour*
> *2 cups sugar*
> *2 tsp baking soda*
> *pinch salt (optional)*
> *2 cups cold water*
> *2 tbsp vinegar*
> *2/3 cup vegetable oil*
> *2 tsp vanilla*

1. Preheat oven to 350.
2. Mix all the dry ingredients together.
3. Add the water, vinegar, vegetable oil and vanilla.
4. Mix thoroughly. Then bake at 350 oven for 25 to 35 minutes.

	Ordinary Ingredients	Low-Protein Ingredients
Calories		542
Protein		0
Fat		22
Phosphorus		24
Potassium		9

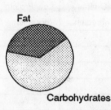

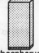

Gary And Dianne Dulin's
Dressing

- ✦ **low-protein bread**
- ✦ **onion**
- ✦ **celery**

Preparation time: *10 minutes*   **Cooking time:** *5 minutes*
Servings: *2*

3 slices low protein bread, toasted
1 tbsp chopped celery
1 tbsp chopped onion
1 tbsp margarine
¼ tsp poultry seasoning
1 low sodium chicken bouillon cube
½ cup hot water

1. Cut the toasted low protein bread into small pieces.
2. Microwave the chopped celery and onion in the margarine on high for 30 seconds.
3. Combine the bread, celery and onion and seasoning.
4. Dissolve the chicken bouillon in the hot water, and pour it over the dressing mixture.
5. Cook in the microwave at high for 2-3 minutes.

	Ordinary Ingredients	Low-Protein Ingredients
Calories		194
Protein		1
Fat		11
Phosphorus		17
Potassium		101

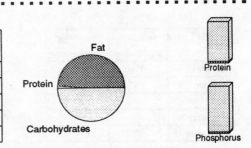

Pasta and Summer Vegetables

- -

✦ **Onion**   ✦ **Chili pepper**
✦ **Zucchini**   ✦ **Tomatoes**

Preparation Time: *10 minutes* **Cooking Time:** *25 minutes*
Servings: *4*

1 onion, chopped
1 fresh green chili pepper, seeds removed, chopped (if you like spicy food)
2 small zucchini, peeled or not, quartered, sliced thinly
2 fresh ripe tomatoes, chopped
2 cloves garlic, minced
3 tbsp olive oil, or other oil
2 cups pasta, (ziti, rigatoni, or similar)
1 bouillon cube dissovled in a cup of hot water

1. Heat the oil over medium heat in a pan deep enough to hold all the ingredients. Add the chopped onion and minced garlic, and stir occasionally, cooking until the onions are softened. (Add the chopped chili pepper, if you like a spicy dish. If you like it *extra spicy*, don't remove the seeds before you chop the pepper.) Meantime, cook the pasta.
2. When the onions are softened, after about 10 or 15 minutes over medium heat, add the bouillon broth. Simmer for about 5 minutes.
3. Add the sliced zucchini and the chopped tomatoes. Simmer for about 10 or 15 minutes, stirring occasionally.
4. Add the drained pasta to the vegetables. Stir thoroughly to mix with the sauce and the vegetables.

- -

	Ordinary Ingredients	Low-Protein Ingredients
Calories	456	
Protein	12	
Fat	15	
Phosphorus	159	
Potassium	576	

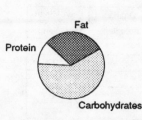

Mediterranean Spaghettini

◆ **Tomatoes**   ◆ **Chili pepper**
◆ **Spaghettini**   ◆ **Cured black olives**

Preparation Time: *10 minutes* **Cooking Time:** *15 minutes*
Servings: *4*

4 tbsp olive oil (extra virgin is best)
2 tsp finely minced jalapeno pepper, or 1 green chili pepper minced, or 1 small dried chili pepper, crumbled
2 large cloves garlic, peeled and finely minced
4 tbsp finely minced fresh parsley
4 large ripe tomatoes, chopped, or 1 2-pound can of tomatoes
½ cup cured black olives, pitted and diced (Canned California ripe olives are nearly tasteless. Some supermarkets or delis sell good olives.)
1 to 2 tsp fresh lemon rind, finely grated
1 ½ tbsp capers, drained (Italian capers packed in brine are best.)
¾ pound spaghettini

1. In a heavy skillet, sauté the chili pepper for 2 or 3 minutes. If you like a spicy sauce, leave the pepper in the pan. If not, remove and discard it once the oil has been flavored.

2. Add the garlic to the chili oil and cook for a minute or two without browning it. Add the parsley and tomatoes, bring to a boil and simmer, stirring often, for about 5 or 10 minutes to reduce the liquid slightly. (Don't reduce it too much. It should be quite juicy.)

3. Add the olives, lemon rind, and capers to the tomato mixture and mix thoroughly. Cover the skillet and keep it warm over low heat.

4. Bring a large pot of salted water to a boil for the spaghettini (or other pasta.) Cook the pasta for about 8 or 10 minutes, until it is just tender. Drain it thoroughly and add it to the skillet. Toss gently and season with salt and pepper.

	Ordinary Ingredients	Low-Protein Ingredients
Calories	480	
Protein	12	
Fat	17	
Phosphorus	144	
Potassium	462	

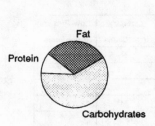

Pan Baked
Potatoes and Onions

● ●

✦ **Potatoes**
✦ **Onions**

Preparation Time: *10 minutes* **Cooking Time** *1¼ hour*
Servings: *5*

5 tbsp butter
2 tbsp olive oil
3 large yellow or red onions, peeled, quartered and thinly sliced
1 tbsp fresh thyme leaves, or 1 tsp dried
4 large baking potatoes, about 2 ¼ pounds, peeled and sliced thinly
2 bouillon cubes dissovled in 2 cups hot water

1. Heat half the butter and all of the olive oil in a skillet then add the onions, and cook over medium heat for about 10 minutes, stirring frequently.
2. Reduce the heat to low, add the thyme and cook, partially covered, for about 20 minutes, until the onions are soft and browned.
3. Add the sliced potatoes and 2 tablespoons of butter to the onions in the skillet, stirring thoroughly.
4. Coat a baking dish with some butter or oil. Spoon the potato and onion mixture into the baking dish. Add the bouillon broth. (If there isn't enough to cover the potatoes and onions, add some more.)
5. Cover the baking dish with aluminum foil and bake it in the oven for about an hour, until the potatoes are tender and the liquid has been absorbed.

● ●

	Ordinary Ingredients	Low-Protein Ingredients
Calories	450	
Protein	6	
Fat	21	
Phosphorus	149	
Potassium	1,097	

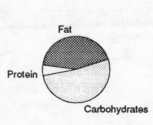

Appendix 6

Mail Order Sources
of Low-Protein Products

Dietary Specialities, Inc.
P.O. Box 227
Rochester, NY 14601
(716) 263-2787

ENER-G Foods, Inc.
P. O. Box 84487
Seattle, Washington 98124-5787
(800) 331-5222

Med Diet
1409 Fairfield Road, South
Minnetonka, Minnesota 55343
(800) 633-3438

Bibliography

Introduction

Papers

Eggers, P.W. Mortality rates among dialysis patients in medicare's end-stage renal disease program. *Am J Kid Dis*. 15:5:414-421, 1990.

Schrier, RW, and Klahr, S. The future of nephrology. *Am J Kid Dis*. 16:6:590-593, 1990.

Pamphlets

American Kidney Fund. Kidney disease: a guide for patients and their families; in Garella, S, Mattern W.D (eds): *American Kidney Fund Public Information Series*. Rockville, 1987.

National Kidney Foundation, Inc. *Your kidneys: master chemists of the body*. New York: 1989.

National Kidney Foundation, Inc. *What everyone should know about kidneys and kidney diseases*. New York: 1990.

Chapter One

Books

Giovannetti, S. *The Nutritional Treatment of Chronic Renal Failure*. Norwell: Kluwer Academic Publisher, 1989.

Mitch, W., et al (eds). *The Progressive Nature of Renal Disease*. New York: Churchill Livingstone, 1986.

Mitch W., and Klahr, S (eds). *Nutrition and the Kidney*. Boston: Little, Brown and Company, 1988.

U.S. Renal Data System, USRDS 1990 Annual Report, The National Institutes of Health, National Institute of Diabetes and Digestive and Kidney Diseases, Bethesda, August, 1990.

Walser, M., et al. *Nutritional Management*. Philadelphia: W. B. Saunders Company, 1984.

Papers

Bergström, J. Discovery and rediscovery of low protein diet. *Clin. Nephrol*. 21:1:29-35, 1984.

Klahr, S: Overview of the pathophysiology of chronic renal disease and uremia; in Alterman P, Gastel B, Eliastam M (eds): End-Stage Renal Disease: Pathophysiology, Dialysis, and Transplantation. U. S. Department of Health and Human Services, 1981, pp 1-9.

Striker, Gary E. Measuring kidney function. *Am J Kid Dis* 16:5:504-505, 1990.

Pamphlets

National Institutes of Health. National Kidney and Urologic Diseases Advisory Board 1990 Long-Range Plan: Window on the 21st Century. March, 1990.

Chapter Two

Books

Beale, L.S. *Kidney Diseases, Urinary Deposits, and Calculous Disorders; Their Nature and Treatment.* Philadelphia: Lindsay and Blakiston, 1869.

Berkow, Robert (ed). *The Merck Manual.* Rahway:Merck Sharp & Dohme Research Laboratories, 1987.

Nissenson, Allen, R. Fine, Richard N., Gentile, Dominick. *Clinical Dialysis; 2nd Edition.* Norwalk: Appleton & Lange. 1990.

Payer, Lynn. *Medicine and Culture.* New York: Penguin Books, 1988.

U.S. Renal Data System, USRDS 1990 Annual Report, The National Institutes of Health, National Institute of Diabetes and Digestive and Kidney Diseases, Bethesda, August, 1990.

Papers

Alexander, J.W. The cutting edge: a look to the future in transplantation.*Transplantation.* 49:2:237-240, 1990.

Eggers, P.W. Health care policies/economics of the geriatric renal population. *Am J Kid Dis.* 16:4:384-391, 1990.

El Nahas, A.M., and Coles, G.A. Dietary treatment of chronic renal failure: ten unanswered questions. *Lancet.* March 15, 1986:597-600.

Evans, R.W. Organ donation: facts and figures. *Dial & Trans.* 19:5:234-237, 1990.

Gentile, M.G., et al. Preliminary experience on dietary management of chronic renal failure. *Contr Nephrol.* 53:102-108, 1986.

Giovannetti, S. Low protein diet in chronic uremia: a historical survey. *Contr Nephrol.* 53:1-6, 1986.

Giovannetti, S. Dietary treatment of chronic renal failure: why is it not used more frequently? *Nephron.* 40:1-12, 1985.

Hall, P.M. Can progression of renal disease be prevented? *PostGrad Med.* 86:1:113-120, 1989.

Klahr, S. The modification of diet in renal disease study. *N Engl J Med.* 320:13:864-866, 1989.

Klahr, S. Rationing of health care and the end-stage renal diseae program. *Am J Kid Dis.* 16:4:392-395, 1990.

Kolata, G. American Transplant Pioneers Win Nobel Prize in Medicine. *The New York Times.* October 9, 1990:C3.

Lamm, R.D. High technology health care. *Am J Kid Dis.* 16:4:378-383, 1990.

Mitch, W., and Walser, M: Nutritional therapy of the uremic patient; in Brenner B, Rector F (eds): *The Kidney.* Philadelphia, W.B. Saunders, 1991, pp 2186-2222.

Monaco, A.P. Transplantation: the state of the art. *Trans Proc.* 22:3:896-901, 1990.

O'Dell, K. Ethical issues with ESRD patients. *Dial & Trans.* 19:1:18,21, 1990.

Peterson, C.A. How do federal cuts hurt the ESRD program? *Dial & Trans.* 19:9:476-481, 1990.

Schiffman, J.R. Health Costs: Can a low-protein diet put off costly dialysis? *Wall Street Journal.* January 31, 1990:B1.

Schrier, R. W. and Klahr, S. The future of nephrology. *Am J Kid Dis.* 16:6:590-593, 1990

Scribner, Belding H. A personalized history of chronic hemodialysis. *Am J Kid Dis* 16:6:511-519, 1990

Starzl, T.E. In a small Iowa town. *Trans Proc.* 19:12-17, 1987.

Starzl, T.E. Introduction. *Trans Proc.* 22:1:Suppl 1:5, 1990.

Walser, M. Ketoacids in the treatment of uremia. *Clin Nephrol.* 3:180-186, 1975.

Pamphlets

American Kidney Fund. Kidney disease: a guide for patients and their families; in Garella, S, Mattern W.D (eds): American Kidney Fund Public Information Series. Rockville, 1987.

National Kidney Foundation, Inc. *What everyone should know about kidneys and kidney diseases.* New York: 1990.

Chapter Three

Books

Cameron, S. *Kidney Disease: The Facts.* Oxford: Oxford University Press, 1986.

U.S. Renal Data System, USRDS 1990 Annual Report, The National Institutes of Health, National Institute of Diabetes and Digestive and Kidney Diseases, Bethesda, August, 1990.

Papers

Eggers, P. Health care policies/economics of the geriatric renal population. *Am J Kid Dis.* 16:4:384-391, 1990.

Gordon, D. Racial differences in ESRD. *Dial & Trans.* 19:3:114-116, 1990.

Jacobs, C: Treatment of terminal renal failure in the western european countries; in Klinkmann H, Smeby LC (eds): Terminal Renal Failure: Therapeutic Problems, Possibilities, and Potentials. *Contrib Nephrol.* Basel, Karger, 1990, vol 78, pp 174-177.

Kishimoto, T: Present status of ESRD treatment in Japan: report from the Patient Registries of Dialysis and Kidney Transplantation; in Klinkmann H, Smeby LC (eds): Terminal Renal Failure: Therapeutic Problems, Possibilities, and Potentials. *Contrib Nephrol.* Basel, Karger, 1990, vol 78, pp 178-180.

Klahr, S: Potential factors responsible for the progression of renal failure; in D'Amico G, Colasanti G (eds): Psychological and Physiological Aspects of Chronic Renal Failure. *Contrib Nephrol.* Basel, Karger, 1990, vol 77, pp 77-85.

Klahr, S., and Harris, K. Role of dietary lipids and renal eicosanoids on the progression of renal disease. *Kidney Int.* 36:27:S–27-S–31, 1989.

Klahr, S. Preventing progression of renal disease. *Dial & Trans.* 19:9:503, 511, 1990.

Klahr, S: Overview of the pathophysiology of chronic renal disease and uremia; in Alterman P, Gastel B, Eliastam M (eds): End-Stage Renal Disease: Pathophysiology, Dialysis, and Transplantation. U. S. Department of Health and Human Services, 1981, pp 1-9.

Klahr, S. The kidney in hypertension–villain and victim. *N Engl J Med*. 320:11:731-733, 1989.

Rosansky, SJ., et al. Comparative incidence rates of end-stage renal disease treatment by state. *Am J Nephrol*. 10:198-204, 1990.

Rostand, S., et al. Renal insufficiency in treated essential hypertension. *N Engl J Med*. 320:11:684-688, 1989.

Sadler, J: Quantity and quality of ESRD treatment in the United States of America; in Klinkmann H, Smeby LC (eds): Terminal Renal Failure: Therapeutic Problems, Possibilities, and Potentials. *Contrib Nephrol*. Basel, Karger, 1990, vol 78, pp 181-185.

Taraba, I: Treatment of ESRD in eastern europe; in Klinkmann H, Smeby LC (eds): Terminal Renal Failure: Therapeutic Problems, Possibilities, and Potentials. *Contrib Nephrol*. Basel, Karger, 1990, vol 78, pp 186-190.

Pamphlets

National Center for Health Statistics. *Current Estimates from the National Health Interview Survey*. U.S. Department of Health and Human Services, 1987.

National Institutes of Health. *National Kidney and Urologic Diseases Advisory Board 1990 Long-Range Plan: Window on the 21st Century*. March, 1990.

Chapter Four

Books

Heimlich, Jane. *What Your Doctor Won't Tell You*. New York: Harper Perennial, 1990.

Horowitz, Lawrence C. *Taking Charge Of Your Medical Fate*. New York: Random House, 1988.

Jarvis, D.C. *Folk Medicine*. New York:Fawcett Crest, 1958.

Kowalski, Robert E. *The 8-Week Cholesterol Cure*. New York: Harper & Row, 1989.

The Kidneys: Balancing the Fluids. New York: Torstar Books, 1985.

Trowell, H.C., and Burkitt, D.P. *Western Diseases:Their Emergence and Prevention*. Cambridge:Harvard University Press, 1981.

Papers

Leaf, A, and Ryan, T.J. Prevention of coronary artery disease; a medical imperative. *N Engl J Med*. 323:20:1419, 1990.

Lewis, C. E. et al. The counseling practices of internists. *Ann Intern Med*. 114:1:54-58, 1991.

Lundberg, George D. Countdown to millennium—balancing the professionalism and business of medicine. *JAMA*. 263:1:86, 1990.

Mitch, W: Nutritional therapy and the progression of renal insufficiency; in Mitch W, Klahr, S (eds): *Nutrition and the Kidney*. Boston: Little, Brown and Company, 1988, pp 154-179.

Mitch, W., and Walser, M: Nutritional therapy of the uremic patient; in Brenner BM, Rector FC (eds): *The Kidney, 4th Edition*. Philadelphia: W.B. Saunders, 1991.

Pamphlets

American Kidney Fund. Kidney disease: a guide for patients and their families; in Garella, S, Mattern W.D (eds): American Kidney Fund Public Information Series. Rockville, 1987.

Boylan, C.R. *Kidneys for Kids*. Rockville: American Kidney Fund, 1988.

Charytan, C., et al. *The Dialysis Patient: An Informative Guide For The Dentist*. Rockville: American Kidney Fund, 1987.

Diamond, L.H (ed). *High Blood Pressure And Its Effects On The Kidneys*.Rockville: American Kidney Fund, 1987.

Dining Out With Confidence: A Guide for Renal Patients. New York: National Kidney Foundation, Inc., 1990.

Directory of Public/Professional Education Materials. Rockville: American Kidney Fund, 1987.

Fitness After Kidney Failure...Building Strength Through Exercise. New York: National Kidney Foundation, Inc., 1986.

Garella, S., and Mattern, W.D (eds). *Kidney Disease: A guide for patients and their families*. Rockville: American Kidney Fund, 1987.

Mattern, W.D (ed). *Facts About Kidney Diseases and Their Treatment*. Rockville: American Kidney Fund, 1987.

Moser, M. *High blood pressure & What you can do about it*. Bethesda: The High Blood Pressure Information Center, 1985.

National Kidney Foundation, Inc. *What everyone should know about kidneys and kidney diseases*. New York: 1990.

Nutrition And Changing Kidney Function. New York: National Kidney Foundation, Inc.,1990.

Pak, C (ed). *Facts About Kidney Stones*. Rockville: American Kidney Fund, 1987.

What Everyone Should Know About Kidneys and Kidney Diseases. New York: National Kidney Foundation, Inc.,1990.

Working With Kidney Disease: Rehabilitation and Employment. New York: National Kidney Foundation, Inc., 1990.

You And Your Blood Pressure. New York: National Kidney Foundation, Inc.,1990.

Your Kidneys: Master Chemists of the Body. New York: National Kidney Foundation, Inc., 1989.

Chapter Five

Papers

Fine, L.G. A proposal to improve the attractiveness of nephrology as a subspecialty choice for residents in internal medicine. *Am J Kid Dis*. 15:4:302-302, 1990.

Chapter Six

Books

Anderton, J. L., Parsons, F. M., Jones, D. E. *Living with renal failure*. Baltimore: University Park Press, 1978.

Callahan, Daniel. *What Kind Of Life*. New York:Simon And Schuster, 1990.

Cogan, Martin G., and Garovoy, Marvin R. *Introduction To Dialysis*. New York: Churchill Livingstone, 1985.

Czaczkes, J. W., and De-Nour, A. K. *Chronic Hemodialysis As A Way Of Life*. New York: Brunner/Mazel, 1978.

Fox, Renée C., and Swazey, Judith P. *The Courage To Fail*. Chicago: The University of Chicago Press, 1978.

Kurtzman, Joel, and Gordon, Phillip. *No More Dying*. New York:Dell Publishing, 1976.

Levy, Norman B. *Psychonephrology Two: Psychological Problems in Kidney Failure and Their Treatment*. New York: Plenum Medical Book Company, 1983.

Levy, Norman B. *Living Or Dying: Adaptation To Hemodialysis*. Springfield: Charles C. Thomas, 1974.

Nissenson, Allen, R. Fine, Richard N., Gentile, Dominick. *Clinical Dialysis; 2nd Edition*. Norwalk: Appleton & Lange, 1990.

Plough, A.L. *Borrowed Time: Artificial Organs and the Politics of Extending Lives*. Philadelphia: Temple University Press, 1986.

The Kidneys: Balancing the Fluids. New York: Torstar Books, 1985.

U.S. Renal Data System, USRDS 1990 Annual Report, The National Institutes of Health, National Institute of Diabetes and Digestive and Kidney Diseases, Bethesda, August, 1990.

Papers

Bennett, William M., et al. An EPO progress report. *Dial & Trans*. 19:6:280-283, 1990.

Bremer, B.A., and Wrona, R.M. Quality of life in end-stage renal disease: a reexamination. *Am J Kid Dis*. 13:3:200-209, 1989.

Butera, E. Huge demand for nurses persists. *Dial & Trans*. 18:12:691-692, 1989.

Calland, C.H. Iatrogenic problems in end-stage renal failure. *N Engl J Med*. 287:7:334-336, 1972.

Campbell, J.D., et al. The social and economic costs of end-stage renal disease. *N Engl J Med*. 299:8:386-392, 1978.

Chazan, J.A. Elective withdrawal from dialysis: an important cause of death among patients with chronic renal failure. *Dial & Trans*. 19:10:530-553, 1990.

Churchill, D.N. Results of the Canadian morbidity study in end-stage renal disease patients treated by hemodialysis. *Semin Nephrol*. 10:2:Suppl 1:66-72, 1990.

David, D.S. The agony and the ecstasy of the nephrologist. *JAMA*. 222:5:584-585, 1972.

Dial, K.J., and Aguilar, E.S. Growing challenges for the renal dietitian. *Dial & Trans*. 18:12:696-700, 1989.

Eggers, P.W. Mortality rates among dialysis patients in medicare's end-stage renal disease program. *Am J Kid Dis*. 15:5:414-421, 1990.

Eggers, P.W. Health care policies/economics of the geriatric renal population. *Am J Kid Dis*. 16:4:384-391, 1990.

Hamburger, R.J., et al. A dialysis modality decision guide based on the experience of six dialysis centers. *Dial & Trans*. 19:2:66-84, 1990.

Held, P.J., et al. Five-year survival for end-stage renal disease patients in the United States, Europe, and Japan, 1982 to 1987. *Am J Kid Dis*. 15:5:451-457, 1990.

Held, P.J., et al. Survival analysis of patients undergoing dialysis. *JAMA*. 257:5:645-650, 1987.

Henrich, W.L. A clinical review. *Dial & Trans*. 18:12:688, 1989.

Holley, J.L., et al. Continuous cycling peritoneal dialysis is associated with lower rates of catheter infections than continuous ambulatory peritoneal dialysis. *Am J Kid Dis.* 16:2:133-136, 1990.

Hudson, M. Techs need more cohesiveness. *Dial & Trans.* 18:12:692-693, 1989.

Hull, A.R., and Parker III, T.F. Introduction and summary. *Am J Kid Dis.* 15:5:375-383, 1990.

Jahnke, A. Blood and money. *Boston Magazine.* December, 1988:185-249.

Kjellstrand, C.M. et al. Mortality on dialysis—On the influence of early start, patient characteristics, and transplantation and acceptance rates. *Am J Kid Dis.* 15:5:483-490, 1990.

Klein, J. Social workers attempting to thrive despite cuts. *Dial & Trans.* 18:12:694-696, 1989.

Kochavi, S. Implementing a pre-dialysis education program for patients and families. *Dial & Trans.* 19:10:526-527, 1990.

La Greca, G. Concluding remarks. *Contrib Nephrol.* 84:97-98, 1990.

La Greca, G., et al: Updating on continuous ambulatory peritoneal dialysis; in Scarpioni LL, Ballocchi S (eds): Evolution and Trends in Peritoneal Dialysis. *Contrib Nephrol.* Basel, Karger, 1990, vol 84, pp 1-9.

Levy, N.B. Psychonephrology's past and future. *Dial & Trans.* 18:12:693-694, 1989.

Luckenbaugh, P.R. A patient's view of survival. *Dial & Trans.* 19:3:140-147, 1990.

Lundin, P. A personal experience of twenty-four years of dialysis. *Trans Proc.* 222:3:957-958, 1990.

Nolph, K.D. Comparison of continuous ambulatory peritoneal dialysis and hemodialysis. *Kidney Int.* 33:24:S–123-S–131, 1988.

Nolph, K.D., et al. Continuous ambulatory peritoneal dialysis. *N Engl J Med.* 318:24:1595-1600, 1988.

Penner, B.S., et al. Renal failure patients: our perception of their psychological symptoms. *Kidney Int.* 33:24:S–18-S–20, 1988.

Plough, A.L. Medical technology and the crisis of experience: the costs of clinical legitimation. *Soc Sci & Med.* 15F:89-101, 1981.

Reilly, G.S. A questionnaire for dialysis patients on treatment cessation issues. *Dial & Trans.* 19:10:533-545, 1990.

Rettig, R. A. Study of the medicare end-stage renal disease program. *Am J Kid Dis.* 15:5:491-493, 1990.

Roy, D.J. Dignity, dialysis, and dying. *Dial & Trans.* 19:1:19-21, 1990.

Sargent, J.A. Shortfalls in the delivery of dialysis. *Am J Kid Dis.* 15:5:500-510, 1990.

Sekkarie, M.A., et al. Recovery from end-stage renal disease. *Am J Kid Dis.* 15:1:61-65, 1990.

Shaldon, S: Panel discussion: treatment of terminal renal failure in the western european countries; in Klinkmann H, Smeby LC (eds): Terminal Renal Failure: Therapeutic Problems, Possibilities, and Potentials. *Contrib Nephrol.* Basel, Karger, 1990, vol 78, pp 191-197.

Soskolne, V., and De-Nour, A.K. The psychosocial adjustment of patients and spouses to dialysis treatment. *Soc Sci Med.* 29:4:497-502, 1989.

Toledo-Pereyra, L.H. The transplantation vision. *Dial & Trans.* 18:12:689-691, 1989.

Twardowski, Z.J., et al. Renal replacement in the next decade. *Dial & Trans.* 18:12:688-689, 1989.

Vollmer, W.M., et al. Survival with dialysis and transplantation in patients with end-stage renal disease. *N Engl J Med.* 308:26:1553-1557, 1983.

Ward, E. Death or dialysis—a personal view. *Brit Med J.* 289:1712-1713, 1984.

Williams, G.H. Book Review: *Borrowed Time*: artificial organs and the politics of extending time. *Soc Sci Med*. 26:7:770-772, 1988.

Witten, E. EPO's first year: an overview. *Dial & Trans*. 19:6:279-283, 1990.

Wolfe, R.A., et al. A comparison of survival among dialytic therapies of choice: in-center hemodialysis versus continuous ambulatory peritoneal dialysis at home. *Am J Kid Dis*. 15:5:433-440, 1990.

Chapter Seven

Books

Brent, Leslie, and Sells, Robert A. (eds): *Organ Transplantation: Current Clinical and Immunological Concepts*. London: Baillière Tindall, 1989.

Fox, Renée C., and Swazey, Judith P. *The Courage To Fail*. Chicago: The University of Chicago Press, 1978.

U.S. Bureau of the Census, *Statistical Abstract of the United States*: 1989 (109th edition.) Washington, DC, 1989.

U.S. Renal Data System, USRDS 1990 Annual Report, The National Institutes of Health, National Institute of Diabetes and Digestive and Kidney Diseases, Bethesda, August, 1990.

Papers

Alexander, J.W. The cutting edge: a look to the future in transplantation.*Transplantation*. 49:2:237-240, 1990.

Burnet, F.M. The new approach to immunology *N Engl J Med*. 264:1:24-34, 1961.

Cook, Daniel J., and Terasaki, Paul I.: Renal transplantation on the American continent; in Brent L and Sells RA. *Organ Transplantation: Current Clinical and Immunological Concepts*. London: Baillière Tindall, 1989.

Dowie, M. Maverick surgeon. *Amer Health*. June, 1989:87-97.

Interchangeable parts. *Newsweek*. September, 12, 1988:61.

Kolata, G. American Transplant Pioneers Win Nobel Prize in Medicine. *The New York Times*. October 9, 1990:C3.

Lamm, R.D. Health care as economic cancer. *Dial & Trans*. 16:8:432, 1987.

Schrier, R.W. and Klahr, S. The future of nephrology. *Am J Kid Dis* 16:5:590-593, 1990.

Starzl, T.E. The development of clinical renal transplantation. *Am J Kid Dis* 16:6:548-556, 1990.

Starzl, T.E. In a small Iowa town. *Trans Proc*. 19:12-17, 1987.

Starzl, T.E. et al. Long-term (25-year) survival after renal homotransplantation—the world experience. *Trans Proc* 22:5:2361-2365, 1990.

Starzl, T.E. New options. *Dial & Trans*. 16:8:432-433, 1987.

Vollmer, W.M., et al. Survival with dialysis and transplantation in patients with end-stage renal disease. *N Engl J Med*. 308:26:1553-1557, 1983.

Yaes, R. letter. *New York Times Magazine*. November 4, 1990, p. 12.

Chapter Eight

Books

Cerilli, G. J. et al. *Organ Transplantation and Replacement*. Philadelphia: J. B. Lippincott, 1988.

Glasser, Ronald J. *The Body Is The Hero*. New York: Bantam Books, 1976.

Gutkind, Lee. *Many Sleepless Nights*. New York: W.W. Norton & Company, 1988.

The Kidneys: Balancing the Fluids. New York: Torstar Books, 1985.

Payer, Lynn. *Medicine and Culture*. New York: Penguin Books, 1988.

U.S. Renal Data System, USRDS 1990 Annual Report, The National Institutes of Health, National Institute of Diabetes and Digestive and Kidney Diseases, Bethesda, August, 1990.

Papers

Alexander, J.W. The cutting edge: a look to the future in transplantation.*Transplantation*. 49:2:237-240, 1990.

Andrykowski, M.A., et al. The quality of life in adult survivors of allogeneic bone marrow transplantation. *Transplantation*. 50:3:399-406, 1990.

Ascher, N.L. Appendix B: The pros and cons of cyclosporine. *Hearings before the Committee on Labor and Human Resources*, U.S. Senate, October 20, 1983:306-307.

Barr, D.M.J., and Keogh, A.M. Renal donors—how selective should we be? *Trans Proc*. 22:4:2066-2067, 1990.

Bartucci, M.R., and Seller, M.C. A study of donor families' reactions to letters from organ recipients. *Trans Proc*. 20:5:786-790, 1988.

Broad, W.J. Near-Fatal Blow Dealt to the 'Star' of 'Star Wars'. *The New York Times*. October 21, 1990:29.

Calland, C.H. Iatrogenic problems in end-stage renal failure. *N Engl J Med*. 287:7:334-336, 1972.

Cantarovich, F. Values sacrificed and values gained by the commerce of organs: the Argentine experience. *Trans Proc*. 22:3:925-927, 1990.

Catto, G.R.D: Series editor's foreword; in Catto GRD (ed): *New Clinical Applications Nephrology*. Dordrecht, Kluwer Academic Publishers, 1989, pp vii.

Chatterjee, S.N. Book Review: Organ Transplantation and Replacement. *Dial & Trans*. 19:9:504, 1990.

Coates, C. Stormie Jones' Family Plans Public Funeral. *Philadelphia Daily News*. November 13, 1990:13.

Cook, D.J., and Terasaki, P.I: Renal transplantation on the American continent; in Brent L, Sells RA (eds): *Organ Transplantation: Current Clinical and Immunological Concepts*. London: Baillière Tindall, 1989, pp 195-200.

Cutler, R.E. Cyclosporine revisited, part 2: clinical efficacy, toxic complications and optimizing therapy. *Dial & Trans*. 19:9:492-498, 1990.

Dickens, B.M. Human rights and commerce in health care. *Trans Proc*. 22:3:904-905, 1990.

Dossetor, J.B. Innovative treatment versus clinical research: an ethics issue in transplantation. *Trans Proc*. 22:3:966-968, 1990.

Dossetor, J.B. Discussion. *Trans Proc*. 22:3:933-938, 1990.

Dowie, M. Maverick surgeon. *Amer Health*. June, 1989:87-97.

Evans, R.W., and Manninen, D.L. US public opinion concerning the procurement and distribution of donor organs. *Trans Proc.* 20:5:781-785, 1988.

Evans, R.W. Organ donation: facts and figures. *Dial & Trans.* 19:5:234-237, 1990.

Evans, R.W. The private sector vis-a-vis government in future funding of organ transplantation. *Trans Proc.* 22:3:975-979, 1990.

Fitzpatrick, P.M., et al. Long-term outcome of renal transplantation in autosomal dominant polycystic kidney disease. *Am J Kid Dis.*15:6:535-543, 1990.

Five Kidneys and Two Years of Hell. *San Francisco Chronicle.* 107:9, January 11, 1971.

Gil, G. The artificial heart juggernaut. *Hastings Center Report.* March/April, 1989:24-31.

Haberal, M., et al. Is donor nephrectomy a safe procedure in the elderly? *Trans Proc.* 20:5:791-793, 1988.

Hano, A. Incredible ordeal of Chad Calland, M.D. *Redbook.* 137:94, September, 1971.

Harmer, A.W., et al. Preliminary report: dramatic rise in renal allograft failure rate. *Lancet.* 335:1184-1185, 1990.

Johnson, L.W., et al. Mexican-American and Anglo-American attitudes toward organ donation. *Trans Proc.* 20:5:822-823, 1988.

Johny, K.V., et al. Values gained and lost in live unrelated renal transplantation. *Trans Proc.* 22:3:915-917, 1990.

Kasiske, B.L. Risk factors for accelerated atherosclerosis in renal transplant recipients. *Am J Med.* 84:6:985-991, 1988.

Kleffman, G. Book Review: Textbook of Hemodialysis for Patient Care Personnel. *Dial & Trans.* 19:9:504, 1990.

Kolata, G. Rat Immune System Is Taught to Accept Transplant, Researchers Say. *The New York Times.* September 14, 1990:A18.

Kolata, G. American Transplant Pioneers Win Nobel Prize in Medicine. *The New York Times.* October 9, 1990:C3.

Kootstra, G. Will there still be an organ shortage in the year 2000? *Trans Proc.* 20:5:809-811, 1988.

Lazarovits, A.I., and Stiller, C.R: Immunological monitoring; in Catto GRD (ed): *New Clinical Applications Nephrology.* Dordrecht, Kluwer Academic Publishers, 1989, pp 95-115.

Martinez, C. Personal experience with a transplant. *Trans Proc.* 22:3:959-960, 1990.

Mittal, V.K., and Toledo-Pereyra, L.H.: Cadaver transplantation results; in Toledo-Pereyra LH (ed): *Kidney Transplantation.* Philadelphia, F.A. Davis Company, 1988, pp 247-263.

Monaco, A.P. Transplantation: the state of the art. *Trans Proc.* 22:3:896-901, 1990.

Moore, F.D: The doctors' dilemmas; in *Transplant: The Give and Take of Tissue Transplantation.* New York: Simon and Schuster, 1972, pp 313-320.

Morris, R.E., et al. A study of the contrasting effects of cyclosporine, FK 506, and rapamycin on the suppression of allograft rejection. *Trans Proc.* 22:4:1638-1641, 1990.

Murray, J.E. The past, present, and future: renal transplantation before Starzl. *Trans Proc.* 19:339-341, 1987.

Opelz, G: Renal transplantation in Europe; in Brent L, Sells RA (eds): *Organ Transplantation: Current Clinical and Immunological Concepts.* London: Baillière Tindall, 1989, pp 185-193.

Paller, M.S. Cyclosporine nephrotoxicity and the role of cyclosporine in living-related donor transplantation. *Am J Kid Dis.* 16:5:414-416, 1990.

Puschett, J.B., et al. The spectrum of ciclosporin nephrotoxicity. *Am J Nephrol.* 10:296-309, 1990.

Reddy, K.C., et al. Unconventional renal transplantation in India. *Trans Proc.* 22:3:910-911, 1990.

Rolles, K: Summary of clinical data: liver transplantation; in Brent L, Sells RA (eds): *Organ Transplantation: Current Clinical and Immunological Concepts*. London: Baillière Tindall, 1989, pp 201-205.

Ryle, A. Book Review: Health and Lifestyles. *Lancet*. 335:1185-1186, 1990.

Salvatierra, O: Foreword; in Toledo-Pereyra LH (ed): *Kidney Transplantation*. Philadelphia, F.A. Davis Company, 1988.

Salvatierra, O: Living related transplantation results; in Toledo-Pereyra LH (ed): *Kidney Transplantation*. Philadelphia, F.A. Davis Company, 1988, pp 369-378.

Salvatierra Jr., O. Renal transplantation—The Starzl influence. *Trans Proc*. 19:343-349, 1987.

Salvatierra Jr., O. Optimal use of organs for transplantation. *N Engl J Med*. 318:20:1329-1331, 1988.

Schrier, RW, and Klahr, S. The future of nephrology. *Am J Kid Dis*. 16:6:590-593, 1990.

Sells, R.A., and Wing, A.J:The incidence of renal failure worldwide and national statistics for treatment by transplantation; in Brent L, Sells RA (eds): *Organ Transplantation: Current Clinical and Immunological Concepts*. London: Baillière Tindall, 1989, pp 255-268.

Shapiro, R., et al: Cadaveric renal transplantation under the american organ allocation system; in Bonomini V, Scolari MP, Stefoni S, et al (eds): Biotechnology in Renal Replacement Therapy. *Contrib Nephrol*. Basel, Karger, 1989, vol 70, pp 30-40.

Slomowitz, L.A., et al. Evaluation of kidney function in renal transplant patients receiving long-term cyclosporine. *Am J Kid Dis*. 15:6:530-534, 1990.

Spital, A. Living kidney donation: still worth the risk. *Trans Proc*. 20:5:1051-1058, 1988.

Squifflet, J.P., et al. Unrelated living donor kidney transplantation. *Transplant Int*. 3:32-35, 1990.

Starzl, T.E. In a small Iowa town. *Trans Proc*. 19:12-17, 1987.

Starzl, T.E. Introduction. *Trans Proc*. 22:1:Suppl 1:5, 1990.

Starzl, T.E., et al. Kidney transplantation under FK 506. *JAMA*. 264:1:63-67, 1990.

Starzl, T.E. Long-term (25-year) survival after renal homotransplantation—the world experience. *Trans Proc* 22:5:2361-2365, 1990.

Starzl, Thomas E. Personal Reflections on Transplantaion. *Surg Clin North Am*. 58:5:879-893, 1978.

Sumrani, N., et al. HLA-Identical renal transplants: impact of cyclosporine on intermediate-term survival and renal function. *Am J Kid Dis*. 16:5:417-422, 1990.

Thiagarajan, C.M., et al. The practice of unconventional renal transplantation (UCRT) at a single centre in India. *Trans Proc*. 22:3:912-914, 1990.

Thomson, A.W. FK 506 enters the clinic. *Immun Today*. 11:2:35-36, 1990.

Trucco, T. Sales of Kidneys Prompt New Laws and Debate. *The New York Times*. August 1, 1989:C1,C6.

Turcotte, J.G., et al. Global review of transplantation practices. *Trans Proc*. 22:3:906-907, 1990.

Vromen, M.A.M., et al. Short-and long-term results with adult non-heart-beating donor kidneys. *Trans Proc*. 20:5:743-745, 1988.

Werth, B. The Drug That Works in Pittsburgh. *The New York Times Magazine*. September 30, 1990:35,58-60.

White, D.J.G., et al: Immunosuppression; in Catto GRD (ed): *New Clinical Applications Nephrology*. Dordrecht, Kluwer Academic Publishers, 1989, pp 117-133.

Yadav, R.V.S. Transplantation as a health priority in India. *Trans Proc*. 22:3:908-909, 1990.

Chapter Nine

Books

Beale, L.S. *Kidney Diseases, Urinary Deposits, and Calculous Disorders; Their Nature and Treatment*. Philadelphia: Lindsay and Blakiston, 1869.

Giovannetti, S. *The Nutritional Treatment of Chronic Renal Failure*. Norwell: Kluwer Academic Publisher, 1989.

Mitch W., and Klahr, S (eds). *Nutrition and the Kidney*. Boston: Little, Brown and Company, 1988.

Suggested Guidelines for Nutrition Care of Renal Patients. Chicago: The American Dietetic Association, 1986.

Walser, M., et al. *Nutritional Management*. Philadelphia: W. B. Saunders Company, 1984.

Papers

Albertazzi, A., et al: Control of hypertension and progression of chronic renal failure; in Oldrizzi L, Maschio G, Rugiu C, et al. (eds): The Progressive Nature of Renal Disease: Myths and Facts. *Contrib Nephrol*. Basel, Karger, 1989, vol 75, pp 167-176.

Altman, L.K. High blood pressure: an overtreated condition? *The New York Times*. November 8, 1990, pp B25.

Aparicio, M., et al. Proteinuria and progression of renal failure in patients on a low-protein diet. *Nephron*. 51:292-293, 1989.

Attman, P.O., et al: Provision of energy in low-protein diets for treatment of renal failure; in Gretz N, Giovannetti S, Strauch M (eds): Low-Protein Diets in Renal Patients: Composition and Absorption. *Contrib Nephrol*. Basel, Karger, 1989, vol 72, pp 21-35.

Barsotti, G., et al. Protection of renal function and of nutritional status in uremic rats by means of a low-protein, low-phosphorus supplemented diet. *Nephron*. 49:197-202, 1988.

Barsotti, G., et al. Effects of a vegetarian, supplemented diet on renal function, proteinuria, and glucose metabolism in patients with 'overt' diabetic nephropathy and renal insufficiency. *Contr Nephrol*. 65:87-94, 1988.

Bergström, J. Discovery and rediscovery of low protein diet. *Clin. Nephrol*. 21:1:29-35, 1984.

Bergström, J., et al: Is chronic renal disease always progressive?; in Oldrizzi L, Maschio G, Rugiu C, et al. (eds): The Progressive Nature of Renal Disease: Myths and Facts. *Contrib Nephrol*. Basel, Karger, 1989, vol 75, pp 60-67.

Brody, J.E. Huge Study Of Diet Indicts Fat And Meat. *The New York Times*. May 8, 1990:C1,C14.

Ciardella, F., et al. Metabolic effects of a very-low-protein, low-phosphorus diet supplemented with essential amino acids and keto analogues in end-stage renal diseases. *Contr Nephrol*. 65:72-80, 1988.

Close, J.H. The use of amino acid precursors in nitrogen-accumulation diseases. *N. Engl. J. Med*. 290:12:663-667, 1974.

El Nahas, A.M., and Coles, G.A. Dietary treatment of chronic renal failure: ten unanswered questions. *Lancet*. March 15, 1986:597-600.

El Nahas, A.M., Personal Communication, 1990.

Erbersdobler, H.F: Changes due to food processing in low-protein diets for renal patients; in Gretz N, Giovannetti S, Strauch M (eds): Low-Protein Diets in Renal Patients: Composition and Absorption. *Contrib Nephrol*. Basel, Karger, 1989, vol 72, pp 49-65.

Fischer, D. Letter to the editor. *N Engl J Med*. 322:22:1609-1610, 1990.

Gentile, M.G., et al. Effects of dietetic manipulation on the control of blood pressure and on the progression of chronic renal insufficiency. *Scandinavian J Urol Nephrol.* 108:13-15, 1988.

Gentile, M.G., et al. Preliminary experience on dietary management of chronic renal failure. *Contr Nephrol.* 53:102-108, 1986.

Giovannetti, S: Supplemented diet for severe chronic renal failure: some controversial points; in Oldrizzi L, Maschio G, Rugiu C, et al. (eds): The Progressive Nature of Renal Disease: Myths and Facts. *Contrib Nephrol.* Basel, Karger, 1989, vol 75, pp 147-154.

Giovannetti, S. Answers to ten questions on the dietary treatment of chronic renal failure. *Lancet.* November 15, 1986:1140-1142.

Giovannetti, S. Low protein diet in chronic uremia: a historical survey. *Contr Nephrol.* 53:1-6, 1986.

Giovannetti, S. Dietary treatment of chronic renal failure: why is it not used more frequently? *Nephron.* 40:1-12, 1985.

Gretz, N. Low protein diet and progression of chronic renal failure. *Klin Wochenschr.* 66:415-417, 1988.

Gretz, N., et al: Low-protein diets: mineral and electrolyte contents; in Gretz N, Giovannetti S, Strauch M (eds): Low-Protein Diets in Renal Patients: Composition and Absorption. *Contrib Nephrol.* Basel, Karger, 1989, vol 72, pp 36-41.

Gretz, N., et al: Preface; in Gretz N, Giovannetti S, Strauch M (eds): Low-Protein Diets in Renal Patients: Composition and Absorption. *Contrib Nephrol.* Basel, Karger, 1989, vol 72, pp VII-IX.

Gretz, N., et al. Renal function, anemia and blood pressure in patients with chronic renal failure. *Scandinavian J. Urolog. Nephrol.* 108:57-60, 1988.

Gretz, N., et al. Caloric supplements for patients on low-protein diets? *Nephron.* 50:129-132, 1988.

Guarnieri, G., et al: The assessment of nutritional status in chronically uremic patients; in Gretz N, Giovannetti S, Strauch M (eds): Low-Protein Diets in Renal Patients: Composition and Absorption. *Contrib Nephrol.* Basel, Karger, 1989, vol 72, pp 73-103.

Guarnieri, G., et al. Nutritional assessment in patients with early renal insufficiency on long-term low protein diet. *Contrib Nephrol.* 53:40-50, 1986.

Hall, P.M. Can progression of renal disease be prevented? *PostGrad Med.* 86:1:113-120, 1989.

Hunsicker, L.G. Studies of therapy of progressive renal failure in humans. *Semin Nephrol.* 9:4:380-394, 1989.

Ihle, B.U., et al. The effect of protein restriction on the progression of renal insufficiency. *N Engl J Med.* 321:26:1773-1777, 1989.

Klahr, S. Effects of protein intake on the progression of renal disease. *Annu. Rev. Nutr.* 9:87-108, 1989.

Klahr, S. Preventing progression of renal disease. *Dial & Trans.* September, 1990:503,511.

Klahr, S. The modification of diet in renal disease study. *N Engl J Med.* 320:13:864-866, 1989.

Klahr, S. Does dietary protein restriction slow the rate of progression of chronic renal disease? *Inter J Artifical Organs.* 13:2:65-69, 1990.

Kluthe, R., and Fürst, P (chairmen). Workshop: Calcium and phosphate provision of renal patients: nutrition–metabolism–drugs. *Clin Nephrol.* 30:5:288-292, 1988.

Kolata, Gina. Animal Fat Is Tied To Colon Cancer. *The New York Times.* December 13, 1990:1,B20.

Leaf, A, and Ryan, T.J. Prevention of coronary artery disease—a medical imperative. *N Engl J Med.* 323:20:1419, 1990.

Locatelli, F: Controlled study of protein-restricted diet in chronic renal failure; in Oldrizzi L, Maschio G, Rugiu C, et al. (eds): The Progressive Nature of Renal Disease: Myths and Facts. *Contrib Nephrol*. Basel, Karger, 1989, vol 75, pp 141-146.

Loschiavo, C., et al. Effect of protein-restricted diet on serum lipids and atherosclerosis risk factors in patients with chronic renal failure. *Clin Nephrol*. 29:3:113-118, 1988.

Maschio, G., et al: Protein-restricted diet in early chronic renal failure; in Oldrizzi L, Maschio G, Rugiu C, et al. (eds): The Progressive Nature of Renal Disease: Myths and Facts. *Contrib Nephrol*. Basel, Karger, 1989, vol 75, pp 134-140.

Maschio, G., et al. Effects of dietary protein and phosphorus restriction on the progression of early renal failure. *Kidney Int*. 22:371-376, 1982.

Mitch, W: Nutritional therapy and the progression of renal insufficiency; in Mitch W, Klahr, S (eds): *Nutrition and the Kidney*. Boston: Little, Brown and Company, 1988, pp 154-179.

Mitch, W. The influence of the diet on the progression of renal insufficiency. *Ann Rev Med*. 35:249-264, 1984.

Mitch, W., and Walser, M: Nutritional therapy of the uremic patient; in Brenner B, Rector F (eds): *The Kidney*. Philadelphia, W.B. Saunders, 1991, pp 2186-2222.

Oldrizzi, L. Different protein diets in renal failure: a self-controlled study. *Am J Nephrol*. 9:184-189, 1989.

Oldrizzi, L., et al: The optimal protein intake in patients with early chronic renal failure; in Oldrizzi L, Maschio G, Rugiu C, et al. (eds): The Progressive Nature of Renal Disease: Myths and Facts. *Contrib Nephrol*. Basel, Karger, 1989, vol 75, pp 203-208.

O'Neill, M. Eating to Heal: Mapping Out New Frontiers. *The New York Times*. February 2, 1990:C1,C6.

Rosenthal, E. Health risks seen in blood pressure just above normal: signs of organ damage. *The New York Times*. July 18, 1990, pp A1, A19.

Rosman, Johan B., et al. Letter to the editor. *N Engl J Med*. 322:22:1610, 1990.

Rudman, D., and Cohan, M.E. Nutritional causes of renal impairment in old age. *Am J Kid Dis*. 16:4:289-295, 1990.

Schiffman, J.R. Health Costs: Can a low-protein diet put off costly dialysis? *Wall Street Journal*. January 31, 1990:B1.

Schreiner, G.E. Prevention of renal disease and conservation of renal function. *Am J Kid Dis*. 16:4:360-366, 1990.

Smadel, J.E., et al. The effect of diet on the pathological changes in rats with nephrotoxic nephritis. *Am. J. Path*. 15:26:199-221, 1939.

Strauch, M., et al: The 'normal' food intake; in Gretz N, Giovannetti S, Strauch M (eds): Low-Protein Diets in Renal Patients: Composition and Absorption. *Contrib Nephrol*. Basel, Karger, 1989, vol 72, pp 1-10.

Toigo, G., et al: Nutritional and metabolic effects of ten years of protein-restricted diet in patients with early renal failure; in Oldrizzi L, Maschio G, Rugiu C, et al. (eds): The Progressive Nature of Renal Disease: Myths and Facts. *Contrib Nephrol*. Basel, Karger, 1989, vol 75, pp 194-202.

Vito, M., et al: Antihypertensive therapy and progression of renal failure; in Oldrizzi L, Maschio G, Rugiu C, et al. (eds): The Progressive Nature of Renal Disease: Myths and Facts. *Contrib Nephrol*. Basel, Karger, 1989, vol 75, pp 155-166.

Walker, J.D. Restriction of dietary protein and progression of renal failure in diabetic nephropathy. *Lancet*. 2:1411-1415, 1989.

Walser, M: Weighted least square regression analysis of factors contributing to progression of chronic renal failure; in Oldrizzi L, Maschio G, Rugiu C, et al. (eds): The Progressive Nature of Renal Disease: Myths and Facts. *Contrib Nephrol*. Basel, Karger, 1989, vol 75, pp 127-133.

Walser, M. Ketoacids in the treatment of uremia. *Clin Nephrol*. 3:180-186, 1975.

Walser, M. Nutritional support in renal failure: future directions. *Lancet*. February 12, 1983:340-342.

Walser, M. Progression of chronic renal failure in man. *Kidney Int*. 37:1195-1210, 1990.

Zeller, Kathleen, et al. Effect of restricting dietary protein on the progression of renal failure in patients with insulin-dependent diabetes mellitus. *N Engl J Med*. 324:2:78-84, 1991.

Pamphlets

American Kidney Fund. Kidney disease: a guide for patients and their families; in Garella, S, Mattern W.D (eds): American Kidney Fund Public Information Series. Rockville, 1987.

National Institutes of Health. *National Kidney and Urologic Diseases Advisory Board 1990 Long-Range Plan: Window on the 21st Century*. March, 1990.

Chapter Ten

Books

Brent L. and Sells R.A. *Organ Transplantation: Current Clinical and Immunological Concepts*. London: Baillière Tindall, 1989.

Horowitz, Lawrence C. *Taking Charge Of Your Medical Fate*. New York: Random House, 1988.

U.S. Renal Data System, USRDS 1990 Annual Report, The National Institutes of Health, National Institute of Diabetes and Digestive and Kidney Diseases, Bethesda, August, 1990.

Papers

Brunner, F.P., and Selwood, N.H. Results of renal replacement therapy in Europe, 1980-1987. *Am J Kid Dis*. 15:5:384-396, 1990.

Calland, C.H. Iatrogenic problems in end-stage renal failure. *N Engl J Med*. 287:7:334-336, 1972.

Cook, Daniel J., and Terasaki, Paul I.: Renal transplantation on the American continent; in Brent L and Sells RA. *Organ Transplantation: Current Clinical and Immunological Concepts*. London: Baillière Tindall, 1989.

Croxson, B.E., and Ashton, T. A cost effectiveness analysis of the treatment of end stage renal failure. *N Zealand Med J*. 103:888:171-174, 1990.

Eggers, P.W. Effect of transplantation on the medicare end-stage renal disease program. *N Engl J Med*. 318:4:223-229, 1988.

Evans, R.W., et al. The quality of life of patients with end-stage renal disease. *N Engl J Med*. 312:553-559, 1985.

Hamburger, R.J., et al. A dialysis modality decision guide based on the experience of six dialysis centers. *Dial & Trans*. 19:2:66-84, 1990.

Kjellstrand, C.M., et al: Late deaths on dialysis and transplantation therapy; in Bonomini V, Scolari MP, Stefoni S, et al (eds): Biotechnology in Renal Replacement Therapy. *Contrib Nephrol*. Basel, Karger, 1989, vol 70, pp 64-74.

Lundin, P. A personal experience of twenty-four years of dialysis. *Trans Proc*. 222:3:957-958, 1990.

Morris, R.E. Treating rejection of transplants in the post-cyclosporine era. *Dial & Trans.* 19:10:544-555, 1990.

Nolph, K.D. Comparison of continuous ambulatory peritoneal dialysis and hemodialysis. *Kidney Int.* 33:24:S–123-S–131, 1988.

Schlesinger, M., et al. The ownership of health facilities and clinical decisionmaking: the case of the ESRD industry. *Medical Care.* 27:3:244-258, 1989.

Sells, R.A. Commerce in human organs: a global review. *Dial & Trans.* 19:1:10,17, 1990.

Simmons, R.G., et al. Comparison of quality of life of patients on continuous ambulatory peritoneal dialysis, hemodialysis, and after transplantation. *Am J Kid Dis.* 4:253-255, 1984.

Showstack, J., et al. The association of cyclosporine with the 1-year costs of cadaver-donor kidney transplants. *JAMA.* 264:14:1818-1823, 1990.

U.S. Renal Data System, USRDS 1990 Annual Report, The National Institutes of Health, National Institute of Diabetes and Digestive and Kidney Diseases, Bethesda, August, 1990.

Youngner, S.J. Brain death and organ procurement: some vexing problems remain. *Dial & Trans.* 19:1:12-14,17, 1990.

Chapter Eleven

Books

Eaton, S., et al. *The Paleolithic Prescription; A Program Of Diet And Exercise And A Design For Living.* New York: Harper & Row, 1988.

Gussow, Joan Dye, and Thomas, Paul R. *The Nutrition Debate.* Palo Alto: Bull Publishing Company, 1986.

Reader, John. *Man On Earth.* Austin: University of Texas Press, 1988.

Tannahill, Reay. *Food In History.* New York: Crown Publishers, Inc., 1988.

The Surgeon General's Report On Nutrition & Health. New York: Warner Communications Company, 1989.

Trowell, H.C., and Burkitt, D.P. *Western Diseases:Their Emergence and Prevention.* Cambridge:Harvard University Press, 1981.

Walford, Roy L. *The 120 Year Diet.* New York: Pocket Books, 1986.

Papers

Altman, Lawrence K. Scientists Link Hormone To High Blood Pressure. *The New York Times.* September 15, 1990:9.

Becker, M.H. The cholesterol saga: whither health promotion? *Ann Intern Med.* 106:4:623-626, 1987.

Booth, W. Age 85 Is The Ceiling For Life Expectancy, A New Study Concludes. *Philadelphia Inquirer.* November 2, 1990:A1,A14.

Brody, J.E. Huge Study Of Diet Indicts Fat And Meat. *The New York Times.* May 8, 1990:C1,C14.

Brody, J.E. After 4,000 Years, Medical Science Considers Garlic. *The New York Times.* November 4, 1990:C1,C10.

Brody, J.E. As Its Virtues Emerge, The Potato Goes Global. *The New York Times.* October 9, 1990:C1,C11.

Castelli, W.P. Diet, smoking, and alcohol: influence on coronary heart disease risk. *Am J Kid Dis.* 16:4:Suppl 1:41-46, 1990.

Connor, W.E. Dietary fiber—nostrum or critical nutrient? *N Engl J Med.* 322:3:193-195, 1990.

Crawford, P. The nutrition connection: why doesn't the public know? *AJPH.* 78:9:1147-1148, 1988.

Friedewald, W.T., and Thom, T.J. Decline of coronary heart disease mortality in the United States. *Israel J Med Sciences.* 22:307-312, 1986.

Georges, C.J. Studies Find a Link Between Aggressiveness and Cholesterol Levels. *The New York Times.* September 11, 1990:C3.

Goleman, D. New Study Says Diet Can Heal Arteries. *The New York Times.* November 15, 1988:C1,C11.

Hegsted, D.M. Nutrition: the changing scene. *Nutr Rev.* 43:12:357-367, 1985.

Herrin, A. New U.S. Guidelines Take More Relaxed View of Diet, Weight. *Philadelphia Inquirer.* November 6, 1990:A1.

Hilts, P.J. U.S. Dietary Guides Sets Fat and Alcohol Limits. *The New York Times.* November 6, 1990:C9.

Holusha, J. Packaging and Public Image: McDonald's Fills a Big Order. *The New York Times.* November 2, 1990:A1,D5.

Johnson, G.T. Restoring trust between patient and doctor. *N Engl J Med.* 322:3:195-197, 1990.

Kannel, W.B. Nutrition and the occurrence and prevention of cardiovascular disease in the elderly. *Nutr Rev.* 46:2:68-78, 1988.

Kolata, G. Study Disputes Coffee's Tie to Heart Disease Risk. *The New York Times.* October 11, 1990:B12.

Kolata, G. Study Offers First Evidence That Cutting Cholesterol Levels Saves Lives. *The New York Times.* October 4, 1990:B21.

McGinnis, J.M. and Nestle, M. The Surgeon General's report on nutrition and health: policy implications and implementation strategies. *Am J Clin Nutr.* 49:23-8, 1989.

O'Neill, M. Eating to Heal: Mapping Out New Frontiers. *The New York Times.* February 2, 1990:C1,C6.

Reuters. Has Science Stretched Life Expectancy About as Far as It Can Go? *The New York Times.* November 2, 1990:A17.

Rhoads, G.G. Reliability of diet measures as chronic disease risk factors. *Am J Clin Nutr.* 45:1073-1079, 1987.

Rosenthal, E. Sticky Blood Newly Linked To Heart Risk. *The New York Times.* October 16, 1990:C1.

Stacey, M. Reinventing The Egg. *The New Yorker.* October 1, 1990:73-88.

Stevens, W.K. Global Climate Changes Seen As Force in Human Evolution. *The New York Times.* October 16, 1990:C1.

Tobian, Louis. Potassium and hypertension. *Nutr Rev.* 46:8:273-283, 1988.

Trevisan, M., et al. Consumption of olive oil, butter, and vegetable oils and coronary heart disease risk factors. *JAMA.* 263:5:688-692, 1990.

Trowell, H. Book Review: Pritikin: The Man Who Healed America's Heart. *Am J Clin Nutr.* 48:174, 1988.

Truswell, A.S. Evolution of dietary recommendations, goals, and guidelines. *Am J Clin Nutr.* 45:1060-1072, 1987.

Yudkin, J. Book Review: The Paleolithic Prescription: A Program of Diet & Exercise and a Design for Living. *Nature.* 336:282, 1988.

Chapter Thirteen

Papers

Caggiula, Arlene W., et al. *Dietary compliance patterns in the modification of diet in renal disease (MDRD) study, phase III*. National Institute of Diabetes and Digestive and Kidney Diseases, Bethesda, MD.

Chapter Fourteen

Books

Encyclopedia Of Food. Emmaus. Prevention Publishers, 1990.

Tannahill, Reay. *Food in History*. New York: Crown Publishers, Inc., 1988.

Papers

O'Neill, Molly. The New Nutrition: Protein On The Side. *The New York Times*. November 28, 1990:C1.

Pamphlets

You Can Control Your Cholesterol: A Guide to Low-Cholesterol Living. Merck Sharp & Dohme, 1989.

Chapter Fifteen

Books

Killilea, Marie: Mutual help organizations: Interpretations in the literature; in Caplan G, Killilea M (eds): *Support Systems And Mutual Help*. New York: Grune & Stratton, 1976.

Middleton, Lillian. *Alzheimer's Family Support Groups: A Manual For Group Facilitators*. Tampa: Suncoast Gerontology Center, 1984.

Zarit, Steven H., et al. *Working With Families Of Dementia Victims: A Treatment Manual*. Los Angeles: UCLA/USC Long-term Care Gerontology Center, 1983.

Papers

Baron, Robert, et al. Social support and immune function among spouses of cancer patients. *J Pers Soc Psych*. 59:2:344-352, 1990.

Fawzy, FI., et al. A structured psychiatric intervention for cancer patients; changes over time in immunological measure. *Arch Gen Psych*. 47:8:729-735, 1990.

Goleman, D. Support Groups May Do More In Cancer Than Relieve The Mind. *The New York Times*. October 18, 1990:B12.

Spiegel, David, et al. Effect of psychosocial treatment on survival of patients with metastatic breast cancer. *Lancet*. 14:2(8668):888-891, 1989.

Trojan, Alf. Benefits of self-help groups: a survey of 232 members from 65 disease-related groups. *Soc Sci Med.* 29:2:225-232, 1989.

Chapter Sixteen

Books

Abramson, Leonard. *Healing Our Health Care System.* New York: Grove Weidenfeld, 1990.

Califano, Joseph A., Jr. *America's Health Care Revolution; Who Lives? Who Dies? Who Pays?* New York: Random House, 1986.

Callahan, Daniel. *What Kind Of Life; The Limits Of Medical Progress.* New York: Simon and Schuster, 1990.

Carson, Rachael. *Silent Spring.*Boston: Houghton Mifflin Company, 1962.

Kuhn, Thomas S. *The Structure Of Scientific Revolutions.* 2nd Edition. Chicago: University of Chicago Press, 1970.

National Center for Health Statistics. Health, United States, 1990. Hyattsville, Maryland: Public Health Service. 1991.

Ornish, Dean. *Dr. Dean Ornish's Program For Reversing Heart Disease.* New York: Random House, 1990.

U.S. Renal Data System, USRDS 1990 Annual Report, The National Institutes of Health, National Institute of Diabetes and Digestive and Kidney Diseases, Bethesda, August, 1990.

Papers

Calland, C.H. Iatrogenic problems in end-stage renal failure. *N Engl J Med.* 287:7:334-336, 1972.

Lamm, Richard D. Health care as economic cancer. *Dial & Trans.* 16:6:432-433, 1987.

McNeill Lehrer Report. PBS. December 28, 1990.

Reuben, Carolyn. Lobbying for alternatives. *L.A. Weekly.* 10:45. 1988.

Warsh, David. Point Of View On Historic Recognition For A Model Scholar's Theory. *Washington Post.* December 26, 1990:F3.

Notes

Introduction

1. National Kidney Foundation, Inc. *Your kidneys: master chemists of the body*. New York: 1989.
2. American Kidney Fund. Kidney disease: a guide for patients and their families; in Garella, S, Mattern W.D (eds): *American Kidney Fund Public Information Series*. Rockville, 1987.
3. Eggers, P.W. Mortality rates among dialysis patients in medicare's end-stage renal disease program. *Am J Kid Dis*. 15:5:414-421, 1990.
4. Schrier, RW, and Klahr, S. The future of nephrology. *Am J Kid Dis*. 16:6:590-593, 1990.

Chapter One

1. U.S. Renal Data System, USRDS 1990 Annual Report, The National Institutes of Health, National Institute of Diabetes and Digestive and Kidney Diseases, Bethesda, August, 1990.
2. National Institutes of Health. National Kidney and Urologic Diseases Advisory Board 1990 Long-Range Plan: Window on the 21st Century. March, 1990.
3. Striker, Gary E. Measuring kidney function. *Am J Kid Dis* 16:5:504-505, 1990.
4. Bergström, J. Discovery and rediscovery of low protein diet. *Clin. Nephrol*. 21:1:29-35, 1984.
5. Striker, Gary E. Measuring kidney function. *Am J Kid Dis* 16:5:504-505, 1990.
6. Walser, M. Ketoacids in the treatment of uremia. *Clin Nephrol*. 3:180-186, 1975.
7. Giovannetti, S. Personal Communication, November, 1990.
8. U.S. Renal Data System, USRDS 1990 Annual Report, The National Institutes of Health, National Institute of Diabetes and Digestive and Kidney Diseases, Bethesda, August, 1990.
9. Mitch W.E., and Klahr, S (eds). *Nutrition and the Kidney*. Boston: Little, Brown and Company, 1988.

Chapter Two

1. U.S. Renal Data System, USRDS 1990 Annual Report, The National Institutes of Health, National Institute of Diabetes and Digestive and Kidney Diseases, Bethesda, August, 1990.
2. Alexander, J.W. The cutting edge: a look to the future in transplantation.*Transplantation*. 49:2:237-240, 1990.
3. U.S. Renal Data System, USRDS 1990 Annual Report, The National Institutes of Health, National Institute of Diabetes and Digestive and Kidney Diseases, Bethesda, August, 1990.
4. Hall, P.M. Can progression of renal disease be prevented? *PostGrad Med*. 86:1:113-120, 1989.
5. Mitch, W., and Walser, M: Nutritional therapy of the uremic patient; in Brenner B, Rector F (eds): *The Kidney*. Philadelphia, W.B. Saunders, 1991, pp 2186-2222.
6. El Nahas, A.M., and Coles, G.A. Dietary treatment of chronic renal failure: ten unanswered questions. *Lancet*. March 15, 1986:597-600.
7. Schrier, RW, and Klahr, S. The future of nephrology. *Am J Kid Dis*. 16:6:590-593, 1990.
8. Gentile, M.G., et al. Preliminary experience on dietary management of chronic renal failure. *Contr Nephrol*. 53:102-108, 1986.
9. American Kidney Fund. Kidney disease: a guide for patients and their families; in Garella, S, Mattern W.D (eds): American Kidney Fund Public Information Series. Rockville, 1987.
10. National Kidney Foundation, Inc. *What everyone should know about kidneys and kidney diseases*. New York: 1990.
11. Klahr, S. The modification of diet in renal disease study. *N Engl J Med*. 320:13:864-866, 1989.

12. Mitch, W., and Walser, M: Nutritional therapy of the uremic patient; in Brenner B, Rector F (eds): *The Kidney.* Philadelphia, W.B. Saunders, 1991, pp 2186-2222.

13. Scribner, Belding H. A personalized history of chronic hemodialysis. *Am J Kid Dis* 16:6:511-519, 1990

14. Payer, Lynn. *Medicine and Culture.* New York: Penguin Books, 1988.

15. U.S. Renal Data System, USRDS 1990 Annual Report, The National Institutes of Health, National Institute of Diabetes and Digestive and Kidney Diseases, Bethesda, August, 1990.

16. Starzl, T.E. In a small Iowa town. *Trans Proc.* 19:12-17, 1987.

17. Kolata, G. American Transplant Pioneers Win Nobel Prize in Medicine. *The New York Times.* October 9, 1990:C3.

18. Berkow, Robert (ed). *The Merck Manual.* Rahway:Merck Sharp & Dohme Research Laboratories, 1987.

19. Hall, P.M. Can progression of renal disease be prevented? *PostGrad Med.* 86:1:113-120, 1989.

20. Starzl, T.E. In a small Iowa town. *Trans Proc.* 19:12-17, 1987.

21. Nissenson, Allen, R. Fine, Richard N., Gentile, Dominick. *Clinical Dialysis; 2nd Edition.* Norwalk: Appleton & Lange. 1990.

22. Evans, R.W. Organ donation: facts and figures. *Dial & Trans.* 19:5:234-237, 1990.

23. Monaco, A.P. Transplantation: the state of the art. *Trans Proc.* 22:3:896-901, 1990.

24. Beale, L.S. *Kidney Diseases, Urinary Deposits, and Calculous Disorders; Their Nature and Treatment.* Philadelphia: Lindsay and Blakiston, 1869.

25. Walser, M. Ketoacids in the treatment of uremia. *Clin Nephrol.* 3:180-186, 1975.

26. Walser, M. Personal communication, 1990.

27. Klahr, S. The modification of diet in renal disease study. *N Engl J Med.* 320:13:864-866, 1989.

28. Walser, M. Personal communication, 1990.

29. Schrier, R. W. and Klahr, S. The future of nephrology. *Am J Kid Dis.* 16:6:590-593, 1990

30. Klahr, Saulo. Personal Communication, April, 1991.

31. Doolittle, Russell. Biotechnology—the enormous cost of success. *N Engl J Med.* 324:19:1360-1361, 1991.

32. U.S. Renal Data System, USRDS 1990 Annual Report, The National Institutes of Health, National Institute of Diabetes and Digestive and Kidney Diseases, Bethesda, August, 1990.

Chapter Three

1. U.S. Renal Data System, USRDS 1990 Annual Report, The National Institutes of Health, National Institute of Diabetes and Digestive and Kidney Diseases, Bethesda, August, 1990.

2. U.S. Renal Data System, USRDS 1990 Annual Report, The National Institutes of Health, National Institute of Diabetes and Digestive and Kidney Diseases, Bethesda, August, 1990.

3. Rosansky, SJ., et al. Comparative incidence rates of end-stage renal disease treatment by state. *Am J Nephrol.* 10:198-204, 1990.

4. Rosansky, SJ., et al. Comparative incidence rates of end-stage renal disease treatment by state. *Am J Nephrol.* 10:198-204, 1990.

5. Jacobs, C: Treatment of terminal renal failure in the western european countries; in Klinkmann H, Smeby LC (eds): Terminal Renal Failure: Therapeutic Problems, Possibilities, and Potentials. *Contrib Nephrol.* Basel, Karger, 1990, vol 78, pp 174-177.

6. Kishimoto, T: Present status of ESRD treatment in Japan: report from the Patient Registries of Dialysis and Kidney Transplantation; in Klinkmann H, Smeby LC (eds): Terminal Renal Failure: Therapeutic Problems, Possibilities, and Potentials. *Contrib Nephrol.* Basel, Karger, 1990, vol 78, pp 178-180.

7. Eggers, P. Health care policies/economics of the geriatric renal population. *Am J Kid Dis.* 16:4:384-391, 1990.

8. U.S. Renal Data System, USRDS 1990 Annual Report, The National Institutes of Health, National Institute of Diabetes and Digestive and Kidney Diseases, Bethesda, August, 1990.

9. Klahr, S. Preventing progression of renal disease. *Dial & Trans.* 19:9:503, 511, 1990.

10. Klahr, S. Preventing progression of renal disease. *Dial & Trans.* 19:9:503, 511, 1990.

11. Klahr, S., and Harris, K. Role of dietary lipids and renal eicosanoids on the progression of renal disease. *Kidney Int*. 36:27:S–27-S–31, 1989.

12. Klahr, S. Preventing progression of renal disease. *Dial & Trans*. 19:9:503, 511, 1990.

13. Klahr, S: Potential factors responsible for the progression of renal failure; in D'Amico G, Colasanti G (eds): Psychological and Physiological Aspects of Chronic Renal Failure. *Contrib Nephrol*. Basel, Karger, 1990, vol 77, pp 77-85.

14. Klahr, S. Preventing progression of renal disease. *Dial & Trans*. 19:9:503, 511, 1990.

15. Klahr, S: Potential factors responsible for the progression of renal failure; in D'Amico G, Colasanti G (eds): Psychological and Physiological Aspects of Chronic Renal Failure. *Contrib Nephrol*. Basel, Karger, 1990, vol 77, pp 77-85.

16. Cameron, S. *Kidney Disease: The Facts*. Oxford: Oxford University Press, 1986.

17. Striker, Gary E. Measuring kidney function. *Am J Kid Dis* 16:5:504-505, 1990.

18. Klahr, S: Overview of the pathophysiology of chronic renal disease and uremia; in Alterman P, Gastel B, Eliastam M (eds): *End-Stage Renal Disease: Pathophysiology, Dialysis, and Transplantation*. U. S. Department of Health and Human Services, 1981, pp 1-9.

19. Cameron, S. *Kidney Disease: The Facts*. Oxford: Oxford University Press, 1986.

20. Cameron, S. *Kidney Disease: The Facts*. Oxford: Oxford University Press, 1986.

Chapter Four

1. Kowalski, Robert E. *The 8-Week Cholesterol Cure*. New York: Harper & Row, 1989.

2. Trowell, H.C., and Burkitt, D.P. *Western Diseases:Their Emergence and Prevention*. Cambridge:Harvard University Press, 1981.

3. American Kidney Fund. Kidney disease: a guide for patients and their families; in Garella, S, Mattern W.D (eds): American Kidney Fund Public Information Series. Rockville, 1987.

4. National Kidney Foundation, Inc. *What everyone should know about kidneys and kidney diseases*. New York: 1990.

5. Mitch, W.E: Nutritional therapy and the progression of renal insufficiency; in Mitch W.E, Klahr, S (eds): *Nutrition and the Kidney*. Boston: Little, Brown and Company, 1988, pp 154-179.

6. Jarvis, D.C. Folk Medicine. New York:Fawcett Crest, 1958.

7. Lewis, C. E. et al. The counseling practices of internists. *Ann Intern Med*. 114:1:54-58, 1991.

8. Leaf, A, and Ryan, T.J. Prevention of coronary artery disease; a medical imperative. *N Engl J Med*. 323:20:1419, 1990.

9. Heimlich, Jane. *What Your Doctor Won't Tell You*. New York: Harper Perennial, 1990.

10. Lundberg, George D. Countdown to millennium—balancing the professionalism and business of medicine. *JAMA*. 263:1:86, 1990.

11. Horowitz, Lawrence C. *Taking Charge Of Your Medical Fate*. New York: Random House, 1988.

Chapter Five

1. Fine, L.G. A proposal to improve the attractiveness of nephrology as a subspecialty choice for residents in internal medicine. *Am J Kid Dis*. 15:4:302-302, 1990.

Chapter Six

1. Callahan, Daniel. *What Kind Of Life*. New York:Simon And Schuster, 1990.

2. Eggers, P.W. Health care policies/economics of the geriatric renal population. *Am J Kid Dis*. 16:4:384-391, 1990.

3. Hull, A.R., and Parker III, T.F. Introduction and summary. *Am J Kid Dis*. 15:5:375-383, 1990.

4. Eggers, P.W. Health care policies/economics of the geriatric renal population. *Am J Kid Dis*. 16:4:384-391, 1990.

5. Eggers, P.W. Health care policies/economics of the geriatric renal population. *Am J Kid Dis.* 16:4:384-391, 1990.

6. U.S. Renal Data System, USRDS 1990 Annual Report, The National Institutes of Health, National Institute of Diabetes and Digestive and Kidney Diseases, Bethesda, August, 1990.

7. Eggers, P.W. Health care policies/economics of the geriatric renal population. *Am J Kid Dis.* 16:4:384-391, 1990.

8. Hull, A.R., and Parker III, T.F. Introduction and summary. *Am J Kid Dis.* 15:5:375-383, 1990.

9. Hull, A.R., and Parker III, T.F. Introduction and summary. *Am J Kid Dis.* 15:5:375-383, 1990.

10. Hull, A.R., and Parker III, T.F. Introduction and summary. *Am J Kid Dis.* 15:5:375-383, 1990.

11. Hull, A.R., and Parker III, T.F. Introduction and summary. *Am J Kid Dis.* 15:5:375-383, 1990.

12. Kurtzman, Joel, and Gordon, Phillip. *No More Dying.* New York:Dell Publishing, 1976.

13. U.S. Renal Data System, USRDS 1990 Annual Report, The National Institutes of Health, National Institute of Diabetes and Digestive and Kidney Diseases, Bethesda, August, 1990.

14. *The Kidneys: Balancing the Fluids.* New York: Torstar Books, 1985.

15. Czaczkes, J.W. and Kaplan De-Nour, A. *Chronic Hemodialysis as a Way of Life* New York, Brunner/Mazel, 1978.

16. Henrich, W.L. A clinical review. *Dial & Trans.* 18:12:688, 1989.

17. Henrich, W.L. A clinical review. *Dial & Trans.* 18:12:688, 1989.

18. Henrich, W.L. A clinical review. *Dial & Trans.* 18:12:688, 1989.

19. U.S. Renal Data System, USRDS 1990 Annual Report, The National Institutes of Health, National Institute of Diabetes and Digestive and Kidney Diseases, Bethesda, August, 1990.

20. Nolph, K.D., et al. Continuous ambulatory peritoneal dialysis. *N Engl J Med.* 318:24:1595-1600, 1988.

21. Nolph, K.D., et al. Continuous ambulatory peritoneal dialysis. *N Engl J Med.* 318:24:1595-1600, 1988.

22. Nolph, K.D., et al. Continuous ambulatory peritoneal dialysis. *N Engl J Med.* 318:24:1595-1600, 1988.

23. Nolph, K.D., et al. Continuous ambulatory peritoneal dialysis. *N Engl J Med.* 318:24:1595-1600, 1988.

24. Levy, N.B. *Psychonephrology Two: Psychological Problems In Kidney Failure And Their Treatment.* New York: Plenum Medical Book Company, 1983.

25. Levy, N.B. Psychonephrology's past and future. *Dial & Trans.* 18:12:693-694, 1989.

26. Levy, N.B. *Psychonephrology Two: Psychological Problems In Kidney Failure And Their Treatment.* New York: Plenum Medical Book Company, 1983.

27. Levy, N.B. Psychonephrology's past and future. *Dial & Trans.* 18:12:693-694, 1989.

28. Bennett, William M., et al. An EPO progress report. *Dial & Trans.* 19:6:280-283, 1990.

Chapter Seven

1. U.S. Renal Data System, USRDS 1990 Annual Report, The National Institutes of Health, National Institute of Diabetes and Digestive and Kidney Diseases, Bethesda, August, 1990.

2. U.S. Renal Data System, USRDS 1990 Annual Report, The National Institutes of Health, National Institute of Diabetes and Digestive and Kidney Diseases, Bethesda, August, 1990.

3. Alexander, J.W. The cutting edge: a look to the future in transplantation.*Transplantation.* 49:2:237-240, 1990.

4. U.S. Renal Data System, USRDS 1990 Annual Report, The National Institutes of Health, National Institute of Diabetes and Digestive and Kidney Diseases, Bethesda, August, 1990.

5. U.S. Renal Data System, USRDS 1990 Annual Report, The National Institutes of Health, National Institute of Diabetes and Digestive and Kidney Diseases, Bethesda, August, 1990.

6. Alexander, J.W. The cutting edge: a look to the future in transplantation.*Transplantation.* 49:2:237-240, 1990.

7. U.S. Renal Data System, USRDS 1990 Annual Report, The National Institutes of Health, National Institute of Diabetes and Digestive and Kidney Diseases, Bethesda, August, 1990.

8. U.S. Renal Data System, USRDS 1990 Annual Report, The National Institutes of Health, National Institute of Diabetes and Digestive and Kidney Diseases, Bethesda, August, 1990.

9. U.S. Renal Data System, USRDS 1990 Annual Report, The National Institutes of Health, National Institute of Diabetes and Digestive and Kidney Diseases, Bethesda, August, 1990.

10. U.S. Renal Data System, USRDS 1990 Annual Report, The National Institutes of Health, National Institute of Diabetes and Digestive and Kidney Diseases, Bethesda, August, 1990.

11. U.S. Renal Data System, USRDS 1990 Annual Report, The National Institutes of Health, National Institute of Diabetes and Digestive and Kidney Diseases, Bethesda, August, 1990.

12. U.S. Renal Data System, USRDS 1990 Annual Report, The National Institutes of Health, National Institute of Diabetes and Digestive and Kidney Diseases, Bethesda, August, 1990.

13. U.S. Renal Data System, USRDS 1990 Annual Report, The National Institutes of Health, National Institute of Diabetes and Digestive and Kidney Diseases, Bethesda, August, 1990.

14. U.S. Renal Data System, USRDS 1990 Annual Report, The National Institutes of Health, National Institute of Diabetes and Digestive and Kidney Diseases, Bethesda, August, 1990.

15. Alexander, J.W. The cutting edge: a look to the future in transplantation.*Transplantation*. 49:2:237-240, 1990.

16. U.S. Bureau of the Census, *Statistical Abstract of the United States*: 1989 (109th edition.) Washington, DC, 1989.

17. U.S. Renal Data System, USRDS 1990 Annual Report, The National Institutes of Health, National Institute of Diabetes and Digestive and Kidney Diseases, Bethesda, August, 1990.

18. Interchangeable parts. *Newsweek*. September 12, 1988:61.

19. Schrier, R.W. and Klahr, S. The future of nephrology. *Am J Kid Dis* 16:5:590-593, 1990.

20. Dowie, M. Maverick surgeon. *Amer Health*. June, 1989:87-97.

21. Starzl, T.E. In a small Iowa town. *Trans Proc*. 19:12-17, 1987.

22. Burnet, F.M. The new approach to immunology *N Engl J Med*. 264:1:24-34, 1961.

23. Starzl, T.E. The development of clinical renal transplantation. *Am J Kid Dis* 16:6:548-556, 1990.

24. Starzl, T.E. In a small Iowa town. *Trans Proc*. 19:12-17, 1987.

25. Brent, Leslie, and Sells, Robert A (eds): *Organ Transplantation: Current Clinical and Immunological Concepts*. London: Baillière Tindall, 1989.

26. Brent, Leslie, and Sells, Robert A (eds): *Organ Transplantation: Current Clinical and Immunological Concepts*. London: Baillière Tindall, 1989.

27. Yaes, R. letter. *New York Times Magazine*. November 4, 1990, p. 12.

28. Starzl, T.E. et al. Long-term (25-year) survival after renal homotransplantation—the world experience. *Trans Proc* 22:5:2361-2365, 1990.

29. Starzl, T.E. et al. Long-term (25-year) survival after renal homotransplantation—the world experience. *Trans Proc* 22:5:2361-2365, 1990.

30. Kolata, G. American Transplant Pioneers Win Nobel Prize in Medicine. *The New York Times*. October 9, 1990:C3.

31. Starzl, T.E. The development of clinical renal transplantation. *Am J Kid Dis*. 16:6:548-556, 1990

32. Dowie, M. Maverick surgeon. *Amer Health*. June, 1989:87-97.

Chapter Eight

1. Kolata, G. American Transplant Pioneers Win Nobel Prize in Medicine. *The New York Times*. October 9, 1990:C3.

2. Murray, J.E. The past, present, and future: renal transplantation before Starzl. *Trans Proc*. 19:339-341, 1987.

3. Starzl, T.E., et al. Kidney transplantation under FK 506. *JAMA*. 264:1:63-67, 1990.

4. Starzl, T.E. In a small Iowa town. *Trans Proc*. 19:12-17, 1987.

5. Gutkind, Lee. *Many Sleepless Nights*. New York: W.W. Norton & Company, 1988.

6. Glasser, Ronald J. *The Body Is The Hero*. New York: Bantam Books, 1976.

7. Starzl, T.E. Long-term (25-year) survival after renal homotransplantation—the world experience. *Trans Proc* 22:5:2361-2365, 1990.

8. Glasser, Ronald J. *The Body Is The Hero*. New York: Bantam Books, 1976.

9. *The Kidneys: Balancing the Fluids.* New York: Torstar Books, 1985.

10. Kolata, G. Rat Immune System Is Taught to Accept Transplant, Researchers Say. *The New York Times.* September 14, 1990:A18.

11. Cerilli, G. J. *Organ Transplantation and Replacement.* Philadelphia: J. B. Lippincott, 1988.

12. Starzl, Thomas E. Personal reflections in transplantation. *Surg Clin North Am.* 58:5:879-893, 1978.

13. Salvatierra Jr., O. Renal transplantation—The Starzl influence. *Trans Proc.* 19:343-349, 1987.

14. Salvatierra Jr., O. Renal transplantation—The Starzl influence. *Trans Proc.* 19:343-349, 1987.

15. Monaco, A.P. Transplantation: the state of the art. *Trans Proc.* 22:3:896-901, 1990.

16. White, D.J.G., et al: Immunosuppression; in Catto GRD (ed): *New Clinical Applications Nephrology.* Dordrecht, Kluwer Academic Publishers, 1989, pp 117-133.

17. Paller, M.S. Cyclosporine nephrotoxicity and the role of cyclosporine in living-related donor transplantation. *Am J Kid Dis.* 16:5:414-416, 1990.

18. Gutkind, Lee. *Many Sleepless Nights.* New York: W.W. Norton & Company, 1988.

19. Paller, M.S. Cyclosporine nephrotoxicity and the role of cyclosporine in living-related donor transplantation. *Am J Kid Dis.* 16:5:414-416, 1990.

20. Schrier, RW, and Klahr, S. The future of nephrology. *Am J Kid Dis.* 16:6:590-593, 1990.

21. Gutkind, Lee. *Many Sleepless Nights.* New York: W.W. Norton & Company, 1988.

22. U.S. Renal Data System, USRDS 1990 Annual Report, The National Institutes of Health, National Institute of Diabetes and Digestive and Kidney Diseases, Bethesda, August, 1990.

23. Payer, Lynn. *Medicine and Culture.* New York: Penguin Books, 1988.

24. Moore, F.D: The doctors' dilemmas; in *Transplant: The Give and Take of Tissue Transplantation.* New York: Simon and Schuster, 1972, pp 313-320.

25. Calland, C.H. Iatrogenic problems in end-stage renal failure. *N Engl J Med.* 287:7:334-336, 1972.

26. Five Kidneys and Two Years of Hell. *San Francisco Chronicle.* 107:9, January 11, 1971.

27. Hano, A. Incredible ordeal of Chad Calland, M.D. *Redbook.* 137:94, September, 1971.

28. Calland, C.H. Iatrogenic problems in end-stage renal failure. *N Engl J Med.* 287:7:334-336, 1972.

29. Werth, B. The Drug That Works in Pittsburgh. *The New York Times Magazine.* September 30, 1990:35,58-60.

30. Werth, B. The Drug That Works in Pittsburgh. *The New York Times Magazine.* September 30, 1990:35,58-60.

31. Werth, B. The Drug That Works in Pittsburgh. *The New York Times Magazine.* September 30, 1990:35,58-60.

32. Starzl, T.E. Long-term (25-year) survival after renal homotransplantation—the world experience. *Trans Proc* 22:5:2361-2365, 1990.

Chapter Nine

1. Mitch W., and Klahr, S (eds). *Nutrition and the Kidney.* Boston: Little, Brown and Company, 1988.

2. Giovannetti, S. *The Nutritional Treatment of Chronic Renal Failure.* Norwell: Kluwer Academic Publisher, 1989.

3. Bergström, J. Discovery and rediscovery of low protein diet. *Clin. Nephrol.* 21:1:29-35, 1984.

4. Bergström, J. Discovery and rediscovery of low protein diet. *Clin. Nephrol.* 21:1:29-35, 1984.

5. Strauch, M., et al: The 'normal' food intake; in Gretz N, Giovannetti S, Strauch M (eds): Low-Protein Diets in Renal Patients: Composition and Absorption. *Contrib Nephrol.* Basel, Karger, 1989, vol 72, pp 1-10.

6. Brody, J.E. Huge Study Of Diet Indicts Fat And Meat. *The New York Times.* May 8, 1990:C1,C14.

7. Beale, L.S. *Kidney Diseases, Urinary Deposits, and Calculous Disorders; Their Nature and Treatment.* Philadelphia: Lindsay and Blakiston, 1869.

8.   O'Neill, M. Eating to Heal: Mapping Out New Frontiers. *The New York Times.* February 2, 1990:C1,C6.

9.   Smadel, J.E., et al. The effect of diet on the pathological changes in rats with nephrotoxic nephritis. *Am. J. Path.* 15:26:199-221, 1939.

10. Bergström, J. Discovery and rediscovery of low protein diet. *Clin. Nephrol.* 21:1:29-35, 1984.

11. Bergström, J. Discovery and rediscovery of low protein diet. *Clin. Nephrol.* 21:1:29-35, 1984.

12. Giovannetti, S. Low protein diet in chronic uremia: a historical survey. *Contr Nephrol.* 53:1-6, 1986.

13. Walser, M. Ketoacids in the treatment of uremia. *Clin Nephrol.* 3:180-186, 1975.

14. Kolata, Gina. Animal Fat Is Tied To Colon Cancer. *The New York Times.* December 13, 1990:1,B20.

15. Leaf, A, and Ryan, T.J. Prevention of coronary artery disease—a medical imperative. *N Engl J Med.* 323:20:1419, 1990.

16. National Institutes of Health. *National Kidney and Urologic Diseases Advisory Board 1990 Long-Range Plan: Window on the 21st Century.* March, 1990.

17. Ihle, B.U., et al. The effect of protein restriction on the progression of renal insufficiency. *N Engl J Med.* 321:26:1773-1777, 1989.

18. Schiffman, J.R. Health Costs: Can a low-protein diet put off costly dialysis? *Wall Street Journal.* January 31, 1990:B1.

19. Fischer, D. Letter to the editor. *N Engl J Med.* 322:22:1609-1610, 1990.

20. Rosman, Johan B., et al. Letter to the editor. *N Engl J Med.* 322:22:1610, 1990.

21. Zeller, Kathleen, et al. Effect of restricting dietary protein on the progression of renal failure in patients with insulin-dependent diabetes mellitus. *N Engl J Med.* 324:2:78-84, 1991.

22. Hall, P.M. Can progression of renal disease be prevented? *PostGrad Med.* 86:1:113-120, 1989.

23. Giovannetti, S. Dietary treatment of chronic renal failure: why is it not used more frequently? *Nephron.* 40:1-12, 1985.

24. Giovannetti, S. Dietary treatment of chronic renal failure: why is it not used more frequently? *Nephron.* 40:1-12, 1985.

25. Giovannetti, S. Dietary treatment of chronic renal failure: why it is not used more frequently? *Nephron.* 40:1-12, 1985.

26. El Nahas, A.M., and Coles, G.A. Dietary treatment of chronic renal failure: ten unanswered questions. *Lancet.* March 15, 1986:597-600.

27. El Nahas, A.M., and Coles, G.A. Dietary treatment of chronic renal failure: ten unanswered questions. *Lancet.* March 15, 1986:597-600.

28. El Nahas, A.M., Personal Communication, 1990.

29. Giovannetti, S. Answers to ten questions on the dietary treatment of chronic renal failure. *Lancet.* November 15, 1986:1140-1142.

30. Bergström, J. Discovery and rediscovery of low protein diet. *Clin. Nephrol.* 21:1:29-35, 1984.

31. Maschio, G., et al: Protein-restricted diet in early chronic renal failure; in Oldrizzi L, Maschio G, Rugiu C, et al. (eds): The Progressive Nature of Renal Disease: Myths and Facts. *Contrib Nephrol.* Basel, Karger, 1989, vol 75, pp 134-140.

Chapter Ten

1.   U.S. Renal Data System, USRDS 1990 Annual Report, The National Institutes of Health, National Institute of Diabetes and Digestive and Kidney Diseases, Bethesda, August, 1990.

2.   U.S. Renal Data System, USRDS 1990 Annual Report, The National Institutes of Health, National Institute of Diabetes and Digestive and Kidney Diseases, Bethesda, August, 1990.

3.   Nolph, K.D. Comparison of continuous ambulatory peritoneal dialysis and hemodialysis. *Kidney Int.* 33:24:S–123-S–131, 1988.

4.   Simmons, R.G., et al. Comparison of quality of life of patients on continuous ambulatory peritoneal dialysis, hemodialysis, and after transplantation. *Am J Kid Dis.* 4:253-255, 1984.

5.   Nolph, K.D. Comparison of continuous ambulatory peritoneal dialysis and hemodialysis. *Kidney Int.* 33:24:S–123-S–131, 1988.

6. Schlesinger, M., et al. The ownership of health facilities and clinical decisionmaking: the case of the ESRD industry. *Medical Care*. 27:3:244-258, 1989.

7. Horowitz, Lawrence C. *Taking Charge Of Your Medical Fate*. New York: Random House, 1988.

8. Hamburger, R.J., et al. A dialysis modality decision guide based on the experience of six dialysis centers. *Dial & Trans*. 19:2:66-84, 1990.

9. Cook, Daniel J., and Terasaki, Paul I.: Renal transplantation on the American continent; in Brent L and Sells RA. *Organ Transplantation: Current Clinical and Immunological Concepts*. London: Baillière Tindall, 1989.

10. U.S. Renal Data System, USRDS 1990 Annual Report, The National Institutes of Health, National Institute of Diabetes and Digestive and Kidney Diseases, Bethesda, August, 1990.

11. Lundin, P. A personal experience of twenty-four years of dialysis. *Trans Proc*. 222:3:957-958, 1990.

Chapter Eleven

1. Gussow, Joan Dye, and Thomas, Paul R. *The Nutrition Debate*. Palo Alto: Bull Publishing Company, 1986.

2. Gussow, Joan Dye, and Thomas, Paul R. *The Nutrition Debate*. Palo Alto: Bull Publishing Company, 1986.

3. Gussow, Joan Dye, and Thomas, Paul R. *The Nutrition Debate*. Palo Alto: Bull Publishing Company, 1986.

4. Gussow, Joan Dye, and Thomas, Paul R. *The Nutrition Debate*. Palo Alto: Bull Publishing Company, 1986.

5. Georges, C.J. Studies Find a Link Between Aggressiveness and Cholesterol Levels. *The New York Times*. September 11, 1990:C3.

6. Kolata, G. Study Offers First Evidence That Cutting Cholesterol Levels Saves Lives. *The New York Times*. October 4, 1990:B21.

7. Trevisan, M., et al. Consumption of olive oil, butter, and vegetable oils and coronary heart disease risk factors. *JAMA*. 263:5:688-692, 1990.

8. Tannahill, Reay. *Food In History*. New York: Crown Publishers, Inc., 1988.

9. Kolata, G. Study Disputes Coffee's Tie to Heart Disease Risk. *The New York Times*. October 11, 1990:B12.

10. Tobian, Louis. Potassium and hypertension. *Nutr Rev*. 46:8:273-283, 1988.

11. Trowell, H. Book Review: Pritikin: The Man Who Healed America's Heart. *Am J Clin Nutr*. 48:174, 1988.

12. Grossman, Robert A. Personal Communication, 1988.

13. Altman, Lawrence K. Scientists Link Hormone To High Blood Pressure. *The New York Times*. September 15, 1990:9.

14. Reader, John. *Man On Earth*. Austin: University of Texas Press, 1988.

15. Eaton, S., et al. *The Paleolithic Prescription; A Program Of Diet And Exercise And A Design For Living*. New York: Harper & Row, 1988.

16. Walford, Roy L. *The 120 Year Diet*. New York: Pocket Books, 1986.

17. Trowell, H.C., and Burkitt, D.P. *Western Diseases:Their Emergence and Prevention*. Cambridge:Harvard University Press, 1981.

Chapter Thirteen

1. Caggiula, Arlene W., et al. *Dietary compliance patterns in the modification of diet in renal disease (MDRD) study, phase III*. National Institute of Diabetes and Digestive and Kidney Diseases, Bethesda, MD.

Chapter Fourteen

1. O'Neill, Molly. The New Nutrition: Protein On The Side. *The New York Times*. November 28, 1990:C1.
2. Tannahill, Reay. *Food in History*. New York: Crown Publishers, Inc., 1988.
3. *Encyclopedia Of Food*. Emmaus: Prevention Publishers, 1990.

Chapter Fifteen

1. Zarit, Steven H., et al. *Working With Families Of Dementia Victims: A Treatment Manual*. Los Angeles: UCLA/USC Long-term Care Gerontology Center, 1983.
2. Trojan, Alf. Benefits of self-help groups: a survey of 232 members from 65 disease-related groups. *Soc Sci Med*. 29:2:225-232, 1989.
3. Killilea, Marie: Mutual help organizations: Interpretations in the literature; in Caplan G, Killilea M (eds): *Support Systems And Mutual Help*. New York: Grune & Stratton, 1976.
4. Killilea, Marie: Mutual help organizations: Interpretations in the literature; in Caplan G, Killilea M (eds): *Support Systems And Mutual Help*. New York: Grune & Stratton, 1976.
5. Killilea, Marie: Mutual help organizations: Interpretations in the literature; in Caplan G, Killilea M (eds): *Support Systems And Mutual Help*. New York: Grune & Stratton, 1976.
6. Middleton, Lillian. *Alzheimer's Family Support Groups: A Manual For Group Facilitators*. Tampa: Suncoast Gerontology Center, 1984.
7. Fawzy, FI., et al. A structured psychiatric intervention for cancer patients; changes over time in immunological measure. *Arch Gen Psych*. 47:8:729-735, 1990.
8. Spiegel, David, et al. Effect of psychosocial treatment on survival of patients with metastatic breast cancer. *Lancet*. 14:2(8668):888-891, 1989.
9. Baron, Robert, et al. Social support and immune function among spouses of cancer patients. *J Pers Soc Psych*. 59:2:344-352, 1990.
10. Goleman, D. Support Groups May Do More In Cancer Than Relieve The Mind. *The New York Times*. October 18, 1990:B12.

Chapter Sixteen

1. U.S. Renal Data System, USRDS 1990 Annual Report, The National Institutes of Health, National Institute of Diabetes and Digestive and Kidney Diseases, Bethesda, August, 1990.
2. Abramson, Leonard. *Healing Our Health Care System*. New York: Grove Weidenfeld, 1990.
3. Callahan, Daniel. *What Kind Of Life; The Limits Of Medical Progress*. New York: Simon and Schuster, 1990.
4. U.S. Bureau of the Census, *Statistical Abstract of the United States*: 1989 (109th edition.) Washington, DC, 1989.
5. National Center for Health Statistics. Health, United States, 1990. Hyattsville, Maryland: Public Health Service. 1991.
6. Califano, Joseph A., Jr. *America's Health Care Revolution; Who Lives? Who Dies? Who Pays?* New York: Random House, 1986.
7. Lamm, Richard D. Health care as economic cancer. *Dial & Trans*. 16:6:432-433, 1987.
8. Califano, Joseph A., Jr. *America's Health Care Revolution; Who Lives? Who Dies? Who Pays?* New York: Random House, 1986.
9. Lamm, Richard D. Health care as economic cancer. *Dial & Trans*. 16:6:432-433, 1987.
10. Kuhn, Thomas S. *The Structure Of Scientific Revolutions*. 2nd edition. Chicago: University of Chicago Press, 1970.
11. Warsh, David. Point Of View On Historic Recognition For A Model Scholar's Theory. *Washington Post*. December 26, 1990:F3.
12. Abramson, Leonard. *Healing Our Health Care System*. New York: Grove Weidenfeld, 1990.

13. Ornish, Dean. *Dr. Dean Ornish's Program For Reversing Heart Disease*. New York: Random House, 1990.
14. *McNeill Lehrer Report*. PBS. December 28, 1990.
15. *McNeill Lehrer Report*. PBS. December 28, 1990.
16. Reuben, Carolyn. Lobbying for alternatives. *L.A. Weekly*. 10:45. 1988.
17. Calland, C.H. Iatrogenic problems in end-stage renal failure. *N Engl J Med*. 287:7:334-336, 1972.
18. Project Cure. Personal Communication, 1990.
19. Lamm, Richard D. Health care as economic cancer. *Dial & Trans*. 16:6:432-433, 1987.
20. Carson, Rachael. *Silent Spring*. Boston: Houghton Mifflin Company, 1962.

INDEX

ABOUT THE AUTHOR

Tim Ahlstrom is a retired high technology inventor, entrepreneur, founder of several companies, and a kidney patient learning to control his chronic disease. He and his wife, Cynthia, have four children and live near Philadelphia. They are among the founders of *The Healing Partnership,* an international non-profit organization of patients, families, doctors and other care-givers working to learn more about the connections between lifestyle and chronic diseases.